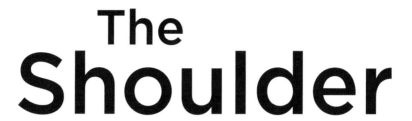

The
Shoulder

AANA Advanced Arthroscopic Surgical Techniques

AANA Advanced Arthroscopic Surgical Techniques
SERIES

SERIES EDITORS, RICHARD K. N. RYU, MD
AND JEFFREY S. ABRAMS, MD

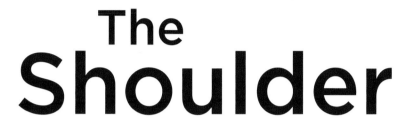

The
Shoulder
AANA Advanced Arthroscopic Surgical Techniques

EDITED BY

RICHARD K. N. RYU, MD
Ryu Hurvitz Orthopedic Clinic
Santa Barbara, California

RICHARD L. ANGELO, MD
President, AANA
ProOrtho, Evergreen Health Medical Center
Kirkland, Washington

JEFFREY S. ABRAMS, MD
Clinical Professor, Department of Surgery
Seton Hall University, School of Graduate Medicine
Orange, New Jersey
Attending Surgeon, Department of Surgery
University Medical Center of Princeton at Plainsboro
Plainsboro Township, New Jersey
Medical Director, Princeton Orthopedic Associates
Princeton, New Jersey

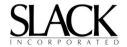

SLACK
INCORPORATED

www.Healio.com/books

ISBN: 978-1-63091-002-0

Published by: SLACK Incorporated
                     6900 Grove Road
                     Thorofare, NJ 08086 USA
                     Telephone: 856-848-1000
                     Fax: 856-848-6091
                     www.Healio.com/books

Contact SLACK Incorporated for more information about other books in this field or about the availability of our books from distributors outside the United States.

Library of Congress Cataloging-in-Publication Data

AANA advanced arthroscopic surgical techniques. The shoulder / edited by Richard K.N. Ryu, Richard L. Angelo, Jeffrey S. Abrams.
     p. ; cm.
    Advanced arthroscopic surgical techniques
    Shoulder
    Preceded by: AANA advanced arthroscopy. The shoulder / [edited by] Richard L. Angelo, James C. Esch, Richard K.N. Ryu. Philadelphia, PA : Saunders/Elsevier, 2010.
    Includes bibliographical references and index.
    ISBN 978-1-63091-002-0 (alk. paper)
    I. Ryu, Richard K. N., editor. II. Angelo, Richard L., editor. III. Abrams, Jeffrey S., 1954- , editor. IV. Arthroscopy Association of North America, issuing body. V. AANA advanced arthroscopy. The shoulder. Preceded by (work): VI. Title: Advanced arthroscopic surgical techniques. VII. Title: Shoulder.
    [DNLM: 1. Shoulder Joint--surgery. 2. Arthroscopy--methods. WE 810]
    RD557.5
    617.5'720592--dc23
                            2015020753

Printed in the United States of America.

Last digit is print number: 10 9 8 7 6 5 4 3 2 1

DEDICATION

To our good buddy, Ben Shaffer; a consummate surgeon, orthopedic whiz kid, family man, and best friend to so many. Rest in peace. We will always miss you.

Rick, Jeff, Rick, and the entire AANA Family

To my inspirational and brilliant mother, Helen; to my loving and patient wife, Linda; and to my three accomplished and delightful daughters, JJ, Alison, and Samantha, I dedicate this textbook. No one gets anywhere alone, and my journey has been meaningful because of you, your companionship, and your unwavering support. Long days and tough hours evaporated with one of your knowing winks. Fortune has smiled upon me, and I am forever grateful to my family and for my blessings.

Richard K. N. Ryu, MD

To Marguerite: Your unfailing love enriches my life beyond measure and your sacrifices enable me to say "yes" to commitments more often than I should;

To Dom, Sam, and Ben: No father could be more proud of his quiver; your incredible talents are too numerous to catalogue, but more importantly, your unselfish hearts direct your passions and pursuits;

To all of you, I give my heartfelt gratitude and love always.

Richard L. Angelo, MD

A journey begins with opportunity and continues with support and guidance. To my parents, Iris and Murry, who provided me with an opportunity to seek education, value integrity, and gain an appreciation for life. To my sister, Belle-Ann, who has taught me that hard work and good humor is the right combination. To Kathleen, my center of the universe, who I walk side by side through an unparalleled life of love, humor, and growth. To Kimberly and Matthew for their love of life, filled with appreciation and generosity. A gift of good fortune, unlimited opportunity, and lifetime relationships…and I am indebted for this amazing journey.

Jeffrey S. Abrams, MD

CONTENTS

Dedication..*v*

Acknowledgments...*ix*

About the Editors...*xi*

Contributing Authors...*xiii*

Foreword by Richard J. Hawkins, MD...*xvii*

Foreword by James R. Andrews, MD...*xix*

Introduction...*xxi*

Chapter 1   Arthroscopic Knot Tying 1
            Robert A. Pedowitz, MD, PhD

Chapter 2   Arthroscopic Anterior Bankart Repair...13
            Frederick S. Song, MD and Jeffrey S. Abrams, MD

Chapter 3   Arthroscopic Humeral Avulsion of the Glenohumeral Ligament Repair 31
            *Gregory C. Mallo, MD, FAAOS; Petar Golijanin; Matthew Doran; and
            Matthew T. Provencher, MD*

Chapter 4   Revision Arthroscopic Shoulder Stabilization 39
            *Brian J. Cole, MD, MBA; Chris R. Mellano, MD; Rachel M. Frank, MD;
            Andrew J. Riff, MD; and Matthew T. Provencher, MD*

Chapter 5   Arthroscopic Single-Row Rotator Cuff Repair 49
            Robert T. Burks, MD and R. Judd Robins, MD

Chapter 6   Arthroscopic Rotator Cuff Mobilization Techniques 61
            Ian Lo, MD, FRCSC

Chapter 7   Arthroscopic Acromioclavicular Joint Repair for Acute Injury 71
            Craig R. Bottoni, MD and Kevin P. Krul, MD

Chapter 8   Arthroscopic Acromioclavicular Joint Reconstruction With
            Allograft/Autograft...81
            Lane N. Rush, MD; Michael J. O'Brien, MD; and Felix H. Savoie III, MD

Chapter 9   Arthroscopic Extracellular Matrix Rotator Cuff Replacement/Augmentation...95
            Nolan R. May, MD and Stephen J. Snyder, MD

Chapter 10   Arthroscopic Hill-Sachs Remplissage 107
            Nathan D. Faulkner, MD; Matthew D. Driscoll, MD; and Mark H. Getelman, MD

Chapter 11   Arthroscopic Capsular Plication....................................123
            Eric Ferkel, MD; Alan Curtis, MD; and Suzanne Miller, MD

Chapter 12   Arthroscopic Linked Double-Row Rotator Cuff Repair 133
            Stephen S. Burkhart, MD and Patrick J. Denard, MD

Chapter 13   Arthroscopic Bony Bankart Repair 147
            Benjamin Shaffer, MD and Matthew Mantell, MD

Chapter 14   Arthroscopic Suprapectoral Biceps Tenodesis 165
            Guillermo Arce, MD

Chapter 15   Arthroscopic Pancapsular Release 181
            Katy Morris, MD and James Esch, MD

Chapter 16   Arthroscopic Anterior Glenoid Bone Block Stabilization 189
Hiroyuki Sugaya, MD

Chapter 17   Arthroscopic Latarjet Stabilization. 199
Ashish Gupta, MBBS, FRACS and Laurent LaFosse, MD

Chapter 18   Arthroscopic Suprascapular Nerve Release: The Transverse Scapular Ligament
and Spinoglenoid Notch 219
Kevin D. Plancher, MD, MS and Stephanie C. Petterson, MPT, PhD

Chapter 19   Arthroscopic Subscapularis Repair: The Extra-Articular Technique 233
Richard K. N. Ryu, MD and Matthew T. Provencher, MD

Chapter 20   Arthroscopic Transtendon Repair of Partial-Thickness Rotator Cuff Tear. . . . 245
Richard L. Angelo, MD

Chapter 21   Arthroscopic Posterior Bankart Repair 257
Steven A. Giuseffi, MD and Larry D. Field, MD

Chapter 22   Arthroscopic Greater Tuberosity Fracture Repair 269
Brody A. Flanagin, MD; Joe Burns, MD; Connor Larose, MD; Raffaele Garofalo, MD;
MAJ Kelly Fitzpatrick, DO, MC, US Army; and Sumant G. Krishnan, MD

Chapter 23   Arthroscopic Bursectomy and Superomedial Angle Resection for the Treatment
of Scapulothoracic Bursitis and Snapping Scapula Syndrome 277
Simon A. Euler, MD; Ryan J. Warth, MD; and Peter J. Millett, MD, MSc

Chapter 24   Arthroscopic Panlabral Repair 285
Jon J. P. Warner, MD; Matthew F. Dilisio, MD; and Stephen A. Parada, MD

Chapter 25   Arthroscopic Superior Labral Anteroposterior Repair. 297
Anthony A. Romeo, MD; Peter N. Chalmers, MD; and Chris R. Mellano, MD

Financial Disclosures. 313
Index 317

ACKNOWLEDGMENTS

We are very grateful for the textbook editors who took on this ambitious project to create a 5-volume surgical technique series that represents the most compelling and current resource available to the arthroscopist. We thank the following editors for their leadership, determination, and expertise: for *The Knee*, Drs. Sgaglione, Provencher, and Lubowitz; for *The Hip*, Drs. Byrd, Bedi, and Stubbs; for *The Elbow and Wrist*, Drs. Savoie, Field, and Steinmann; for *The Foot and Ankle*, Drs. Stone, Kennedy, and Glazebrook; and for *The Shoulder*, Drs. Ryu, Abrams, and Angelo.

That these textbooks are a timely and cogent resource comes as no surprise given the extraordinary quality of the authors who so graciously contributed not only their valuable time, but also their expertise, recognized on a global scale. They were tenacious in following a rigid publication schedule so that the material would represent the most current and cutting-edge concepts and surgical innovations. Their final "product" speaks for itself: concise, masterful, and most importantly, helpful to all that avail themselves of these textbooks. We sincerely thank them for their colossal effort.

Carrie Kotlar, John Bond, and the SLACK Incorporated team were uncompromising in their dedication and commitment to this project. Every endeavor has its highs and lows and their leadership ensured that the highs weren't too high and likewise, the lows were easily surmounted. AANA is grateful for the collaboration, and we, as editors, deeply appreciate their professionalism and courtesies.

James Andrews and Richard Hawkins are two of the greatest shoulder surgeons to grace the orthopedic specialty. That they would take time to write the Foreword for our textbook is meaningful in so many ways, but their imprimatur on our effort can signify no higher value. We remain indebted to Jimmy and Hawk for their mentorship, their leadership, and most importantly, their friendship.

Lastly we want to acknowledge AANA and its leadership for giving us the opportunity to complete this project. In particular, Peter Jokl, a veritable fountain of great ideas, was the "instigator" in this venture. When you listen closely, there is very little that Peter speaks of that isn't pure gold. Finally, all of the editors and authors have transferred all royalties and rights from this 5-volume publication to the AANA Education Foundation. The common goal of promoting world-wide arthroscopic education in an effort to help not only surgeons, but ultimately our patients, reflects the noble and generous nature of all who contributed to what we believe is an outstanding textbook series.

Richard K. N. Ryu, MD
Jeffrey S. Abrams, MD
Richard L. Angelo, MD

ABOUT THE EDITORS

Richard K. N. Ryu, MD is a cum laude graduate of Yale University in New Haven, Connecticut and an Alpha Omega Alpha graduate of UCSF School of Medicine in San Francisco, California. He completed his residency training in Orthopedic Surgery at UCSF and a fellowship in Sports Medicine and Arthroscopy at the Kerlan-Jobe Orthopedic Clinic in Los Angeles, California.

He is Past President of the Arthroscopy Association of North America (AANA) and has also served as their Education and Program Chairman. He is currently Chairman of the AANA Education Foundation and the Journal Board of Trustees, providing oversight for the *Journal of Arthroscopy and Related Research*. He was designated by AANA in 1999 as a Master Shoulder Surgeon at the Orthopedic Learning Center in Chicago

Dr. Ryu is an elected California delegate to the Council of Delegates for the American Orthopedic Society for Sports Medicine and serves on the editorial board for *Operative Techniques in Sports Medicine* and *Orthopedics Today*. He is also a member of the American Shoulder and Elbow Society and the American Academy of Orthopedic Surgeons. He has delivered over 200 lectures, nationally and internationally, and has authored over 70 scientific articles and book chapters while serving as the Series Editor for both the first and second 5-volume editions of the *AANA Advanced Arthroscopic Surgery* textbooks. Dr. Ryu has also been honored as the Wayne O. Southwick Visiting Professor at Yale and as the Verne Inman Lecturer at UCSF.

He resides in Santa Barbara where he has been in private practice since 1986, focusing on athletic knee and shoulder injuries.

Richard L. Angelo, MD is a graduate of the University of Washington Medical School in Seattle, Washington. He completed a surgical internship at the University of California, Irvine and an orthopedic residency at the University of Utah in Salt Lake City. A fellowship in shoulder surgery under Dr. Richard Hawkins at the University of Western Ontario and a second in arthroscopy and sports medicine under Dr. James Andrews completed his training.

He is Past President of the Arthroscopy Association of North America and has also served on their Board of Directors and as their Education and Program Chairman. He is currently serving on the AANA Education Foundation Board and the Journal Board of Trustees for the *Journal of Arthroscopy and Related Research*. He was designated by AANA in 1999 as a Master Shoulder Surgeon at the Orthopedic Learning Center in Chicago.

Dr. Angelo was on the senior advisory board for the 1st and 2nd World Congress on Surgical Training held in Goteborg, Sweden. Formerly, he served as a team physician for the University of Washington Huskies, Clinical Professor for the Department of Orthopedics at the University of Washington, and Chief of Surgery at Evergreen Medical Center in Kirkland, Washington. He was a co-editor of the first and this, the second edition, of the textbook, *AANA Advanced Arthroscopic Surgery—Shoulder Volume*.

Jeffrey S. Abrams, MD is a cum laude graduate from Rensselaer Polytechnic Institute located in Troy, New York, and he graduated from medical school from the State University of New York at Syracuse. He completed his surgical internship in Santa Barbara, California and his orthopedic residency at Thomas Jefferson University Hospital in Philadelphia, Pennsylvania. He completed a shoulder fellowship with Dr. Richard J. Hawkins at the University of Western Ontario in London, sports medicine fellowship in Aspen, Colorado, and a sports medicine fellowship with Dr. James Andrews in Columbus, Georgia.

Dr. Abrams is a Clinical Professor at Seton Hall University, School of Graduate Medicine in South Orange, New Jersey and an attending surgeon at the University Medical Center of Princeton in New Jersey. He has served as the president of the American Shoulder and Elbow Surgeons and is currently the president of the Arthroscopy Association of North America. He has served on the boards for the Orthopedic Learning Center in Rosemont, Illinois and Princeton Orthopedic Associates, serving as a managing partner.

Dr. Abrams has been awarded the Educator of the Year in New Jersey and was initiated into the New Jersey Inventors Hall of Fame as the Innovator of the Year for patent designs for arthroscopic suture anchors. He has lectured over 800 times in the United States and internationally, has published more than 60 scientific articles and book chapters, and has edited 2 textbooks, *Arthroscopic Rotator Cuff Surgery: A Practical Approach to Management* and *Management of The Unstable Shoulder: Arthroscopic and Open Repairs*. He serves on the editorial staff for 5 orthopedic publications and is currently a co-editor of the *The Shoulder: AANA Advanced Arthroscopy Surgical Techniques* Volume, as well as a series editor for the *Second Edition*.

He serves as a consultant to Princeton University, College of New Jersey, Mercer County Community College, International Management Group, and professional and collegiate athletes. He combines an academic with a community practice in Princeton, New Jersey.

CONTRIBUTING AUTHORS

Guillermo Arce, MD (Chapter 14)
Department of Orthopaedic Surgery
Instituto Argentino de Diagnóstico y Tratamiento
Buenos Aires, Argentina

Craig R. Bottoni, MD (Chapter 7)
Chief, Sports Medicine
Director, Residency Research
Orthopaedic Surgery Service
Tripler Army Medical Center
Honolulu, Hawaii

Stephen S. Burkhart, MD (Chapter 12)
The San Antonio Orthopaedic Group
Clinical Associate Professor
Department of Orthopaedic Surgery
University of Texas Health Science Center at
    San Antonio
San Antonio, Texas

Robert T. Burks, MD (Chapter 5)
Robert Metcalf Chair
Professor, Orthopaedic Surgery
Department of Orthopaedics
University of Utah
Salt Lake City, Utah

Joe Burns, MD (Chapter 22)
Southern California Orthopaedic Institute
Van Nuys, California

Peter N. Chalmers, MD (Chapter 25)
Orthopaedic Surgery Resident
Rush University Medical Center
Chicago, Illinois

Brian J. Cole, MD, MBA (Chapter 4)
Department of Orthopaedic Surgery
Rush University Medical Center
Chicago, Illinois

Alan Curtis, MD (Chapter 11)
Orthopedic Surgeon
Boston Sports & Shoulder Center
Waltham, Massachusetts
Medical Director, Bioskills Laboratory
New England Baptist Hospital
Boston, Massachusetts
Assistant Clinical Professor, Orthopedic Surgery
Tufts University
Medford, Massachusetts

Patrick J. Denard, MD (Chapter 12)
Southern Oregon Orthopedics
Medford, Oregon
Department of Orthopaedics and Rehabilitation
Oregon Health and Science University
Portland, Oregon

Matthew F. Dilisio, MD (Chapter 24)
Assistant Professor, Orthopaedic Surgery
Creighton University Orthopaedics/CHI
    Health Shoulder Center
Omaha, Nebraska

Matthew Doran (Chapter 3)
Sports Medicine Service
Boston, Massachusetts

Matthew D. Driscoll, MD (Chapter 10)
Austin Regional Clinic
Austin, Texas

James Esch, MD (Chapter 15)
Orthopaedic Specialists of North County
Oceanside, California
Voluntary Assistant Clinical Professor
Department of Orthopaedics
University of California
San Diego, California

Simon A. Euler, MD (Chapter 23)
The Steadman Clinic
Steadman Philippon Research Institute
Vail, Colorado

Nathan D. Faulkner, MD (Chapter 10)
Colorado Orthopedic Consultants
Aurora, Colorado

Eric Ferkel, MD (Chapter 11)
Attending Orthopaedic Surgeon
Sports Medicine and Foot & Ankle Surgery
Southern California Orthopedic Institute
    (SCOI)
Van Nuys, California

Larry D. Field, MD (Chapter 21)
Mississippi Sports Medicine & Orthopaedic
    Center
Jackson, Mississippi

*MAJ Kelly Fitzpatrick, DO, MC, US Army
    (Chapter 22)*
Blanchfield Army Hospital
Fort Campbell, Kentucky

Brody A. Flanagin, MD (Chapter 22)
The Shoulder Center
Baylor University Medical Center at Dallas
Dallas, Texas

Rachel M. Frank, MD (Chapter 4)
Department of Orthopaedic Surgery
Rush University Medical Center
Chicago, Illinois

Raffaele Garofalo, MD (Chapter 22)
Shoulder Service
Miulli Hospital
Acquaviva delle Fonti (Ba)
Italy

Mark H. Getelman, MD (Chapter 10)
Attending Physician
Co-Director, Sports Medicine Fellowship
Southern California Orthopedic Institute
Van Nuys, California

Steven A. Giuseffi, MD (Chapter 21)
Fellow
Mississippi Sports Medicine & Orthpaedic
    Center
Jackson, Mississippi

Petar Golijanin (Chapter 3)
Sports Medicine Service
Boston, Massachusetts

Ashish Gupta, MBBS, FRACS (Chapter 17)
Orthopaedic Surgeon
Logan Specialist Centre
Brisbane, Australia

Sumant G. Krishnan, MD (Chapter 22)
Medical Director
The Shoulder Center
Baylor University Medical Center at Dallas
Dallas, Texas

Kevin P. Krul, MD (Chapter 7)
Resident, Orthopaedic Surgery Service
Tripler Army Medical Center
Honolulu, Hawaii

Laurent LaFosse, MD (Chapter 17)
Department of Orthopaedic Surgery
Clinique Generale
Annecy, France

Connor Larose, MD (Chapter 22)
Arrowhead Orthopaedics
Sports Medicine
Rancho Cucamonga, California

Ian Lo, MD, FRCSC (Chapter 6)
Clinical Assistant Professor
University of Calgary
Calgary, Alberta, Canada

Gregory C. Mallo, MD, FAAOS (Chapter 3)
Harvard Shoulder Fellow 2014-15
St. Charles Hospital Orthopedics/Orthopedic
    Associates of Long Island
East Setauket, New York

Matthew Mantell, MD (Chapter 13)
Department of Orthopedic Surgery
George Washington University
Washington, DC

Nolan R. May, MD (Chapter 9)
New West Sports Medicine
Kearney, Nebraska

Chris R. Mellano, MD (Chapters 4, 25)
Orthopaedic Surgical Specialists
Torrance, California

Suzanne Miller, MD (Chapter 11)
New England Baptist Hospital
Boston, Massachusetts
Assistant Professor
Tufts University
Medford, Massachusetts

Peter J. Millett, MD, MSc (Chapter 23)
Center for Outcomes-based Orthopaedic
    Research
Steadman Philippon Research Institute
Vail, Colorado

Katy Morris, MD (Chapter 15)
North Oaks Orthopedic Specialty Center
Hammond, Louisiana

Michael J. O'Brien, MD (Chapter 8)
Assistant Professor
Tulane University School of Medicine
Department of Orthopedic Surgery
New Orleans, Louisiana

Stephen A. Parada, MD (Chapter 24)
Chief, Shoulder Surgery
Associate Program Director
Eisenhower Army Medical Center
Fort Gordon, Georgia
Assistant Professor
Uniformed Services University of the Health
    Science
Bethesda, Maryland

Robert A. Pedowitz, MD, PhD (Chapter 1)
Professor Emeritus
University of California
Oakland, California

Stephanie C. Petterson, MPT, PhD (Chapter 18)
Director of Research
Orthopaedic Foundation
Stamford, Connecticut

Kevin D. Plancher, MD, MS (Chapter 18)
Clinical Professor
Albert Einstein College of Medicine
Plancher Orthopaedics and Sports Medicine
New York, New York

Matthew T. Provencher, MD (Chapters 3, 4, 19)
Chief, MGH Sports Medicine Service
Associate Professor, Orthopaedic Surgery
Harvard Medical School
Sports Medicine Service
Boston, Massachusetts

Andrew J. Riff, MD (Chapter 4)
Department of Orthopaedic Surgery
Rush University Medical Center
Chicago, Illinois

R. Judd Robins, MD (Chapter 5)
Assistant Professor, Surgery
Uniformed Services University of the Health
    Sciences
Sports Medicine Service
Department of Orthopaedic Surgery
US Air Force Academy, Colorado

Anthony A. Romeo, MD (Chapter 25)
Professor, Orthopaedic Surgery
Rush University Medical Center
Chicago, Illinois

Lane N. Rush, MD (Chapter 8)
Resident
Tulane University School of Medicine
Department of Orthopedic Surgery
New Orleans, Louisiana

Felix H. Savoie III, MD (Chapter 8)
Ray J. Haddad Professor & Chairman
Tulane University School of Medicine
Department of Orthopedic Surgery
New Orleans, Louisiana

Benjamin Shaffer, MD (Chapter 13)
Deceased

Stephen J. Snyder, MD (Chapter 9)
Southern California Orthopedic Institute
Van Nuys, California

Frederick S. Song, MD (Chapter 2)
Attending Surgeon
Department of Orthopaedic Surgery
University Medical Center of Princeton at
    Plainsboro
Princeton, New Jersey

Hiroyuki Sugaya, MD (Chapter 16)
Director, Shoulder & Elbow Center
Funabashi Orthopaedic Hospital
Funabashi, Japan

Jon J. P. Warner, MD (Chapter 24)
Boston Shoulder Institute
Massachusetts General Hospital/Harvard
    Medical School
Boston, Massachusetts

Ryan J. Warth, MD (Chapter 23)
Upper Extremity Research Assistant
Center for Outcomes-based Orthopaedic
    Research (COOR)
Steadman Philippon Research Institute
Vail, Colorado

FOREWORD

It is indeed a pleasure to be asked to write a foreword in this book on the shoulder in the series of *AANA Advanced Arthroscopic Surgical Techniques*. *The Shoulder* is part of a series of five arthroscopic books; the others being *Elbow and Wrist*, *Foot and Ankle*, *Knee*, and *Hip*. The reason it is such a pleasure for me is because of my relationship with the editors of this book, Dr. Richard K. N. Ryu, Dr. Richard L. Angelo, and Dr. Jeffrey S. Abrams. I've had the privilege of training Drs. Angelo and Abrams as fellows, and Dr. Ryu is a good friend. They all are or have been President of AANA; in fact, Dr. Abrams is also Past President of the American Shoulder and Elbow Surgeons. These editors are all well known in the shoulder world and have gathered an exemplary group of shoulder experts to take on different sections of this book. As organized individuals, they have divided the book into various sections encompassing such aspects as arthroscopic knot tying all the way to the complex surgical procedure, the Latarjet. They have selected the best physical examination signs, chose the appropriate imaging techniques, and even have described the equipment and set up required in the operating room. Included is a step-by-step surgical description with supporting narrated videos. Each section gives the top five technical pearls as well as the postoperative rehabilitation protocols. The format they have adopted is user friendly and will educate those who are in search of better outcomes through innovation. The timeline for completion was 15 months from decision to actual volume in hand. This book will be of great help to shoulder surgeons who want to understand and apply advanced arthroscopic surgical techniques. AANA and these three editors are congratulated for putting this textbook together. It will be exciting to have a copy in hand as we all love to learn with a passionate curiosity, and will benefit from these advanced arthroscopic techniques.

Finally, all of the editors and authors in this book have signed their royalties over to the AANA Educational Foundation. All proceeds will help AANA with their mission of promoting education and research. Because I know these editors so well and many of the contributors, I am humbled and blessed to write a foreword for this book.

Richard J. Hawkins, MD
Steadman Hawkins Clinic of the Carolinas
Greenville, South Carolina

FOREWORD

This 5-volume *AANA Advanced Arthroscopic Surgical Techniques* textbook will certainly be a big addition to those that are inspired to be on the cutting edge for arthroscopic techniques. This series will include just about every joint, including the shoulder, knee, foot and ankle, wrist, elbow, and hip.

There will be special sections on advanced topics as well as routine arthroscopic techniques. Some of the advanced topics that will be discussed and demonstrated include Arthroscopic Management of Greater Tuberosity Fractures, the very difficult technique of Arthroscopic Latarjet Procedure, and also Arthroscopic Free Bone Block Procedure for Recurrent Anterior Dislocation of the Shoulder. It will also include Arthroscopic AC Joint Reconstruction and Suprascapular Nerve Release along with Snapping Scapular, and many other chapters that will stimulate and educate readers.

The most interesting thing about this 5-volume set is the editors and contributors that have put this together. They are all experts in the area of arthroscopy and their particular areas of interests are included in detail in these volumes. Each chapter will include the physical findings and necessary diagnostic imaging tests needed for a particular problem, along with specific equipment lists that should be present for a step-by-step surgical description, which is supported by narrated videos by the contributing authors. It will also include a specific number of technical pearls for each chapter as well as postoperative rehabilitation protocols.

As you can see, this is an all-in-one advanced arthroscopic technique volume that will cover all of the cutting-edge procedures and will obviously be up to date and inclusive.

The other interesting thing about this 5-volume set is that all of the editors and authors have signed their royalties over to the AANA Education Foundation, which is extremely admirable considering the amount of work that went into these volumes. All of the proceeds will help AANA with their mission of promoting education with timely and cutting-edge arthroscopic techniques. I am sure that you, as a reader, will be impressed and stimulated by all of the work that is presented.

James R. Andrews, MD
The Andrews Institute
Gulf Breeze, Florida

INTRODUCTION

The *AANA Advanced Arthroscopic Surgical Techniques Series* represents the very best that AANA has to offer the practicing orthopedic surgeon. With premier arthroscopic surgeons taking the lead, each book in the series presents the latest diagnostic, therapeutic, and reconstructive techniques available in arthroscopic surgery today.

Each technique-based chapter is consistently organized with a user-friendly interface allowing for a quick reference or for prolonged study. Bulleted lists of easily accessed, high-yield information, including preoperative planning, patient selection, equipment checklists, step-by-step descriptions of procedures, and essential technical pearls, in addition to indications, contraindications, postoperative protocols, and potential complications, make this an invaluable resource for surgeons who want to improve not only their skill level, but also their mastery of the fundamentals that define arthroscopic surgery. Well-edited videos, accompanied by narration, further serve to support the materials systematically outlined in each chapter for each volume.

Education and innovation continue to be the top priority for AANA and its leadership. As such, all proceeds from this Series will be donated to the AANA Education Foundation, which, among other endeavors, helps support resident education at the Orthopedic Learning Center, The Traveling Fellowship, the Society of Military Orthopedic Surgeons (SOMOS)–AANA collaboration, resident scholarships to the Annual Meeting, as well as numerous research grants and awards. With the purchase of this textbook series, AANA will also provide free electronic access to the text and videos from the same book in their initial series, *AANA Advanced Arthroscopy* (2010).

We believe that this 5-volume series is a "must have" resource for those who rely on their arthroscopic skills and knowledge to improve patient outcomes. Concise, current, and cogent help describe the impact that these textbooks will have on your practice and in your clinical successes. AANA is delighted to have again taken on this critical leadership position in surgeon education, and is proud of the quality and immediacy of these 5 outstanding volumes.

Richard K. N. Ryu, MD
Jeffrey S. Abrams, MD
Series Co-Editors

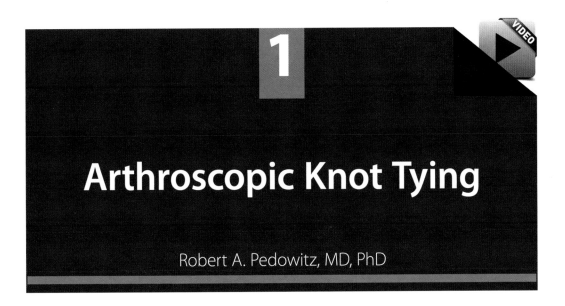

INTRODUCTION

Arthroscopic knot tying is a surgical skill that is difficult to learn and to master. Surgeons must understand basic knot-tying principles in order to create the strongest possible arthroscopic repair. The overall strength of a surgical repair construct, either arthroscopic or open, is defined by the "weakest link" in the chain. In many cases, the biomechanical weak link is the suture knot, as opposed to the suture material, suture anchor, or biological tissue being repaired. Suture materials have unique handling characteristics and knot-tying behaviors. Although "super sutures" decrease the risk of intraoperative suture breakage, high tensile load to failure does not guarantee a secure surgical knot. Surgeons must be diligent and use meticulous operative technique in order to maximize the quality and consistency of arthroscopic knots. Bench-top practice and objective performance feedback can enhance overall proficiency, even for the most experienced surgeon.

INDICATIONS

Most arthroscopic shoulder repair procedures utilize knot-tying skills. The following surgical procedures will be covered in subsequent chapters:

- ▶ Anterior Bankart repair
- ▶ Humeral avulsion of the glenohumeral ligament repair
- ▶ Single-row rotator cuff repair
- ▶ Extracellular matrix rotator cuff augmentation/replacement
- ▶ Hill-Sachs remplissage
- ▶ Capsular plication
- ▶ Transosseous equivalent rotator cuff repair
- ▶ Bony Bankart repair

Ryu RKN, Angelo RL, Abrams JS, eds. *The Shoulder: AANA Advanced Arthroscopic Surgical Techniques* (pp 1-11).
© 2016 AANA.

- Suprapectoral biceps tenodesis
- Anterior glenoid bone block stabilization
- Latarjet stabilization
- Subscapularis repair
- Transtendinous partial rotator cuff tear repair
- Posterior Bankart repair
- Greater tuberosity fracture repair
- Panlabral repair
- Superior labral anteroposterior (SLAP) repair

Alternatives

Some of these surgical procedures can also be performed successfully with knotless fixation devices, per the preference of the operating surgeon:
- Knotless capsulolabral repair
- Knotless SLAP repair
- Knotless rotator cuff repair (eg, double-row repair without medial knots)
- Knotless biceps tenodesis

PRINCIPLES OF ARTHROSCOPIC KNOT TYING

There are a number of basic principles that pertain to the biomechanical performance of surgical knots. It is useful to first consider the primary objective, which is secure apposition that holds tissues in proper position until biologic healing can be achieved. In the absence of healing, all suture constructs will eventually fail under the influence of cyclic load. Thus, treatment represents a race between tissue healing and biomechanical failure (Figure 1-1).

In this context, a few fundamental questions emerge. Foremost, how much "gap" can be tolerated during the healing process since sutures loosen under the influence of postoperative cyclic loads? For example, after an arthroscopic rotator cuff repair, can the local tissues tolerate a small gap between tendon and bone and still achieve successful healing of the cuff? If so, what is the "critical gap" for healing? Additionally, is this critical gap the same for other soft tissue-to-bone repairs, such as the approximation of labrum to glenoid for a SLAP repair? Is the critical gap affected by patient age, systemic disease, or local degeneration (eg, tendinosis)? Should the same threshold apply to suture loops that are tied for tissue-to-tissue repair such as capsular plication to treat multidirectional shoulder instability or side-to-side repair of large rotator cuff ruptures?

At this time, there are no definitive scientific answers to some of these basic questions. However, consider the critical threshold to be less than 3 mm of gap formation to facilitate optimal tissue healing, at least for rotator cuff repair. A 3-mm threshold is a reasonable standard as surgeons practice and test knots in vitro, even though it is an oversimplification to apply the same threshold for all repair conditions.

Tendon-to-bone healing and soft tissue-to-soft tissue healing usually take somewhere between 6 and 12 weeks to achieve a decent modicum of strength at the repair site (under normal physiologic conditions). With a modest estimate of hundreds of loading cycles per day, repair constructs are expected to be subjected to thousands of loading cycles during the healing process. Even under the best conditions of great patient compliance with "passive" rehabilitation protocols (truly

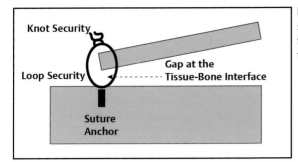

Figure 1-1. Principles of arthroscopic loop security and knot security. Postoperative gap formation can interfere with healing at the tissue-bone interface.

"passive motion" is likely a challenge to achieve after surgical repair), repair constructs will see significant load after surgery and should be able to handle those cyclic loading conditions.

The next logical question pertains to the in vivo loads experienced by arthroscopic repair constructs after surgery. This is a very difficult question to answer since there are little to no biomechanical data from direct postoperative measurement. Most of the available information is based on biomechanical modeling. Loads at the tendon-bone interface after rotator cuff repair are greater with muscle activation compared to passive motion. Local tissue loads would be extremely high during a sudden accidental event, such as a fall, which can cause catastrophic failure of the repair construct.

Based on biomechanical modeling,[1] it is estimated that the force applied via the suture to cuff might be as high as 60 N per suture for an idealized 4-cm long rotator cuff tear (assuming a maximal supraspinatus muscle force of about 300 N and a 3-anchor/3-suture repair). Additional sutures should decrease the load per suture assuming uniform load sharing for all sutures. However, this condition is probably not met in vivo, where it is extremely difficult to achieve a perfectly balanced repair. It seems logical that the "tightest" suture loop would see the greatest initial load, with load transferred to the next tightest loop upon loosening or failure of the first loop. Peak suture-tissue forces are decreased by use of multiple sutures that distribute load evenly to multiple points of tissue fixation. There are disadvantages in the use of an excessive number of sutures. In addition to requiring increased surgical time, those may include local tissue devascularization (which could interfere with healing), excessive bulk (ie, within the joint or in the subacromial space), and tangling of sutures to be tied in relatively tight spaces. Ultimately, arthroscopic suture repair is still about the "balancing act."

Modern "super-sutures" have tensile loads to failure of approximately 300 N (75 lbs), assuming the suture is not nicked or damaged during suture passage and knot tying. Loads in the neighborhood of 300 N would be unusual under most postoperative conditions. However, failure of an arthroscopic knot (defined as greater than or equal to 3 mm of loop expansion) can occur at much lower loads, under the influence of repetitive cyclic loads.

In some cases, the tissue itself is the "weakest link" of the repair construct, but tissue quality is a variable that the surgeon cannot control before or during surgery. Therefore, assuming the use of super-sutures of sufficient tensile strength, surgeons should focus on key technical variables that are within their control during the operation, such as the following:

▶ Snug suture loops (ie, deliberate pretension of the loop in order to remove internal slack)

▶ Tight and strong suture knots

▶ Sufficient number and quality of reversed half-hitches to secure the primary knot

▶ Suture configurations that minimize early loop expansion and/or tissue pull out during postoperative physiologic loading

EQUIPMENT

▶ Knot pusher (single lumen or "sixth finger")

▶ Hemostat (facilitates management of the post limb)

▶ Suture (surgeons should practice with various sutures, such as braided and monofilament)

▶ Suture delivery device and suture anchor, as indicated

▶ Arthroscopic cannula with rubber dam (fluid control)

▶ Specifically for knot-tying practice and assessment of proficiency:

▷ A practice board with knot-tying cylinder or surrogate tissue (ie, the Fundamentals of Arthroscopic Surgery Training [FAST] workstation)

▷ A knot/loop tester to assess biomechanical performance of the construct (ie, the FAST knot tester)

Arthroscopic Knot Pushers and Cannulas

Currently, most arthroscopic surgeons use a single lumen knot pusher that has a distal hole large enough to pass a single limb of suture but small enough to decrease the tendency to drive over the knot being tied. Some surgeons prefer a larger distal hole in the pusher, which allows for deliberate passage over the knot. Some feel that this maneuver assists with proper delivery of half-hitches. Double-holed knot pushers and self-tensioning suture devices are also available, but these have largely fallen out of favor.

Some knot pushers are open-sided, which allows for engagement of the suture limbs within the joint or within the cannula. These knot pushers tend to disengage from the suture limb (which can be a nuisance), and they can occasionally score or fret the suture (which weakens it). Some surgeons prefer to use a "sixth-finger" design, which allows for persistent tension on the knot while half-hitches are delivered, using one instrument to accomplish both tasks. As with everything, there is a learning curve for this device, and practice is required to master the skill.

Controversy remains about whether it is essential to switch the knot pusher from one limb to the other during delivery of reversed hitches on alternating posts. The post is defined by the suture under the most tension. It is not defined by the suture that is being held by the knot pusher. Some surgeons are comfortable flipping posts on sequential throws without changing the knot pusher, simply by preferential pull on one suture strand or the other. Some surgeons prefer to physically swap the knot pusher from one limb to the other, which adds a bit of time to the procedure. Ideally, each surgeon should compare these 2 techniques in their own hands using an objective assessment tool, such as the FAST Knot Tester (see next section). This approach facilitates selection of the best technique by each individual surgeon.

In general, arthroscopic knots should always be delivered down an arthroscopic cannula. Violation of this principle can result in substantial frustration and sometimes technical failure because sutures can encircle nontarget tissues during knot delivery. It is a very good idea to remove all sutures, other than the 2 strands that are being tied, which usually requires use of a loop grasper or crochet hook to deliver sutures out another portal or cannula. It is easy for sutures to become tangled with one another within the cannula during knot tying and, once they become entangled, it can be extremely difficult to correct. Sutures can be "parked" outside of the cannula within the same skin portal, but care should be taken to avoid damage to sutures by the external threads of the cannula itself. Suture protection can be facilitated by using small plastic "straws" as tiny conduits that protect the sutures. The main message is to avoid tangling sutures by keeping only the 2 strands of concern within the cannula during knot tying. This extra step (which requires just a bit of time) will be rewarded by decreased frustration and greater overall surgical efficiency.

Arthroscopic Suture Materials

Arthroscopic sutures can be monofilament or braided, absorbable or nonabsorbable, and standard strength or high strength (so called *super-sutures*). High-tensile strength sutures include Hi-Fi (ConMed Linvatec), Ultrabraid (Smith & Nephew), FiberWire (Arthrex), and Orthocord (DePuy Mitek). Monofilament sutures, such as polydioxanone (PDS [Ethicon]) are relatively easy to pass through tissue, particularly with devices that utilize hollow needles. However, it is more difficult to tie tight arthroscopic knots with monofilament sutures compared to braided sutures due to the inherent "memory" in the material and the fact that monofilament knots have a tendency to unravel or slip. Braided sutures can be delivered by using a shuttling technique. Once a monofilament suture is passed through the tissue, it can be tied around a limb of braided suture with a simple overhand throw. As tension is applied to the other end of the monofilament suture, the braided limb is delivered through the target tissue. Alternatively, commercially available shuttling devices can serve the same purpose.

Antegrade suture-passing tools have made the management of braided sutures much more convenient, whereby braided suture can be advanced in one step through the tissue on the tip of a needle. Some antegrade devices are also self-capturing, which eliminates the need to grasp the suture with an independent device. Care should be taken when using these devices as the sharp needles can cut or nick previously placed sutures. Nicking can weaken the suture, which can result in subsequent breakage.

Super-sutures decrease the incidence of suture breakage during knot tying, which minimizes this previously common experience with standard strength suture. Super-sutures are much more resistant to fraying than conventional suture materials.[2] However, ultra–high-strength does not, in and of itself, guarantee a strong surgical knot. Super-sutures can be quite slippery, and some investigators have reported a tendency for knot slippage without suture breakage with various super-sutures.[3-6] Other investigators have not observed the same differential slip tendency.[7,8] There are substantial variations across high-strength sutures in their weave pattern, which allows some super-sutures to "feel" more like traditional lower-strength braided sutures.[6] Many studies have demonstrated performance differences between knots that are tied with open techniques compared with knots tied using arthroscopic methods. Therefore, it is beneficial for surgeons to practice knot tying with various sutures and various knots in the lab. It is beneficial to take advantage of the objective feedback provided by a knot tester if possible in order to maximize proficiency across the range of materials that are likely to be used in the operating room.

Some super-sutures are so strong that they induce glove tears and finger lacerations during arthroscopic shoulder surgery.[9,10] These tiny finger cuts can be quite painful for the surgeon. More importantly, skin lacerations are a reflection of the amount of force that can be applied by super-sutures across the glove and into the finger. Surgeons should be mindful of glove tears during surgery in order to minimize the risk of bacterial contamination from the skin of the surgeon.

SPECIFIC ARTHROSCOPIC KNOTS (SLIDING AND NONSLIDING)

Many arthroscopic knots are well-described in the literature. It is not necessary for each surgeon to learn every knot. In fact, it makes very little sense to take this educational approach. Common arthroscopic knots include the Duncan loop, Roeder knot, Weston knot, Tennessee slider, Revo-Southern California Orthopedic Institute (SCOI) knot, and the Samsung Medical Center (SMC) knot. Most knots work well as long as the surgeon understands and adheres to fundamental principles of knot security and loop security, including proper use of back up half-hitches. Every arthroscopic surgeon must be comfortable with at least 2 "go-to" knots for the operating room. Knots perform differently for different surgeons,[11,12] so there is no one best knot for all surgeons. It is efficient and effective to become facile and technically consistent with at least one sliding knot, one nonsliding knot, and, if possible, one sliding-locking knot.

Sliding knots are advantageous because the knot is configured outside of the arthroscopic cannula. The knot is then delivered to the target location by the post strand sliding through tissue and the suture anchor. However, in some instances, the suture will not slide through tissue and/ or the anchor. This is not an uncommon occurrence. For example, with a triple-loaded suture anchor, the first 2 sutures may bind on the third suture within the eyelet once they are tied. The only way to utilize the third suture may be to use a nonsliding knot. It is therefore important to routinely assess suture sliding before creating the knot. Sliding knots require a shortened post, which returns to appropriate working length as the knot is delivered and the post is retrieved. In contrast, nonsliding knots should be created on relatively symmetrical limbs. It is critical to assess suture sliding prior to knot selection every time. All arthroscopic surgeons must have the ability to tie a secure nonsliding knot because it will occasionally be required for the operation. Some surgeons prefer to use a nonsliding knot routinely, which is composed of a series of reversed half-hitches on alternating posts.

It is not necessary to learn and master a large number of sliding and nonsliding knots. If arthroscopic knots are backed up properly with at least 3 reversed half-hitches on alternating posts, there is relatively little performance difference between various knots (at physiologic loads). It makes much more sense to master just a few knots. The primary driver of success is meticulous surgical technique and attention to detail, as opposed to specific knot selection.

Sliding knots can be divided into locking and nonlocking variants. There are times during surgery when a sliding-locking knot is advantageous, such as when the repair has a tendency to "spring back" from the target tissue. This tendency can create loop expansion and associated gap formation at the repair site in the brief moment between primary knot placement and half-hitch delivery. The technique for delivering and securing a sliding-locking knot involves 3 sequential steps:

1. Snugging the primary knot and tightening the tissue loop using the knot pusher

2. Slipping the knot pusher (becomes a "puller") past the primary knot

3. Tripping and locking the knot by pulling on the non-post limb

It is important to remove all loop slack by deliberate pretension of the post limb. This step sometimes requires a few assertive pulls on the post limb. Surgical assistants, particularly the person holding the arthroscope, should watch the monitor carefully during this stage of the procedure. It is important to advise the operating surgeon if the loop loosens at any point during knot tying because this is a correctable problem if it is identified before the placement of additional half-hitches. Once additional hitches are delivered, it is difficult (and sometimes impossible) to correct a loose primary loop.

Arthroscopic knot security is achieved by the placement of at least 3 reversed throws on alternating posts to back up the initial knot.[7,13-15] This maneuver essentially locks the primary knot in position. Riboh et al[16] demonstrated that shortcut techniques (tensioning of half-hitches without switching of the knot pusher) can result in decreased knot performance after the placement of a base Tennessee slider. Knot performance was not affected by the method of half-hitch placement after the placement of a base surgeon's knot.[16]

Various suture configurations can be used to stabilize soft tissues during arthroscopic shoulder surgery. In some cases, the soft tissues being repaired are of poor quality (eg, a previously operated and degenerative rotator cuff tendon). In this scenario, solid anchors, strong sutures, and good knots can fail if the suture rips through tissue itself.[17] Complex grasping sutures can help in these situations, but it is important to remove slack from the suture before knot tying because internal slack may convert into early gap formation at the repair site. Gerber and colleagues[18] noted that ultimate tensile strength was significantly increased by the modified Mason-Allen suture with open rotator cuff technique. This grasping suture involves 3 passes of suture through tendon, which provides a self-locking mechanism when tension is applied. However, in a subsequent study of the arthroscopic Mason-Allen technique, they found that this configuration did not increase the strength of an arthroscopic mattress suture configuration.[19] Petit et al[20] noted that mattress suture performed better than simple sutures, but early bone-tendon gap formation was observed consistently with the modified Mason-Allen configuration. This was probably caused by slight slack in the complex suture loops, which created a gap during low-level cyclic load. Therefore, it is important to gently remove slack from sutures, especially from complex grasping sutures, prior to "setting" of the arthroscopic knot.

The massive cuff stitch is created by placing an initial simple loop transverse to the fibers of the rotator cuff. This loop is tied initially, then a simple suture from an anchor is passed medial to the initial suture loop. When the simple suture is tied, tension is partially born by the initial transverse suture loop, which decreases the tendency for tissue cut out. This configuration was noted to be approximately 4 times stronger than a simple suture or horizontal mattress suture and roughly equivalent to the load to failure of an openly placed modified Mason-Allen stitch.[21] Similar objectives can be achieved in poor-quality tissue when using a double-loaded suture anchor. The first suture is placed in horizontal mattress configuration. The second suture is passed as a simple suture medial to the 2 mattress limbs. The mattress is tied first, and when the simple suture is brought under tension, it engages the mattress limbs.

PRACTICE BOARDS AND KNOT TESTER

Recent studies suggest that knot-tying performance and consistency may be less than desired, even in the hands of experienced surgeons.[22] The surgeon's objective is to tie strong knots in an efficient manner that conserves operative time. Technical quality and consistency can be improved with practice. Historically, most training has typically involved practice on knot-tying boards, using written instructions and/or video demonstrations that are emulated by the learner. Evaluation of knot-tying skills is usually limited to subjective observation and assessment by a more experienced mentor. Some investigators describe self-evaluation tools that can augment the effectiveness of knot-tying instruction.[23]

Biomechanical feedback can be particularly useful for learning and for practice; this approach can be of substantial benefit for residents, fellows, and practicing surgeons. Unfortunately, the use of sophisticated material testing devices can be cost-prohibitive and impractical for most learning labs. Recently, the Arthroscopy Association of North America (in conjunction with the American Academy of Orthopaedic Surgeons and the American Board of Orthopaedic Surgery) developed a low-cost device that facilitates knot-tying practice and direct objective measurements of arthroscopic knot performance in vitro (Figures 1-2 through 1-6, the FAST workstation and FAST knot tester, available from Sawbones). Instructional video materials are available online at https://abos.org/ within the basic surgical skills learning modules.

POTENTIAL COMPLICATIONS

Arthroscopic knot tying is a challenging skill. Technical pitfalls can be minimized by practice and attention to detail. Suture tangling can be avoided by careful and preplanned management of sutures in order to keep only the 2 working strands within the working cannula during knot tying. Extra sutures within the cannula substantially increase the risk of entrapment within the knot, which can be difficult to correct. The incidence of suture breakage has been decreased by super-sutures, but rupture can still occur if the surgeon is too rough. Modern sutures are so strong that it is fairly easy to pull the suture anchor out of bone, particularly when osteoporosis is present, or

Figure 1-2. The FAST Program base station, which can be used with rope to learn knot tying.

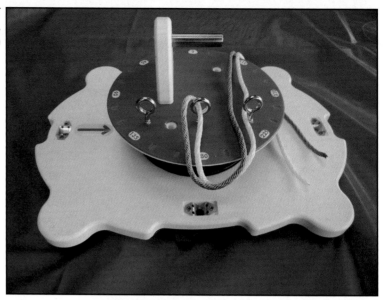

Figure 1-3. The FAST knot-tying mandrel, for practicing knot tying with suture.

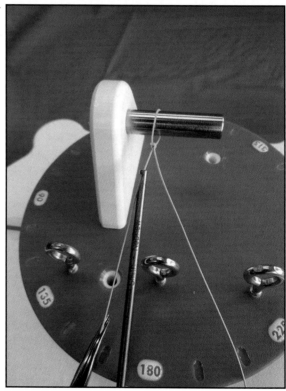

during revision cases when bone integrity may have been compromised by the previous repair. The likelihood of suture breakage increases with nicks and fraying, which can be minimized by taking care with sharp suture passing instruments and "stabber-graspers." A knot can lock within the cannula if half-hitches are not completely delivered to the target. This problem can be minimized by the surgical assistant, noting successful delivery of every half-hitch (and immediate communication to the operating surgeon if the hitch is not visualized). Once this problem is recognized,

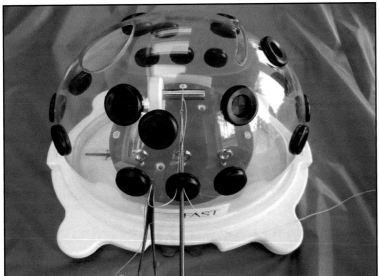

Figure 1-4. A clear dome with multiple portals facilitates practice through cannulas under direct visualization.

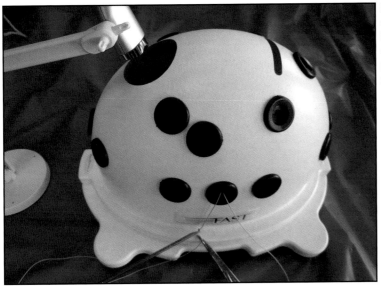

Figure 1-5. An opaque dome can be used with an inexpensive USB camera connected to a laptop computer to practice knot-tying skills under video control.

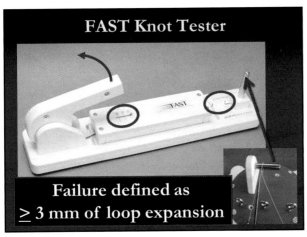

Figure 1-6. The FAST knot tester. The first notch on the loop-sizer matches the knot-tying mandrel of the base station. Gentle pull on the handle applies a 15-lb tensile load to the suture loop, which is remeasured using the loop-sizer. Failure is defined as > 3 mm of loop expansion.

avoid further tightening of the knot. It may be possible to salvage the construct by delivering the knot into the working space without tension on the limbs. Two pairs of loop graspers from different portals may enable the knot to be teased and untied and the separate limbs retrieved. Slippage of the initial knot can increase loop size, which may be associated with gap at the tissue-bone interface. Loop expansion substantially increases the risk of construct failure. This can be avoided by maintaining tension on the post limb, at least until the first back up hitch is delivered and/or the knot is locked securely. At times, an assistant can stabilize the knot or soft tissue with an arthroscopic grasping instrument to gently control spring-back. Knot slippage is probably the most important and common technical pitfall. This can be avoided by meticulous and deliberate surgical technique, including placement of at least 3 reversed hitches on alternating posts behind the primary knot.

TOP TECHNICAL PEARLS FOR THE PROCEDURE

1. Plan the arthroscopic procedure and rehearse each suture shuttling step in your mind. This will minimize the risk of suture tangling.

2. Practice and become proficient with at least one arthroscopic sliding knot, one nonsliding knot, and one sliding-locking knot. Use a knot testing board to assess your skills.

3. During surgery, watch the initial knot and confirm that the loop has not displaced prior to the delivery of half-hitches. Loop expansion can be associated with failure of tissues to heal.

4. Back up the primary knot with at least 3 reversed half-hitches on reversed posts. Do this every time.

5. Super-sutures decrease the risk of breakage, but sutures do not create secure knots on their own. Use meticulous surgical technique and practice your knot-tying skills.

REFERENCES

1. Burkhart SS, Wirth MA, Simonick M, Salem D, Lanctot D, Athanasiou K. Knot security in simple sliding knots and its relationship to rotator cuff repair: how secure must the knot be? *Arthroscopy.* 2000;16(2):202-207.
2. Wüst DM, Meyer DC, Favre P, Gerber C. Mechanical and handling properties of braided polyblend polyethylene sutures in comparison to braided polyester and monofilament polydioxanone sutures. *Arthroscopy.* 2006;22(11):1146-1153.
3. Abbi G, Espinoza L, Odell T, Mahar A. Pedowitz R. Evaluation of 5 knots and 2 suture materials for arthroscopic rotator cuff repair: very strong sutures can still slip. *Arthroscopy.* 2006;22(1):38-43.
4. Barber FA, Herbert MA, Beavis RC. Cyclic load and failure behavior of arthroscopic knots and high strength sutures. *Arthroscopy.* 2009;25(2):192-199.
5. Hughes PJ, Kerin C, Hagan RP, Fisher AC, Frostick SP. The behaviour of knots and sutures during the first 12 hours following a Bankart repair. *Acta Orthop Belg.* 2008;74(5):596-601.
6. Mahar AT, Moezzi DM, Serra-Hsu F, Pedowitz RA. Comparison and performance characteristics of 3 different knots when tied with 2 suture materials used for shoulder arthroscopy. *Arthroscopy.* 2006;22(6):614.e1-2.
7. Ilahi OA, Younas SA, Ho DM, Noble PC. Security of knots tied with ethibond, fiberwire, orthocord, or ultrabraid. *Am J Sports Med.* 2008;36(12):2407-2414.

8. Lo IK, Ochoa E Jr, Burkhart SS. A comparison of knot security and loop security in arthroscopic knots tied with newer high-strength suture materials. *Arthroscopy*. 2010;26(9 Suppl):S120-S126.

9. Kaplan KM, Gruson KI, Gorczynksi CT, Strauss EJ, Kummer FJ, Rokito AS. Glove tears during arthroscopic shoulder surgery using solid-core suture. *Arthroscopy*. 2007;23(1):51-56.

10. Martinez A, Han Y, Sardar ZM, et al. Risk of glove perforation with arthroscopic knot tying using different surgical gloves and high-tensile strength sutures. *Arthroscopy*. 2013;29(9):1552-1558.

11. Hughes PJ, Hagan RP, Fischer AC, Holt EM, Frostick SP. The kinematics and kinetics of slipknots for arthroscopic Bankart repair. *Am J Sports Med*. 2001;29(6):738-745.

12. Livermore RW, Chong AC, Prohaska DJ, Cooke FW, Jones TL. Knot security, loop security, and elongation of braided polyblend sutures used for arthroscopic knots. *Am J Orthop (Belle Mead NJ)*. 2010;39(12):569-576.

13. Kim SH, Yoo JC, Wang JH, Choi KW, Bae TS, Lee CY. Arthroscopic sliding knot: how many additional half-hitches are really needed? *Arthroscopy*. 2005;21(4):405-411.

14. Loutzenheiser TD, Harryman DT, Yung SW, France MP, Sidles JA. Optimizing arthroscopic knots. *Arthroscopy*. 1995;11(2):199-206.

15. Lo IK, Burkhart SS, Chan KC, Athanasiou K. Arthroscopic knots: determining the optimal balance of loop security and knot security. *Arthroscopy*. 2004;20(5):489-502.

16. Riboh JC, Heckman DS, Glisson RR, Moorman CT 3rd. Shortcuts in arthroscopic knot tying: do they affect knot and loop security? *Am J Sports Med*. 2012;40(7):1572-1577.

17. Cummins CA, Murrell GA. Mode of failure for rotator cuff repair with suture anchors identified at revision surgery. *J Shoulder Elbow Surg*. 2003;12(2):128-133.

18. Gerber C, Schneeberger AG, Beck M, Schlegel U. Mechanical strength of repairs of the rotator cuff. *J Bone Joint Surg Br*. 1994;76(3):371-380.

19. Schneeberger AG, von Roll A, Kalberer F, Jacob HA, Gerber C. Mechanical strength of arthroscopic rotator cuff repair techniques: an in vitro study. *J Bone Joint Surg Am*. 2002;84-A(12):2152-2160.

20. Petit CJ, Boswell R, Mahar A, Tasto J, Pedowitz RA. Biomechanical evaluation of a new technique for rotator cuff repair. *Am J Sports Med*. 2003;31(6):849-853.

21. Ma CB, MacGillivray JD, Clabeaux J, Lee S, Otis JC. Biomechanical evaluation of arthroscopic rotator cuff stitches. *J Bone Joint Surg Am*. 2004;86-A(6):1211-1216.

22. Hanypsiak BT, DeLong JM, Simmons L, Lowe W, Burkhart S. Knot strength varies widely among expert arthroscopists. *Am J Sports Med*. 2014;42(8):1978-1984. [Epub ahead of print]

23. Wong IH, Denkers MR, Urquhart NA, Farrokhyar F. Systematic instruction of arthroscopic knot tying with the ArK Trainer: an objective evaluation tool. *Knee Surg Sports Traumatol Arthrosc*. 2015;23(3):912-918. doi: 10.1007/s00167-013-2567-z. Epub 2013 Jun 27.

Please see videos on the accompanying website at

www.ArthroscopicTechniques.com

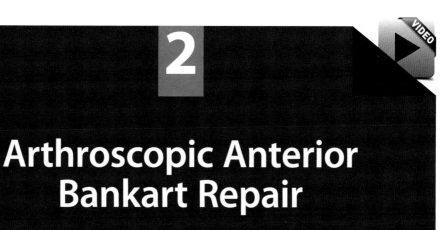

2

Arthroscopic Anterior Bankart Repair

Frederick S. Song, MD and Jeffrey S. Abrams, MD

INTRODUCTION

Anterior glenohumeral dislocation rates in the general population range from 17 to 23.9 per 100,000.[1] According to the National Collegiate Athletic Association Injury Surveillance System,[2] the rate among collegiate athletes is estimated to be 0.12 per 1000 exposures with even higher rates among male collision athletes (ie, football, wrestling, hockey). The young male athlete is known to be at greatest risk for anterior shoulder dislocation and recurrent instability with rates nearly 3-fold higher when compared with females.[3] The anteroinferior labral tear associated with anterior dislocations was originally described by Bankart as the essential lesion.[4] The question regarding whether to surgically correct this lesion and, if so, by which technique has been debated.

Natural history studies of acute anterior shoulder dislocations have revealed varying degrees of success with nonoperative treatment.[5-7] The majority of studies demonstrate a significantly higher risk of recurrent instability in the younger, more active patient population.[5-7] It is in this higher-risk group of patients where surgery is more likely to be required. A recent systematic review performed by Longo et al[8] evaluating a total of 2813 shoulders in 31 studies found a significantly reduced recurrence rate in young, active patients that were treated for anterior dislocations of the shoulder with surgical management compared to those who received conservative treatment.[8]

The risk of recurrent instability also has been correlated with an increase in the development of glenohumeral osteoarthritis. Hovelius and Saeboe[9] reported a 39% incidence of subsequent osteoarthritis in this population, while Ogawa et al[10] have documented increased rates of degenerative disease with recurrent instability. Habermeyer et al,[11] in their series of unstable shoulders, have demonstrated that subsequent recurrent instability led to progressive damage of the labrum-ligament complex.

Traditional open procedures have been associated with good outcomes and a low recurrence rate.[12,13] Despite this, advances in arthroscopic techniques and suture anchor technology have led to a shift from open to arthroscopic treatment. The advantages of an arthroscopic approach include the preservation of the subscapularis; less postoperative pain; greater functional range of motion; and the ability to visualize, diagnose, and treat concomitant pathology. Although early

Ryu RKN, Angelo RL, Abrams JS, eds. *The Shoulder: AANA Advanced Arthroscopic Surgical Techniques* (pp 13-29). © 2016 AANA.

arthroscopic attempts at stabilization had an unacceptable rate of recurrence, technical advances in arthroscopic repair of simple Bankart lesions have yielded overall satisfactory results, similar to those reported for open procedures.[14-17] There is, however, still some debate regarding which procedure will lead to the best clinical outcomes. A recent randomized trial by Mohtadi et al[18] compared open versus arthroscopic stabilization for recurrent anterior shoulder instability. The observed failure rate was significantly higher in the arthroscopic versus the open procedure cohort (22% vs 11%).[18]

In circumstances that involve combined or isolated glenoid or humeral head bone loss, the results of arthroscopic Bankart repair have not been as reliable. Burkhart and DeBeer's[19] case series of 194 patients undergoing arthroscopic Bankart repair demonstrated that arthroscopic results can be inadequate in the face of bone loss. They observed failure rates as high as 67% in cases of significant bone loss and as high as 89% when bone loss was combined with contact sports.[19] In these complex clinical settings, adjunctive arthroscopic procedures, such as the remplissage,[20] have been implemented to improve the success rates. McCabe et al[21] reviewed 30 patients with an engaging Hill-Sachs lesion and less than 25% glenoid bone loss who were treated with a capsulolabral repair coupled with a remplissage procedure, resulting in a 0% failure rate at 2-year follow-up.

Arthroscopic Bankart repair continues to evolve as a procedure. The primary labral pathology, as well as associated tissue damage, is better understood and appreciated, while adjunctive techniques, such as the remplissage and additional inferior capsular tensioning, have been developed to not only promote an anatomic repair, but to provide additional stability in selected circumstances.

INDICATIONS

▶ Recurrent subluxation or dislocation with failure of conservative treatment
▶ First time dislocation in the high-risk population
▶ Instability and associated rotator cuff tear

Controversial Indications

▶ Recurrent instability with significant bone loss
▶ Humeral avulsion of the glenohumeral ligament (HAGL) lesion
▶ Young (age < 22 years), male contact athlete

PERTINENT PHYSICAL FINDINGS

▶ Apprehension test[22]: With the patient in the supine position, the arm is taken to 90 degrees of abduction with the elbow in 90 degrees of flexion. The shoulder is then progressively externally rotated with an anterior force applied. A positive test is demonstrated when the patient demonstrates an apprehensive feeling, indicating instability.
▶ Relocation test[23]: This test is carried out in conjunction with and immediately after the apprehension test. During a positive apprehension test, a force is directed posteriorly to the humeral head. A reduction in apprehensive symptoms and the ability to further externally rotate the shoulder denotes a positive test.
▶ Release (surprise) test[24]: This test immediately follows the relocation test. With the shoulder in continued external rotation, the posterior-directed force on the humeral head is released. A positive test is demonstrated when the patient experiences a sudden feeling of apprehension.

▶ Load and shift test[25,26]: The patient can be in the seated or supine position. The examiner uses one hand to stabilize the scapula and shoulder girdle, while the other hand grasps the arm. The patient's shoulder is typically placed in 0 degrees of abduction and neutral rotation or, alternatively, in 45 degrees of abduction and 45 degrees of external rotation. An axial load is placed to center and load the humeral head on the glenoid. Stress is applied anteriorly and posteriorly to assess the amount of translation. This test can be performed with increased angles of abduction to further isolate the inferior glenohumeral ligaments (IGHL). It is important to always test and compare the contralateral shoulder.

▶ Anterior drawer test[27]: With the patient in the supine position, the scapula is stabilized by placing pressure on the coracoid process. The humeral head is then grasped and an anterior force is applied. The patient's arm is held between 80 to 120 degrees of abduction, 0 to 20 degrees of forward flexion, and 0 to 30 degrees of external rotation. A positive test occurs if there is excessive anterior translation compared with the contralateral shoulder, or the patient exhibits apprehension.

▶ Hyperabduction test[28]: The examiner stands behind the seated or standing patient. The patient's shoulder girdle is stabilized and his or her arm is abducted. If arm abduction is greater than 105 degrees or apprehension is demonstrated by the patient, then the test is positive.

PERTINENT IMAGING

▶ Plain radiographs including anteroposterior, glenoid, scapular-Y, and axillary views

  ▷ Stryker notch view: Patient is in the supine position. The palm of the patient's hand on his or her affected side is placed on top of the head with fingers directed toward the back of the head. The x-ray beam is then aimed 10 degrees cephalad with respect to the shoulder. This view is useful for evaluating any Hill-Sachs lesions.

  ▷ West point view: The patient is in the prone position. The shoulder is raised off the table approximately 7 to 8 cm with a pad. The patient's arm is at 90 degrees of abduction with the forearm hanging off the table. The x-ray beam is then aimed into the axilla with 25 degrees of abduction from the midline and 25 degrees downward from the horizontal. This gives a tangential view of the anteroinferior glenoid rim to help evaluate for glenoid bone loss.

  ▷ Bernageau view: The patient is either standing or seated. The affected arm is abducted 135 degrees with the hand resting on the head. The x-ray beam is directed toward the posterior aspect of the shoulder with a 30-degree caudal tilt. This view is used to evaluate the anteroinferior glenoid rim.

▶ Magnetic resonance imaging (MRI; initial injury) vs MR arthrography

▶ Following plain radiographs, if labral or capsular pathology is suspected based on the patient's history and physical exam and there is a low suspicion of bone loss, an MRI is the next study of choice. Besides evaluation for any labral pathology, an MRI can demonstrate any concomitant pathology, such as biceps and rotator cuff lesions. Intra-articular contrast can further discern and identify labral pathology as well as any capsular detachments. Three-dimensional computed tomography imaging with reconstructions and humeral head subtraction studies should be included in the workup if significant glenoid bone loss is suspected. This imaging modality is also advocated in any failed surgery/revision setting.

EQUIPMENT

- ► Large transparent cannulas (8 to 8.5 cm)
- ► Curved suture hooks (45 degrees right and left)
- ► Small glenoid suture anchors (single- and double-loaded)
- ► Monofilament suture or shuttle
- ► Piercing retrieving instruments
- ► 30-degree arthroscopic viewing instrumentation
- ► Water/saline pump
- ► Suture management instruments: knot tying, cutting, and retrieving

STEP-BY-STEP DESCRIPTION OF THE PROCEDURE

Step 1: Examination Under Anesthesia

In a supine position, shoulder range of motion is recorded. An anterior load and shift test in neutral rotation, and with the arm at 45 degrees abduction and 45 degrees external rotation, is performed. Unstable shoulders will have a palpable endpoint if the shoulder is positioned at 90 degrees of abduction with external rotation. At lesser degrees of abduction and rotation, translation and subluxation may be more easily detected as the remaining glenohumeral ligaments are placed in a less taut configuration. Crepitus and locking are other important palpable findings that may reflect the quality of the static restraints and articular surface. The sulcus sign and posterior translation measurements are important to appreciate joint laxity and may be useful when compared to the contralateral shoulder.

Step 2: Positioning and Portals

The lateral decubitus position is preferred for anterior instability surgery, orienting the glenoid parallel to the floor. Visualization and access to the critical inferior quadrant are essential for a successful repair, and viewing from an anterosuperior portal permits direct visualization of this region. Use of a commercially available arm holder can facilitate proper positioning of the shoulder in addition to the balanced suspension required during the procedure. Direct plication of inferior pouch and supporting capsular ligament bands is best achieved with glenohumeral distraction, permitting direct access to the inferior pouch. With the beach chair position, the weight of the anesthetized arm can create a potential obstacle to overcome when attempting to retension the IGHL. The posterior viewing portal is created initially with a spinal needle, followed by joint inflation. The skin landmark is 2 cm inferior to the lateral edge of junction of the posterior acromion with the spine of the scapula. This is 1 to 2 cm lateral to the customary posterior viewing portal (Figure 2-1). The advantage of this portal placement is the ability to visualize anteromedially with a 30-degree scope, and to avoid levering on the glenoid rim.

The most common technique utilizes dual anterior portals that enter the joint through the rotator interval. The anterosuperior portal is placed inferior to the acromioclavicular joint and enters directly behind the biceps at the upper border of the rotator interval. This portal can be utilized for viewing as well as assisting in the shuttling process and suture management.

The anteroinferior portal is created 2 cm lateral to the coracoid, entering the joint above the superior border of the subscapularis tendon. This will provide an optimal angle for suture anchor placement along the anteroinferior glenoid quadrant. This usually requires a larger cannula to

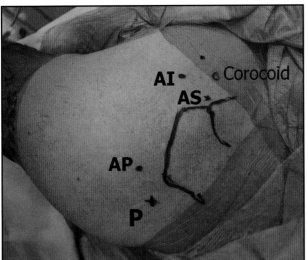

Figure 2-1. Portals commonly used for arthroscopic Bankart repair. AI, anteroinferior; AP, accessory posterior; AS, anterosuperior; P, posterior.

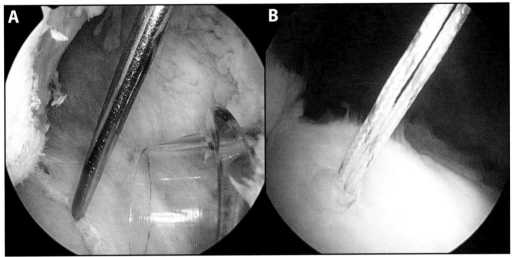

Figure 2-2. Placement of a posteroinferior anchor through an accessory posterior portal to plicate the inferior pouch. (A) Percutaneous location using a spinal needle. (B) Suture anchor insertion.

permit suture hook insertion. When creating this portal, a spinal needle is inserted while viewing from the posterior portal. A gentle posterior force can be applied to the humerus to create additional space, thereby minimizing the risk of abrasion to the humeral head. Additional portals may be helpful to complete an arthroscopic Bankart repair. A 6 o'clock or posteroinferior anchor can be used to directly treat the inferior capsule (Figure 2-2). This accessory posterior portal entry point is made with a spinal needle 2 cm posterior and 2 cm lateral to the typical posterior portal. An unobstructed entry point can be accomplished while the humeral head subluxes along the anteroinferior rim, a common finding in the unstable shoulder. After identifying the optimal angle of entry with a spinal needle, a narrow diameter drill guide is inserted. It is usually unnecessary to place a working cannula in this portal as suturing can be accomplished through the standard posterior portal already established. Concern for the axillary nerve is of paramount importance; however, careful placement of the drill guide under direct visualization should obviate this potential complication.

Figure 2-3. Accessory anterior trans-subscapularis portal in patients with difficult access to the anteroinferior glenoid rim.

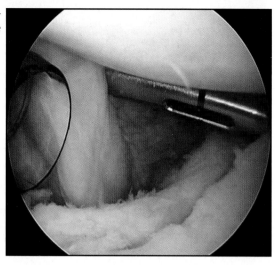

Additional portals can be added in selected cases. An anteroinferior portal (5 o'clock portal) through the subscapularis can be helpful in a bony bridge Bankart repair in which an anchor must be placed medially on the neck of the glenoid and in those HAGL lesions that are amenable to an arthroscopic repair. This is made approximately 2 to 3 cm inferior to the anteroinferior portal, passing dilating instruments through the intra-articular portion of the subscapularis until an appropriately sized cannula can be introduced (Figure 2-3).

Placing larger diameter cannulas both anteriorly and posteriorly can facilitate the insertion of angled suture hooks in the most efficient and ergonomically fashion, enhancing the ability to capture and shift compromised labroligamentous capsule.

Step 3: Diagnostic Arthroscopy

The diagnostic arthroscopy begins with carefully evaluating the entire joint in a systematic fashion. A significant humeral head defect or Hill-Sachs lesion can be measured and quantified to establish if the glenoid track is insufficient and requires a more aggressive approach.[29] Confirmation of the anterior labral tear and identifying potential superior and inferior extensions of the lesion are completed prior to creating the 2 anterior working portals described previously (Figure 2-4). The anteroinferior portal and the posterior portals typically accommodate larger diameter cannulae to allow for passing instrumentation, especially the suture hooks. The optimal view of the anteroinferior pathology is achieved with the arthroscope in the anterosuperior portal (Figure 2-5). Confirmation of an engaging Hill-Sachs lesion is easily achieved while viewing from this portal while the shoulder is rotated and translated.

Step 4: Tissue Mobilization

A critical step in the Bankart repair is capsular mobilization. Through the anterior and posterior portals, an elevator is used to liberate the labral pathology so that the tissue is easily shifted from inferior to superior in addition to closing the defect. Visualizing the subscapularis muscle through the mobilized labral-ligamentous complex indicates a satisfactory degree of soft tissue liberation (Figure 2-6). Not uncommonly, the labral pathology can extend to and beyond the 6 o'clock position on the glenoid. If so, the full extent of the labral abnormalities must be recognized and mobilized, and additional anchors are used to address extended lesions. The glenoid neck and reattachment margins are prepared with a shaver, avoiding any aggressive burring that risks increased bone loss (Figure 2-7). At the completion of the step, the entire IGHL hammock can be easily positioned in the anticipated repair site.

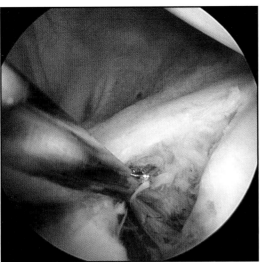

Figure 2-4. Anterior Bankart lesion visualized from the posterior portal.

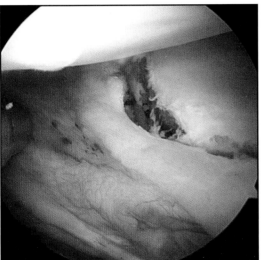

Figure 2-5. Anterior and inferior Bankart lesion visualized from the anterosuperior portal.

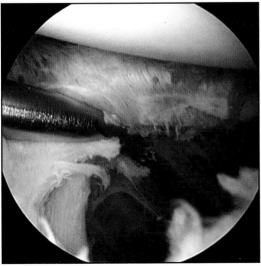

Figure 2-6. Capsular mobilization and separation from the glenoid neck and underlying subscapularis muscle.

Figure 2-7. Gentle glenoid neck debridement prior to suture anchor repair.

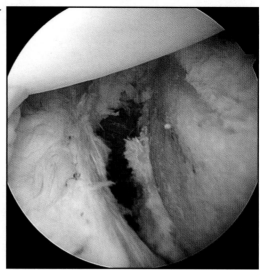

Figure 2-8. A mattress suture was created through a suture anchor placed at 7 o'clock to re-establish the posterior band of the IGHL.

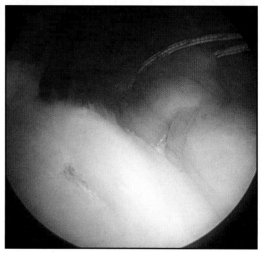

Step 5: Posteroinferior Suture Anchor

Inferior capsular plication is an important step in repairing the unstable shoulder. One distinct advantage of arthroscopy is the ability to visualize the entire IGHL insertion. Capsular stretching combined with labral detachments are commonly found in the recurrent dislocator. Direct capsule labral repair can be performed with a series of sutures or anchors placed along the inferior rim. The 30-degree scope will visualize this from the anterosuperior portal.

Create an accessory portal 2 cm anterior and 2 cm lateral to the posterior portal after visualizing the angle of entry with a spinal needle. The posterior cannula may need to be partially removed to avoid crowding for this step. If the spinal needle can access the appropriate portions of the glenoid, then a drill guide can be inserted. A single- or double-loaded suture anchor can be inserted.

The posterior cannula can be reinserted if it has been removed for the previous step. Thirty-degree curved suture hooks can be inserted to retension the posterior band of the IGHL. This can be accomplished with simple or mattress sutures (Figure 2-8). These sutures can be tied at this time or following the anteroinferior anchor placement in tight shoulders. Additional plication sutures can be added if a large inferior pouch is determined. An absorbable monofilament suture

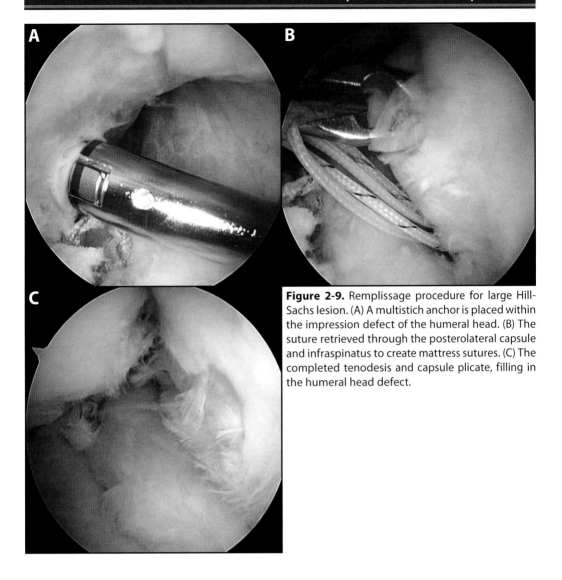

Figure 2-9. Remplissage procedure for large Hill-Sachs lesion. (A) A multistich anchor is placed within the impression defect of the humeral head. (B) The suture retrieved through the posterolateral capsule and infraspinatus to create mattress sutures. (C) The completed tenodesis and capsule plicate, filling in the humeral head defect.

can be placed using the suture hook, creating tension with simple sutures, reducing the capacity of the inferior pouch.

Step 6: Remplissage Augmentation

When a significant humeral head defect is considered large and potentially problematic, a remplissage procedure may be an important adjunctive intervention. The purpose of the remplissage in which the lateral aspect of the infraspinatus is tenodesed into the Hill-Sachs lesion is to render the defect extra-articular while also providing for translational control.[20,21] Performing this procedure before the anterior labral repair offers much better visualization and working space. The remplissage sutures can be tied at the conclusion of the completed anteroinferior labral repair.

Selected patients with humeral head defect felt to be "at risk" for engagement have this step added prior to the anterior repair. After debridement of the defect through the posterior cannula, a drill can be inserted into a hole placed in the central region of the Hill-Sachs defect. A multistitched rotator cuff anchor with threads can be placed (Figure 2-9).

Figure 2-10. An anteroinferior suture anchor is placed on the articular margin of the glenoid through the anteroinferior portal using a drill guide.

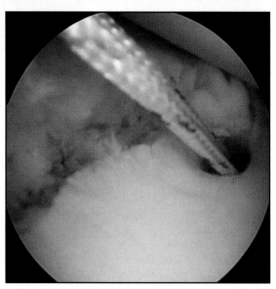

The cannula is partially withdrawn, allowing the posterior capsule and infraspinatus to close in front of the opening of the cannula when visualized from an anterior portal. Creating a lateral-to-medial trajectory, a piercing retrieving instrument is introduced through the cannula and sutures are individually retrieved, creating a mattress suture effect. Special care to avoid medial capsule penetration near the glenoid will avoid overtensioning the posterior capsule. As sutures are retrieved, the knots can be tied on the bursal surface of the infraspinatus and upper teres minor. If this step is completed prior to anterior suture anchor placement, the tied sutures are left and can be used to apply gentle traction during the anterior repair. Some surgeons prefer to tie these sutures after the anteroinferior anchor is placed and secured for maximal visualization.

Step 7: Anteroinferior Suture Anchor

The anterior and inferior suture anchor is placed through a drill guide entering the shoulder through the anteroinferior cannula. The placement of this anchor is best visualized from the anterosuperior portal, and the drill guide permits posterior displacement of the humeral head during the insertion, allowing for the drill hole and anchor to be located approximately 2 mm from the edge of the articular margin (Figure 2-10). Some surgeons have elected to visualize from the posterior portal with either a 70- or 30-degree arthroscope. A single- or multistitched suture anchor can be selected. If the quality of the capsule is robust, a mattress suture configuration can be constructed. If the tissue is thin or deficient, a simple suture configuration is more secure.

After anchor placement, a 30-degree curved suture hook is placed in the anteroinferior cannula. The capsule is penetrated inferior to the anchor to create a superior shift when secured (Figure 2-11). This step is repeated if a mattress suture is being performed. In glenoids in which a multistitch anchor is placed, a mattress suture is placed first but not tied. The second stitch can be a simple stitch placed medially to create reinforcement to the tissue fixation (Figure 2-12). The suture hook penetrates the capsule and can manually be drawn superiorly as it enters the articulation under the detached labrum, creating a plication effect (Figure 2-13). The sutures are tied prior to placement of the next suture anchor.

Step 8: Anterior Mid-Glenoid Anchor

The second anterior suture anchor is placed approximately 8 to 10 mm superior from the inferior anchor. The ideal drill hole is performed using a drill guide through the anteroinferior portal

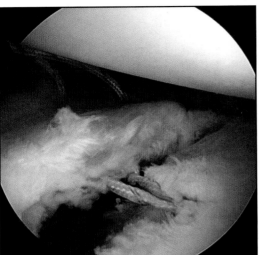

Figure 2-11. Puncturing the capsule inferior to the suture anchor will create a superior shift as the sutures are tied.

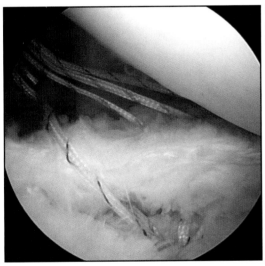

Figure 2-12. Multistitch anchors can be used to create additional fixation. A mattress suture and simple suture combination reinforces the repair site.

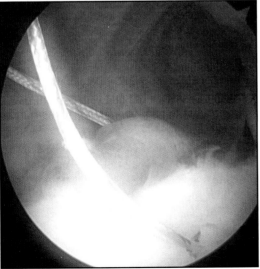

Figure 2-13. A capsular plication and simple suture can be created when the suture hook creates separate penetration of the capsule and labrum.

Figure 2-14. The middle anchor reinforces the upper third of the IGHL with a reinforced mattress suture.

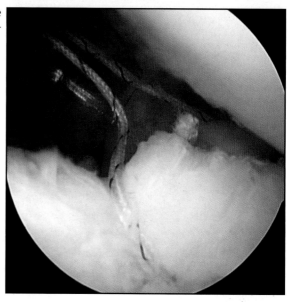

and visualization through the anterosuperior or posterior portals. The multistitched suture anchor is ideal for reinforcing the superior band of the IGHL. Using a 30-degree curved suture hook, the capsule is penetrated and the individual sutures are retrieved using monofilament sutures tied to the anchor sutures. A mattress suture is created. Prior to tightening, the suture hook is reintroduced medially to grasp the superior border of the IGHL and retrieve the second stitch within the anchor. The mattress sutures are secured and tied through the anteroinferior cannula. The second simple stitch configuration is secured, creating secure attachment of the upper portions of the IGHL (Figure 2-14).

Step 9: Anterosuperior Anchor

The third anchor is located adjacent or slightly above the glenoid fovea on the articular margin. The drill guide will need to be readjusted to penetrate the articular surface at a near perpendicular angle of entry. A single suture anchor is often used and a simple suture configuration is chosen due to thinning tissue along the middle and inferior capsular ligament junction. After retrieving a suture with a 30-degree suture hook, the upper border of the IGHL and portions of the middle glenohumeral ligament (MGHL) are secured to the glenoid (Figure 2-15).

Step 10: Rotator Interval Plication

The rotator interval closure has been added to select shoulders that are considered lax prior to their dislocation history. Using the anteroinferior cannula and removing the anterosuperior cannula allows placement of a suture hook through the upper portion of the MGHL along with fibers of the subscapularis. This is best performed approximately halfway from the glenoid margin to the articular insertion and is visualized from the posterior portal (Figure 2-16). A monofilament suture can be selected as this will come in contact with the humeral head articular surface during extension. The larger cannula is partially withdrawn and a penetrating retriever is placed through the superior glenohumeral ligament The suture is retrieved, creating a vertical mattress suture. This is knotted extra-articularly through the anteroinferior cannula.

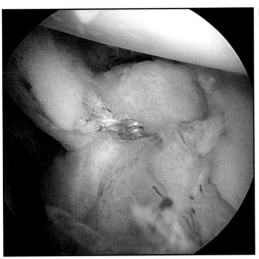

Figure 2-15. The superior suture anchor is placed using a simple suture.

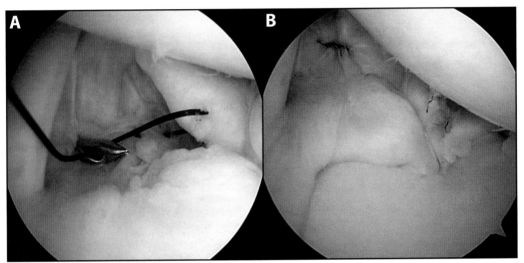

Figure 2-16. The rotator interval closure is performed combining portions of the MGHL, upper border of the subscapularis, and superior glenohumeral ligament. (A) Suture introduction and retrieval. (B) Closed rotator interval.

Step 11: Bracing

Portals are closed with monofilament nylon sutures and dressings are secured. A pillow splint is applied in the operating room, placing the arm in modest internal rotation.

POSTOPERATIVE PROTOCOL

► Initial week:
  ▷ Protective sling brace
  ▷ Elbow flexion and extension
  ▷ Forearm, wrist, and grip strength
  ▷ Scapular posturing exercise

- ▶ Weeks 2 through 5:
  - ▷ Pendulum exercises
  - ▷ Scapular retraction
  - ▷ External rotate assist to 20 degrees with elbow at the side
  - ▷ Lower body conditioning
- ▶ Weeks 5 through 8:
  - ▷ Begin forward flexion to 150 degrees
  - ▷ External rotate at side to 40 degrees
  - ▷ Scapular stabilizing exercises
  - ▷ Core strength
  - ▷ Wean from sling
- ▶ Weeks 8 through 12:
  - ▷ Approach terminal elevation
  - ▷ Increase external rotation to 50 degrees
  - ▷ Rotator cuff strengthening
  - ▷ Scapular strengthening
  - ▷ Increase general conditioning
- ▶ Weeks 12 through 16:
  - ▷ Critical increases in motion to apply to desired sports
  - ▷ Closed-chain exercises for strength and coordination
  - ▷ Overhead throwing motion allowed, but without the ball
- ▶ Week 16 through 6 months:
  - ▷ Begin weightbearing loads, gradual and not ballistic
  - ▷ Avoid contact and collision until shoulder approaches symptom free. May begin overhead throwing as maturity of healing is confirmed
- ▶ Months 4 through 8:
  - ▷ Return to sport if symptoms free, with protective strength and appropriate conditioning

POTENTIAL COMPLICATIONS

Surgical complications can follow operative stabilization of the unstable shoulder. The most common complication is recurrent instability. This includes subluxation with a spontaneous reduction or a complete dislocation that requires assistance with reduction apprehension in abduction and external rotation. There are several identified risk factors for a failed Bankart procedure, including but not limited to younger age, significant bone loss, contact sports, associated ligamentous laxity, and the male gender. Balg and Boileau have introduced the instability severity index score as a means of quantifying the risk of recurrence after an arthroscopic Bankart procedure.[30]

A less common complication of arthroscopic Bankart is stiffness. Although loss of maximal external rotation is a common outcome of any surgical repair of the anterior capsular ligaments, severe restriction is not an anticipated outcome. On occasion, a surgical release of adhesions or overtightening may be appropriate. Inadvertent stabilization of an anatomic variant such as a sublabral foramen in the anterosuperior quadrant can result in significant and disabling losses in external rotation and the overhead-throwing motion.

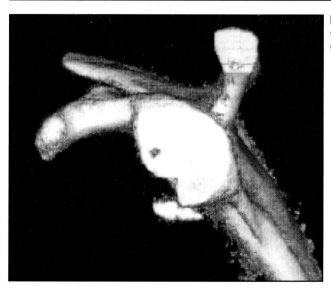

Figure 2-17. Glenoid rim fracture through prior suture anchor holes due to subsequent trauma.

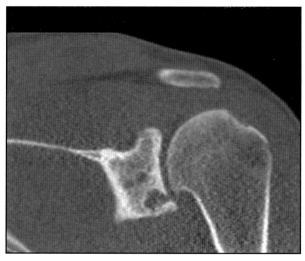

Figure 2-18. Glenoid cysts can be problematic if revision surgery is needed.

Sutures and suture anchors are required in repairing the damaged, avulsed capsulolabral tissue. The introduction of foreign material always carries a risk. Abrasion due to prominent knots can injure the articular cartilage. Patients may complain of a "squeaky" shoulder. Special attention to the placement of sutures and knots can reduce the risk of this phenomenon. Utilizing mattress sutures or alternating mattress and simple sutures can help prevent migration of suture material to the articular margin.

Anterior glenoid rim fractures have occurred as a result of a traumatic anterior re-dislocation after a suture anchor repair (Figure 2-17). Multiple suture anchor holes can create a stress-riser structural weakness, leading to this vulnerability. Maintaining appropriate spacing of the anchors while using implants with narrow diameter drill holes can mitigate this risk.

Suture anchors have been devised using multiple sources including PEEK (polyetheretherketone/plastic), sutured-based material, biologically absorbable compounds, and metallics. Cystic changes in response to these materials have been reported (Figure 2-18). If suspected, the appropriate evaluation would include x-rays, 3D computed tomography imaging, as well as testing for occult infection. In symptomatic patients, an arthroscopic debridement and hardware removal might be prudent, although uncommon.

TOP TECHNICAL PEARLS FOR THE PROCEDURE

1. Avoid cannula crowding, which can limit working space around the 2 anterior cannulas. Insert the cannulas at the most superior and inferior borders of the rotator interval. The inferior cannula is placed immediately adjacent to the superior border of the subscapularis, while the superior cannula enters the joint directly behind the biceps tendon.

2. Adequate capsulolabral mobilization includes liberation of the tissue from the glenoid margin while visualizing the underlying subscapularis muscle belly. The IGHL must be easily retensioned in an inferior-to-superior shift along the articular margin of the glenoid.

3. Use the inferior (6 o'clock) anchor to directly address the inferior capsule. The accessory posteroinferior portal allows placement of this suture anchor, while subsequent suture hook passage through the inferior capsule can be accomplished through either the anteroinferior or standard posterior working portals.

4. The remplissage can be a significant addition to the "at risk" shoulder due to bone loss. In patients with mild changes to the glenoid width and more significant deficiency of the humeral head due to a large, deep Hill-Sachs lesion, this additional step can reduce the risk of recurrence.

5. The rotator interval closure can be added to create additional capsular tension and reduce anterior translation. Simple capsule plications have had mixed results. Incorporating the upper border of the subscapularis with the MGHL will create a robust support to the anterior repair. This is not recommended in overhead-throwing athletes due to undesirable loss of terminal external rotation.

REFERENCES

1. Robinson CM, Seah M, Akhtar MA. The epidemiology, risk of recurrence, and functional outcome after an acute traumatic posterior dislocation of the shoulder. *J Bone Joint Surg Am*. 2011;93:1605-1613.
2. Owens BD, Angel J, Mountcastle SB, et al. Incidence of glenohumeral instability in collegiate athletics. *Am J Sports Med*. 2009;37(9):1750-1754.
3. Zacchilli MA, Owens BD. Edpidemiology of shoulder dislocations presenting to emergency departments in the United States. *J Bone Joint Surg Am*. 2010;92(3):542-549.
4. Bankart AS. Recurrent or habitual dislocation of the shoulder-joint. *Br Med J*. 1923;2(3285):1132-1133.
5. Hovelius L, Olofsson A, Sandström B, et al. Nonoperative treatment of primary anterior shoulder dislocation in patients forty years of age and younger: a prospective twenty-five year follow-up. *J Bone Joint Surg Am*. 2008;90(5):945-952.
6. Sachs RA, Lin D, Stone, ML, et al. Can the need for future surgery for acute traumatic anterior shoulder dislocation be predicted? *J Bone Joint Surg Am*. 2007;89(8):1665-1674.
7. Robinson CM, Howes J, Murdoch H, et al. Functional outcome and risk of recurrent instability after primary traumatic anterior shoulder dislocation in young patients. *J Bone Joint Surg Am*. 2006;88(11):2326-2336.
8. Longo UG, Lappini M, Rizzello G, et al. Management of primary acute anterior shoulder dislocation: systematic review and quantitative synthesis of the literature. *Arthroscopy*. 2014;30(4):506-522.
9. Hovelius L, Saeboe M. Neer Award 2008: Arthropathy after primary anterior shoulder dislocation. 223 shoulders prospectively followed up for twenty-five years. *J Shoulder Elbow Surg*. 2009;18(3):338-347.

10. Ogawa K, Yoshida A, Matsumoto H, et al. Outcome of the open Bankart procedure for shoulder instability and development of osteoarthritis: a 5- to 20-year follow-up study. *Am J Sports Med.* 2010;38(8):1549-1557.

11. Habermeyer P, Gleyze P, Rickert M. Evolution of lesions of the labrum-ligament complex in posttraumatic anterior shoulder instability: a prospective study. *J Shoulder Elbow Surg.* 1999;8(1):66-74.

12. Rowe CR, Zarins B, Ciullo JV. Recurrent anterior dislocation of the shoulder after surgical repair: apparent causes of failure and treatment. *J Bone Joint Surg Am.* 1984;66(2):159-168.

13. Pagnani MJ. Open capsular repair without bone block for recurrent anterior shoulder instability in patients with and without bony defects of the glenoid and/or humeral head. *Am J Sports Med.* 2008;36(9):1805-1812.

14. Brophy RH, Marx RG. The treatment of traumatic anterior instability of the shoulder: nonoperative and surgical treatment. *Arthroscopy.* 2009;25(3):298-304.

15. Owens BD, DeBerardino TM, Nelson BJ, et al. Long-term follow-up of acute arthroscopic Bankart repair for initial anterior shoulder dislocations in young athletes. *Am J Sports Med.* 2009;37(4):669-673.

16. Ozturk BY, Maak TG, Fabricant P, et al. Return to sports after arthroscopic anterior stabilization in patients aged younger than 25 years. *Arthroscopy.* 2013;29(12):1922-1931.

17. Harris JD, Gupta AK, Mall NA, et al. Long-term outcomes after Bankart shoulder stabilization. *Arthroscopy.* 2013;29(5):920-933.

18. Mohtadi, NG, Chan DS, Hollinshead RM, et al. A randomized clinical trial comparing open and arthroscopic stabilization for recurrent traumatic anterior shoulder instability. *J Bone Joint Surg Am.* 2014;96(5):353-360.

19. Burkhart SS, DeBeer J. Traumatic glenohumeral bone defects and their relationship to failure of arthroscopic Bankart repairs: significance of the inverted pear glenoid and the humeral engaging Hill-Sachs lesion. *Arthroscopy.* 2000;16(7):677-694.

20. Purchase RJ, Wolf EM, Hobgood ER, et al. Hill-Sachs remplissage: an arthroscopic solution for the engaging Hill-Sachs lesion. *Arthroscopy.* 2008;24:723-726.

21. McCabe MP, Weinberg D, Field LD, et al. Primary versus revision arthroscopic reconstruction with remplissage for shoulder instability with moderate bone loss. *Arthroscopy.* 2014;30(4):444-450.

22. Rowe CR, Zarins B. Recurrent transient subluxation of the shoulder. *J Bone Joint Surg Am.* 1982;63:863-872.

23. Jobe FW, Kvitne RS, Giangarra CE. Shoulder pain in the overhand or throwing athlete. The relationship of anterior instability and rotator cuff impingement. *Orthop Rev.* 1989;18:963-975.

24. Gross ML, Distefano MC. Anterior release test. A new test for occult shoulder instability. *Clin Orthop Relat Res.* 1997;339:105-108.

25. Silliman JF, Hawkins RJ. Classification and physical diagnosis of instability of the shoulder. *Clin Orthop Relat Res.* 1993;291:7-19.

26. Abrams JS. Arthroscopic anterior instability repair. In: Levine WN, Blaine TA, Ahmad CS, eds. *Minimally Invasive Shoulder and Elbow Surgery.* New York, NY: Informa Healthcare; 2007:91-104.

27. Gerber A, Ganz R. Clinical assessment of instability of the shoulder. With special reference to anterior and posterior drawer tests. *J Bone Joint Surg Br.* 1984;66:551-556.

28. Gagey OJ, Gagey N. The hyperabduction test. *J Bone Joint Surg Br.* 2001;83:69-74.

29. DiGiacomo G, Itoi E, Burkhart SS. Evolving concept of bipolar bone loss and the Hill-Sachs lesion: from "engaging/non-engaging" lesion to "on-track/off-track" lesion. *Arthroscopy.* 2014;30(1): 90-98.

30. Balg F, Boileau P. The instability index score. A simple pre-operative score to select patients for arthroscopic or open shoulder stabilization. *J Bone Joint Surg Br.* 2007;89(11):1470-1477.

Please see videos on the accompanying website at

www.ArthroscopicTechniques.com

3

Arthroscopic Humeral Avulsion of the Glenohumeral Ligament Repair

Gregory C. Mallo, MD, FAAOS; Petar Golijanin;
Matthew Doran; and Matthew T. Provencher, MD

INTRODUCTION

Shoulder instability after trauma often involves injury to both the labrum and the capsule. Typically, this pathology is attributed to separation of the labrum from the anteroinferior glenoid (Bankart lesion) or to plastic deformation of the capsule. However, in some instances, especially with traumatic injury to the arm that is positioned in hyperabduction and external rotation, an avulsion of the inferior glenohumeral ligament (IGHL) from its humeral insertion can occur. Nicola[1] and Bach et al[2] have termed this a *humeral avulsion of the glenohumeral ligament (HAGL) lesion*. Although believed to be relatively uncommon, Wolf et al[3] found a 9.3% incidence of HAGL lesions in 64 patients, while Bokor et al[4] noted a 7.5% incidence in 547 shoulders with instability. The HAGL lesion has been shown to result in persistent anterior instability as well as pain, decreased athletic performance, and lack of strength in the absence of instability symptoms.[5] One must therefore maintain a high index of suspicion for an HAGL lesion based on mechanism of injury, persistence of symptoms, and preoperative magnetic resonance (MR) arthrography.

INDICATIONS

Patients with limited function or athletic performance secondary to symptoms of pain and/or instability and who have failed a trial of conservative treatment should be considered surgical candidates. Identifying an HAGL lesion on preoperative MR arthrogram and confirming this at the time of surgery as well as those primarily identified during diagnostic arthroscopy should be repaired. Surgeons should have a high index of suspicion for younger patients after a shoulder injury with persistent pain, shoulder dysfunction, and complaints that the shoulder is not working well. These findings may herald an HAGL lesion.

Ryu RKN, Angelo RL, Abrams JS, eds. *The Shoulder: AANA Advanced Arthroscopic Surgical Techniques* (pp 31-37).
© 2016 AANA.

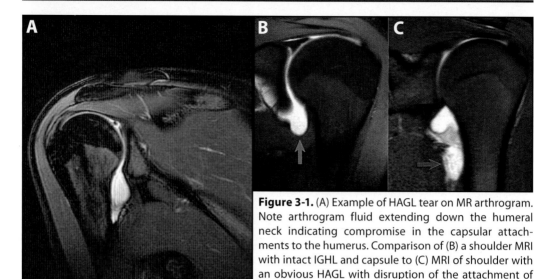

Figure 3-1. (A) Example of HAGL tear on MR arthrogram. Note arthrogram fluid extending down the humeral neck indicating compromise in the capsular attachments to the humerus. Comparison of (B) a shoulder MRI with intact IGHL and capsule to (C) MRI of shoulder with an obvious HAGL with disruption of the attachment of the inferior capsule to the humerus.

Controversial Indications

Relative contraindications include the presence of significant glenoid bone loss or of an engaging Hill-Sachs lesion, which should be addressed in addition to HAGL repair. The role of a concomitant HAGL repair during procedures to address glenoid or humeral bone loss has not been clearly established.

PERTINENT PHYSICAL FINDINGS

There is no specific clinical test to clinically differentiate an HAGL lesion from a more standard Bankart lesion, however anterior instability in the absence of crepitus as the humeral head slides over the labrum is suggestive of an HAGL. However, this subtle finding is not easily appreciated on examination.

PERTINENT IMAGING

The most useful preoperative test for the evaluation of a suspected HAGL lesion is an MR arthrogram. The MR imaging (MRI) characteristics of HAGL include signal intensity and thickening of the inferior capsule, extravasation of contrast material of joint effusion along the medial humeral neck, and a J-shaped axillary pouch ("J" sign) as opposed to the normal U-shaped structure (Figure 3-1).[6,7]

EQUIPMENT

► A standard 4.0-mm arthroscope with a 30-degree lens is commonly used; however, a 70-degree arthroscope should be readily available to assist in viewing

► Complete set of arthroscopic instruments including suture lassos, graspers, bone preparation tools (rasps, cutters), and metal switching sticks

▶ A 3.5- or 4.5-mm full radius bony cutting shaver should be available to abrade capsule and debride necessary labral tissue without aggressive excision of tissue

▶ A set of clear cannulas to allow for instrument passage and knot tying: 5.25 and 8.25 mm

▶ 3.5- or 4.5-mm knotless anchor, or screw-in anchor 3.5 mm or greater

POSITIONING AND PORTALS

Positioning

Patients are placed in the lateral decubitus position under general or laryngeal mask airway anesthesia and an intraoperative examination under anesthesia is performed.

The patient is then prepped and draped in the usual sterile fashion and the arm is placed in 10 lbs of balanced suspension. The limb is positioned in 15 degrees of forward flexion and 50 degrees of abduction in order to gently expose the glenohumeral joint.

Portals

▶ Posterior portal: A standard posterior viewing portal is initially created by identifying the interval between the infraspinatus and the teres minor, which is usually located 1.5 to 3 cm distal and in line with the lateral edge of the acromion.

▶ Anterosuperior portal: This portal is created using an outside-in technique under direct visualization. This is created high in the rotator interval and is used for viewing during creation of the accessory posterolateral portal at the 7 o'clock position. It is located approximately 1 cm laterally to the anterolateral border of the acromion, often just above biceps.

▶ Accessory posterolateral (7 o'clock) portal: This portal is created while viewing from the anterosuperior portal using an 18-gauge spinal needle for localization. It is typically located 4 cm directly lateral to the posterior corner of the acromion. A cannula is then introduced atraumatically over a smooth metal rod.

▶ Anterior mid-to-low glenoid portal: With the camera switched back to the posterior portal, the anterior mid-to-low glenoid portal is established directly above the subscapularis tendon. An 18-gauge spinal needle is used to identify the proper trajectory and angle of approach to the humeral bed and anterior glenoid as needed.

▶ 5 o'clock portal: The 5 o'clock portal is established about 1 cm inferiorly and 2 to 3 cm laterally to the anterior portal through the most lateral portion of the subscapularis tendon, which is helpful for the placement of suture anchors into the humerus. This "killer angle," as noted by Huberty and Burkhart, can only be achieved through the 5 o'clock portal and placing the arm in abduction and external rotation.[8]

STEP-BY-STEP DESCRIPTION OF THE PROCEDURE

After reviewing the preoperative imaging, the surgeon positively identifies the patient and general or laryngeal mask airway anesthesia is initiated. An intraoperative exam under anesthesia is then performed to confirm the diagnosis of instability or to access additional pathology.

The patient is then placed in the lateral decubitus position with a well-padded roll under the down-facing axilla. The patient is then prepped and draped in the usual sterile fashion with the arm hanging in 10 lbs of balanced suspension. The limb is positioned in 15 degrees of forward flexion and 50 degrees of abduction in order to distend the joint and separate the humeral head from the glenoid.

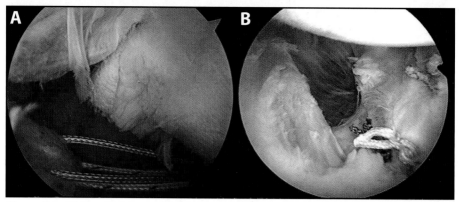

Figure 3-2. (A) Part 2 of the reverse HAGL. Two horizontal sutures are placed (4 passes into the capsule) to be utilized for capsular repair back to the humerus. (B) The Bankart is repaired in a bipolar lesion (both HAGL and labral Bankart tear) and the HAGL will then be repaired.

The standard posterior portal is made and a diagnostic arthroscopy is then initiated. An anterior portal is established in the superior aspect of the rotator interval using an outside-in or inside-out technique. A clear 5.25-mm cannula is then placed and the arthroscope is switched to this location to complete the diagnostic arthroscopy.

Next, while viewing from the anterosuperior portal, an 18-gauge spinal needle is used for localization and establishing the accessory posterolateral or 7 o'clock portal. The needle insertion and portal site is typically located 4 cm directly lateral to the posterior corner of the acromion. A cannula is introduced over a smooth metal rod.[9] Establishing the 7 o'clock portal is a critical element of the arthroscopic HAGL repair technique.

Next, the arthroscope is returned to the posterior portal and a mid-to-low glenoid portal is established directly above the subscapularis tendon. The proper position for this portal is determined using an 18-gauge spinal needle. This portal is necessary for the proper angle of approach to the humeral bone bed as well as the anterior glenoid if necessary (Figure 3-2).[10]

Once the portals are established, the HAGL pathology is further evaluated (Figure 3-3). The anterior glenohumeral ligaments are inspected from their glenoid/labral origin to their attachment on the humeral neck.

Typically, an HAGL presents with an avulsion of all or part of the middle and IGHL complexes from their humeral insertion and may be anterior, inferior, posterior, or a combination of all three. A 70-degree scope in the posterior portal provides excellent visualization of the humeral insertion of this complex. Alternatively, visualization can be achieved with a 30-degree scope placed in the anterosuperior portal (Figure 3-4). A probe is then placed through the anterior mid-to-low glenoid portal to assess the competency of the ligaments.

Concomitant Pathology: Bone Loss or Labral Injury

If a large, engaging Hill-Sachs lesion or significant glenoid bone defect is identified, the treatment plan is changed to an alternative procedure to address the area of bone deficiency. If a Bankart lesion is identified along with an HAGL, the glenohumeral ligaments are first reduced to the humeral neck with a grasper to assess the tension of the capsule. The HAGL is then repaired first to avoid overtightening of the capsule medially. A burr is placed through the anterior mid-glenoid portal and the original humeral insertion site of the IGHL complex is gently debrided to create a bleeding bony bed for reattachment. The Bankart repair is completed in standard fashion using glenoid suture with care taken not to overtension the repair so there is sufficient tissue left to anchor the capsule to the humeral neck avulsion site.

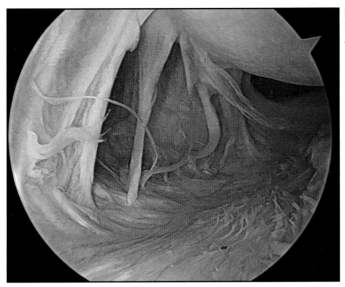

Figure 3-3. HAGL tear of the antero-inferior capsule demonstrating classic striations and tear off the humeral head.

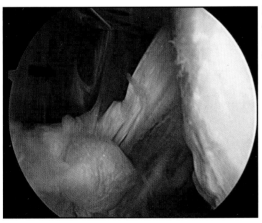

Figure 3-4. An example of a reverse HAGL or a tear of the posterior inferior capsule off the humerus. Note the rotator cuff (infraspinatus) muscle now exposed due to the capsular tear (arrow).

Steps for Humeral Avulsion of the Glenohumeral Ligament Repair

Attention is then turned toward percutaneous suture anchor insertion onto the medial neck of the humerus at the previously prepared footprint. Under direct visualization, an 18-gauge needle is used to establish the correct path for suture anchor placement. The approximate starting point is between the standard posterior portal and the accessory posterolateral portal (7 o'clock). This is obtained in a percutaneous fashion with the anchor-inserting device and drill. Once the appropriate path is established, an appropriate suture anchor is placed and one of the suture limbs is retrieved from the anterosuperior portal. The remaining suture limb is left outside the skin. A straight suture repair device is advanced through a cannula in the 7 o'clock portal and passed through the inferior/lateral capsule just inside of the avulsion borders for shuttling. This can be repeated to create a mattress suture configuration, which is then tied through the 7 o'clock portal with a knot pusher. As the repair continues anteriorly, an accessory low anterior portal is required for correct anchor placement. This portal is created in a trans-subscapularis fashion, staying lateral to the humerus to minimize the risk of axillary nerve injury. This portal can be used to place an anchor percutaneously or a small 5-mm cannula can be used. It is important to use the rotation of the humerus to help control access to all areas of the humeral capsular avulsion site. Once the anchor is in place, sutures are passed through the torn capsule in a similar fashion as described previously using a corkscrew suture-passing device. The sutures are shuttled and brought out of the anterior midlateral portal. In general, sutures are passed in a mattress fashion, allowing the knot to be placed outside of the capsule (see Figure 3-2).

POSTOPERATIVE PROTOCOL

Initially, the arm is placed into a sling for approximately 4 weeks, during which the patient is instructed to perform supine well-arm forward elevation to 90 degrees; passive external rotation with arm at the side to 30 degrees; grip strength; and hand, wrist, and elbow range of motion exercises. Deltoid and rotator cuff isometrics are begun within a few days of the surgery. From 4 to 6 weeks postoperatively, active and active-assisted forward elevation to 140 degrees and external rotation with arm at the side to 40 degrees is begun, deltoid/rotator cuff isometrics are progressed, and scapular-stabilizing exercises are begun. At 8 weeks, full range of motion in all directions, gentle stretching at end range of motion, and progressive light resistance training is permitted. Deltoid and rotator cuff exercises are progressed to isotonic. External rotation in 45 degrees of abduction is started at 10 to 12 weeks postoperatively. After 3 months, or when the patient has pain-free symmetric active range of motion, a strengthening program is initiated and progressed as tolerated. Return to sport is determined after completing an isokinetic and functional test assessment, but is usually 5 to 6 months postoperatively.

POTENTIAL COMPLICATIONS

Complications of HAGL repair include stiffness and nerve injury; however, attention to surgical technique, portal placement, portal trajectory, as well as correct placement of anchors can minimize the chance of having the following complications:

► Stiffness and potential loss of motion after surgical repair of HAGL lesion: This may be due to overtightening the capsule or just the consequence of the injury. The tear itself may predispose to having a capsular constriction after the surgery because sometimes, in order to incorporate quality tissue into the repair, one moves medially into the capsule, thus creating a tension and the potential for overconstraint. A grasping device can be used to access tissue mobility and the goal should be anatomic repair.

► Potential nerve injury: The main concern is injury to the axillary nerve. Care should be taken to avoid anteroinferior and deep anterior or inferior portals where the axillary nerve is at highest risk. It is also at risk laterally, approximately 5 cm lateral to the acromion, although this is highly variable and individualized in patients. Positioning in the lateral decubitus position may afford some protection; however, avoiding injury to the axillary nerve is paramount.

► Implant complications: The humeral head bone is softer than that of the glenoid and care should be taken to choose an anchor that provides adequate fixation into the humeral head for optimized pullout strength. Usually, this is a small rotator cuff type of screw-in anchor. Tap-in type of compression implants may also provide adequate fixation but should be of sufficient diameter (usually greater than 3.5 mm) to maximize strength in the slightly weaker cancellous bone of humerus.

► Failure to recognize bipolar components of the injury: In one series, 43% of patients had both HAGL injury and combined Bankart or labral tear. Care should be taken to address both of these pathologies. Typically, the HAGL is repaired first followed by the labrum, but regardless, both pathologic conditions require treatment to ensure good, stable surgical outcome.

Top Technical Pearls for the Procedure

1. Assess the anterior labrum for a Bankart lesion, significant glenoid bone loss, or an anterior labroligamentous periosteal sleeve avulsion lesion.

2. Elevation of the capsule should be between the plane of the capsule and the underlying subscapularis.

3. Obtaining the correct oblique angle of approach for placement of suture anchors into the humerus can be achieved by using a 5 o'clock portal or a 7 o'clock portal and placing the arm in abduction and external rotation. The arm should be held in this position for preparation of the bone bed and placement of anchors.

4. After passing the suture, the ligaments must be visually confirmed to be reduced back to the proximal humerus and must be maintained in this position as the arthroscopic knots are tied.

5. Avoid suture passage through the subscapularis and be sure that all knots are tied in the plane between the lateral capsule and subscapularis.

References

1. Nicola T. Anterior dislocation of the shoulder; the role of the articular capsule. *J Bone Joint Surg Am*. 1942;24(3):614-616.
2. Bach RB, Warren RF, Fronek J. Disruption of the lateral capsule of the shoulder. A cause of recurrent dislocation. *J Bone Joint Surg Am*. 1988;70(2):274-276.
3. Wolf EM, Cheng JC, Dickson K. Humeral avulsion of glenohumeral ligaments as a cause of anterior shoulder instability. *Arthroscopy*. 1995;11(5):600-607.
4. Bokor DJ, Conboy VB, Olson C. Anterior instability of the glenohumeral joint with humeral avulsion of the glenohumeral ligament. A review of 41 cases. *J Bone Joint Surg Br*. 1999;81(1):93-96.
5. Provencher MT, McCormick F, Gaston T, LeClere L, Solomon DJ, Dewing C. A prospective outcome evaluation of humeral avulsions of the glenohumeral ligament (HAGL) tears in an active population. *Arthroscopy*. 2014;30(S):e5. doi:10.1016/j.arthro.2014.04.017.
6. Bui-Mansfield LT, Dean T, Uhorchak JM, Tenuta JJ. Humeral avulsions of the glenohumeral ligament: imaging features and a review of the literature. *AJR Am J Roentgenol*. 2002;179(3):649-655.
7. Stoller DW. MR arthrography of the glenohumeral joint. *Radiol Clinic North Amer*. 1997;35(1):97-116.
8. Huberty DP, Burkhart SS. Arthroscopic repair of anterior humeral avulsion of the glenohumeral ligaments. *Tech Shoulder Elbow Surg*. 2006;7(4):186-190.
9. Davidson PA. The 7-o'clock posteroinferior portal for shoulder arthroscopy. *Am J Sports Med*. 2002;30(5):693-696.
10. Richards DP, Burkhart SS. Arthroscopic humeral avulsion of the glenohumeral ligaments (HAGL) repair. *Arthroscopy*. 2004;20:134-141.

Please see videos on the accompanying website at

www.ArthroscopicTechniques.com

4

Revision Arthroscopic Shoulder Stabilization

Brian J. Cole, MD, MBA; Chris R. Mellano, MD; Rachel M. Frank, MD;
Andrew J. Riff, MD; and Matthew T. Provencher, MD

INTRODUCTION

Multiple demographic, anatomic, and technical factors have been targeted as risk factors for recurrent instability following surgical stabilization. Demographic factors that are highly predictive of recurrent instability include younger patient age, participation in overhead or contact sports, and male gender. Among the intrinsic patient factors that have been implicated, younger patient age is the most well-delineated factor leading to recurrent instability. Voos and colleagues reported a recurrence rate of 37.5% for patients younger than 20 years of age compared with 15.3% for patients older than 20 years.[1] Similarly, Porcellini et al demonstrated a recurrence rate of 13.3% in patients aged 22 years and younger compared with 6.3% in patients older than 22 years.[2] Participation in contact or overhead sports also dramatically increases a patient's risk of recurrent instability. Owens and colleagues reported mean 11.7-year follow-up data on 39 contact athletes managed with arthroscopic Bankart repair.[3] At final follow-up, 14.3% had experienced a recurrent dislocation, 21.4% had experienced a subluxation event, and 14.3% had undergone revision stabilization surgery. Male gender has also been demonstrated to be a risk factor for recurrent instability. Balg and Boileau demonstrated a recurrence rate of 17% in men compared to 2% in women at an average of 31.2 months after arthroscopic Bankart repair.[4]

Anatomic factors that commonly contribute to recurrent instability include significant glenoid bone loss, the presence of an engaging Hill-Sachs lesion, and increased ligamentous laxity. Glenoid bone loss involving more than 25% of the glenoid surface has been demonstrated to be highly predictive of failure for primary repair attempts.[5] In the revision setting, glenoid bone loss more than 20% has a high rate of failure with revision arthroscopic repair.[6] Moreover, the presence of both an engaging Hill-Sachs lesion and glenoid bone loss of greater than 25% confers nearly a 10-fold increased risk of recurrence compared to those without (51.5% vs 5.5%). Higher rates of failure have also been shown in patients with ligamentous laxity. Balg and Boileau demonstrated that patients with shoulder hyperlaxity (defined by external rotation [ER] > 85 degrees with the shoulder adducted) had a recurrence rate of 18.9% compared with 4.9% in those without hyperlaxity.[4]

Ryu RKN, Angelo RL, Abrams JS, eds. *The Shoulder: AANA Advanced Arthroscopic Surgical Techniques* (pp 39-48).

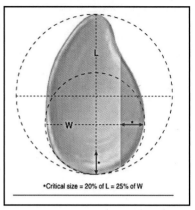

Figure 4-1. Evaluation of glenoid bone loss based on 3D computed tomography reconstruction. The gray area represents bone loss. In a revision setting, if the glenoid bone loss is >10%, then consideration should be given to an open bone block stabilization procedure.

In patients with failed primary stabilization, the surgical technique must be thoroughly evaluated to determine the etiology of failure. In a series of 16 patients, Arce et al found that 75% of primary failures were attributable to a suboptimal surgical technique.[7] Technical missteps can be subdivided into preoperative, intraoperative, and postoperative errors. Preoperatively, failure to recognize posterior instability, multidirectional instability, significant glenoid bone loss, an engaging Hill-Sachs lesion, or humeral avulsion of the glenohumeral ligaments (HAGL lesion) may lead to inadequate restoration of the anatomy and compromise the stability of the joint. Intraoperatively, failure to sufficiently mobilize the labrum and attached capsule will not restore proper capsular tension and glenoid concavity compression. Additionally, inappropriate placements of the anchor medially on the glenoid neck will malreduce the capsulolabral complex and, in turn, compromise the stability of the construct. Postoperatively, patients must be strongly cautioned regarding the risks of contact sports and the importance of avoiding "at-risk" positions.

A 10-point preoperative instability severity index score (ISIS) has been created to stratify patients with regard to risk of recurrent instability and to guide surgical decision making in primary shoulder instability surgery.[4] The score is based on patient age, level of sport, type of sport, presence of hyperlaxity, presence of a Hill-Sachs lesion, and presence of glenoid bone loss. In Balg and Boileau's study, patients with a score of 3 or less had a recurrence rate of 5%, whereas those with a score of more than 6 had a recurrence rate of 70%. The authors recommended that patients with scores >6 be managed with an open bone block procedure. Certainly, treatment of patients with ISIS of 4 to 6 with arthroscopic vs open stabilization remains controversial.

INDICATIONS

▶ Recurrent instability in patients with minimal glenoid bone loss and satisfactory capsular tissue

Controversial Indications

▶ Recurrent instability in patients with 15% to 20% glenoid bone loss
▶ Isolated large, engaging Hill-Sachs lesion requiring concurrent remplissage

Contraindications

▶ Glenoid bone loss >20% (Figure 4-1)
▶ Engaging, "off-track" Hill-Sachs lesion and glenoid bone loss
▶ Poor capsular tissue due to genetic, traumatic, or prior surgery

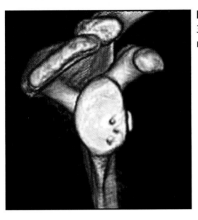

Figure 4-2. Failed previous Bankart repair of a 17-year-old male. 3D computed tomography shows minimal anterior inferior glenoid bone loss and 3 previously placed anchors.

▶ Voluntary dislocations, secondary gain
▶ Patients with multiple risk factors for recurrence (ie, elevated ISIS)

Pertinent Physical Findings

▶ The contralateral shoulder should be examined to establish baseline range of motion (ROM), stability, and laxity.
▶ The posterior jerk test should be performed carefully to rule out posterior instability.
▶ Gagey sign, the presence of hyperabduction > 20 degrees compared to contralateral shoulder, can be seen in inferior capsular laxity or MDI.
▶ Passive ER, with the shoulder adducted, greater than 85 degrees is suggestive of anterior capsular hyperlaxity. A sulcus sign may also suggest capsular laxity.
▶ Other joints should be examined for signs of hyperlaxity (eg, finger hyperextension, elbow hyperextension, ability to passively oppose each thumb to the flexor surface of the arm, etc).
▶ Rotator cuff strength should be assessed.
▶ A careful neurologic examination should be performed to rule out iatrogenic or injury-related compromise of the axillary nerve or brachial plexus.
▶ Concomitant injuries to the biceps tendon, superior labral anteroposterior, and acromioclavicular joint should be ruled out.

Pertinent Imaging

▶ If available, review of initial preoperative imaging including radiographs and advanced imaging is helpful to confirm correct initial diagnosis and surgical indication.
▶ If available, review index procedure arthroscopic images.
▶ If available, previous operative reports should be reviewed to determine previous anchor number, size, position, and composition (eg, biocomposite, PEEK, metal) to anticipate intraoperative challenges.
▶ Post-failure magnetic resonance arthrogram to assess the extent of soft tissue pathology
▶ Post-failure 3D reconstruction computed tomography with humeral head subtraction to quantitate glenoid bone loss and localize prior anchor positions (Figure 4-2).

Equipment

When performing a revision arthroscopic stabilization with augmentation, the standard shoulder arthroscopic Bankart repair equipment is adequate with few modifications. The standard instruments include the following:

▶ Power, arthroscopic rasp to prepare the capsule, arthroscopic periosteal elevator (45 degrees) to elevate the labrum

▶ Wissinger rods (pointed switching stick)

▶ Small hooded burr to prepare the bone bed

▶ Suture-passing device with multiple angles and an absorbable monofilament passing suture (#1 PDS [polydioxanone])

▶ Suture retriever

▶ Arthroscopic knot pusher

▶ Arthroscopic suture cutter

▶ Cannulas with sufficient diameter to accommodate all instruments needed for each step of the surgery (6- to 9-mm diameter)

▶ Appropriately sized dilators are often necessary for cannula insertion over Wissinger rods, especially if penetrating the intra-articular fibers of the subscapularis

▶ Knotless suture anchors (2.9 mm) with broad, low-profile suture (1.5 mm) to avoid suture abrasion on the humeral articular cartilage and to preserve load to failure characteristicss[8]

▶ Alternatively, single- or double-loaded suture anchor (2.4 or 3 mm) can be used if knot fixation is preferred

Positioning and Portals

The authors' preference is to perform all arthroscopic stabilization procedures in the lateral decubitus position with arm-weighted suspension. Other surgeons may prefer a beach chair position for the advantages of anatomic orientation. The authors' experience has been that lateral decubitus position consistently provides adequate arthroscopic visualization regardless of patient body habitus and allows the surgical assistant to assist with the surgical procedure instead of constantly modifying the arm position. Care should be taken to limit duration of weighted suspension to avoid neurologic injury. The authors' preference is to use 10 lbs to suspend the arm in 35 to 40 degrees of abduction and 10 to 20 degrees of forward flexion (FF).

Precise portal positioning is paramount to a successful revision arthroscopic shoulder stabilization procedure. To perform a revision stabilization with augmentation, the authors' preference is to use 4 portals, including a standard posterior viewing portal, a rotator interval portal with an 8.25-mm cannula, a posteroinferior 7 o'clock portal with an 8.25- or 9-mm cannula, and often a percutaneous trans-subscapularis 5 o'clock portal (Figure 4-3).

Step-by-Step Description of the Procedure

Step 1: Diagnostic Arthroscopy

While in the lateral decubitus position, a load and shift test can be performed before weighted suspension is applied. To begin, a standard posterior viewing portal is created slightly more

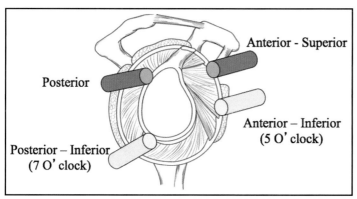

Figure 4-3. Portal placement for revision arthroscopic stabilization. Standard posterior viewing port, rotator interval anterosuperior portal, trans-rotator cuff 5 o'clock portal, and posteroinferior 7 o'clock portal.

lateral than in a beach chair position. Subsequently, an anterior portal is established in the rotator interval directly above the rolled border of the subscapularis following localization with a spinal needle in an outside-in fashion lateral to the coracoid process. An 8.25-mm cannula is introduced. Diagnostic arthroscopy is now performed with a probe through the posterior and anterior cannulas to evaluate the rotator cuff, bicep tendon, superior labrum, and presence of retained hardware. The capsule is assessed for overall tissue quality and for the presence of an HAGL lesion. The amount of anteroinferior glenoid bone loss is then evaluated by the technique described by Burkhart and colleagues.[9] The articular cartilage is then evaluated for the presence of a glenolabral articular disruption lesion for prognostic purposes. The humeral head is inspected for the presence and size of a Hill-Sachs defect. If concern exists for a possible engaging Hill-Sachs lesion, the arm can be taken out of weighted suspension and brought into abduction and ER under arthroscopic visualization. In the rare situation where an engaging Hill-Sachs lesion is present without associated significant glenoid bone loss, then an arthroscopic remplissage procedure is typically performed in addition to anterior Bankart repair. If concern exists for a posterior capsulolabral injury, the arthroscope can be placed through the anterior cannula, and a probe introduced through the posterior portal can palpate the posterior labrum. Once the diagnostic arthroscopy is complete and the diagnosis is confirmed to be an isolated failed Bankart repair with minimal glenoid bone loss and adequate capsular tissue integrity, the surgeon may proceed with the revision arthroscopic Bankart repair with a posteroinferior capsulolabral plication augmentation.

Step 2: Establish a Posteroinferior 7 o'clock Portal

In a revision situation, it is the authors' preference to perform an inferior and posteroinferior capsulolabral plication as an augmentation to the anteroinferior Bankart repair. For a right shoulder, a posteroinferior 7 o'clock portal provides excellent access to the 6 and 7 o'clock position on the glenoid. The 7 o'clock portal location is typically 2 fingerbreadths distal and 2 fingerbreadths lateral to the standard posterior viewing portal, or roughly 4 cm distal to the posterolateral edge of the acromion. A spinal needle is introduced under direct visualization. The spinal needle should hug the humeral head as it enters the joint at a steep trajectory while aiming at the 6 o'clock glenoid position. This steep trajectory will be helpful for eventual anchor insertion at the 6 and 7 o'clock glenoid position. Once the spinal needle position and trajectory are satisfactory, a Wissinger rod replaces the spinal needle. Care is taken to aim toward the axillary pouch when piercing the capsule with the rod to avoid iatrogenic glenoid articular damage. An 8.25- or 9-mm cannula is inserted over the Wissinger rod after dilating with sequential dilators.

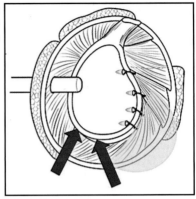

Figure 4-4. Revision arthroscopic Bankart repair requires an inferior and posteroinferior capsulolabral augmentation. Suture anchors are typically placed at the red arrows to help reduce the IGHL capsular laxity and create an internal sling.

Step 3: Capsule and Bone Preparation

While viewing from the standard posterior viewing portal, a rasp is introduced through the anterior cannula to gently prepare the anterior and inferior capsule surfaces. The rasp is then inserted into the 7 o'clock portal to prepare the inferior and posteroinferior capsule. Retained hardware and suture from prior surgery is removed by tightly wrapping the free suture ends around a suture grasper in an "alligator roll" fashion. Next, an arthroscopic periosteal elevator is introduced through the anterior cannula and the anterior and anteroinferior labrum is elevated off the glenoid sharply to create one large sleeve. This step is particularly important in the presence of an anterior labrum periosteal sleeve avulsion or a labrum that was previously "fixed" inferior to the glenoid rim. A grasper placed through the 7 o'clock portal can attempt a trial reduction of the elevated labrum onto the rim of the glenoid to confirm adequate elevation. As the capsulolabral injury often continues posteroinferiorly, the elevator can be used through the 7 o'clock portal to elevate this portion of the labrum as well. To confirm adequate elevation of the anterior capsulo-labral sleeve, some surgeons prefer to view from the anterior portal or an anterosuperior portal to see the subscapularis fibers, but in the authors' experience, this has often not been necessary. Using a 70-degree arthroscope through the posterior portal may also be utilized to view the anterior capsule and subscapularis. Once the injured capsulolabral tissue is adequately elevated, the glenoid bone must be gently decorticated to promote healing. It is important to avoid injury to the adjacent labrum and capsule by using a hooded burr while carefully limiting the amount of bone resection.

Step 4: The 6 o'clock Anchor Placement—The Inferior Capsular Sling Augmentation

To begin the revision repair with inferior capsular augmentation, it is the authors' preference to first create the inferior and posteroinferior capsulolabral plication augmentation. To do this, an anchor is placed at the 6 o'clock or 6:30 position (Figure 4-4). A 90-degree curved suture-passing device is introduced through the 7 o'clock portal and used to shuttle the PDS suture under the capsule and labrum at the 6 o'clock position. Care is taken to avoid the axillary nerve by staying superficial once the tip of the suturing device passes through the capsule. The PDS suture is retrieved through the anterior cannula with a suture retriever. One end of a broad suture (LabralTape 1.5 mm [Arthrex]) is then attached to the PDS suture outside of the cannula and retrograded under the labrum and out the 7 o'clock portal. A suture retriever is then introduced in the 7 o'clock portal to retrieve the other end of the labral tape so that both ends are out of the 7 o'clock portal in a simple suture fashion. Next, a drill sleeve is introduced into the 7 o'clock portal and placed at the 6 o'clock or 6:30 glenoid position. Care is taken to place the drill sleeve up onto the articular surface in front of the labrum and as perpendicular to the articular surface as possible

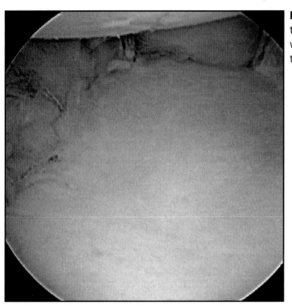

Figure 4-5. Right shoulder lateral position posterior viewing portal. Revision Bankart repair with posterior and posteroinferior augmentation with knotless suture anchors.

to avoid skiving with the drill. While the surgeon holds the drill sleeve and the arthroscope, the assistant drills the glenoid through the drill sleeve. The drill sleeve is removed from the cannula while the arthroscopic view remains fixed on the glenoid drill site to maintain visualization of the anchor insertion site. Next, the assistant passes the 2 ends of the labral tape through the knotless anchor (2.9 mm) islet. The assistant then holds the camera and maintains an arthroscopic view of the glenoid insertion site while the surgeon inserts the anchor into the drilled site. A mallet is used to fully seat the anchor to avoid articular damage from prominent hardware. A suture cutter is used to cut the labral tape flush with the glenoid surface to avoid prominent suture (Figure 4-5).

Depending on surgeon preference, the inferior capsulolabral plication augmentation can be extended posteriorly with an additional anchor at the 7 o'clock or 7:30 position. This would be performed in the same manner as the 6 o'clock anchor described previously. Of note, after this step, when clinically indicated, an arthroscopic remplissage procedure can be performed to address an engaging Hill-Sachs lesion. In a setting with minimal anteroinferior bone deficiency (ie, less than 15%) with a suitable Hill-Sachs lesion, remplissage remains an additional option to reduce the incidence of recurrence. Typically, the bony bed of the lesion is prepared and 1 or 2 double-loaded suture anchors are placed transtendinously through a percutaneous technique. The anchors are placed along the top margin of the defect and a tissue penetrator placed percutaneously is used through the cuff into the joint to retrieve a single suture limb of each suture. The sutures are tied while visualizing through the subacromial space to avoid inadvertent capture of the subdeltoid fascia.

Step 5: Anteroinferior Anchor Insertion Through a Trans-Subscapularis (5 o'clock) Portal

It is the authors' opinion that the low anteroinferior capsulolabral repair is vital to successful revision Bankart repair. Attempting to place this anteroinferior anchor from the anterior cannula in the rotator interval often leads to skiving of the drill or inadequate bony fixation of the anchor, complications that are increasingly likely in a revision setting with compromised bony anatomy. In order to obtain optimal anchor insertion trajectory, it is often necessary to place the anchor through a trans-subscapularis portal (5 o'clock portal for right shoulder). The axillary nerve is below the inferior border of the subscapularis and should be safely 2 to 3 cm away from the

5 o'clock portal site if placed in the middle of the subscapularis fibers.[10] A spinal needle is used first to optimize the portal location and trajectory. To avoid injury to the subscapularis, this anchor can be placed either percutaneously or through a narrow 4-mm metal cannula. A large cannula is not routinely placed through the subscapularis. Once the anchor is introduced through the trans-subscapularis 5 o'clock portal, suturing and knot tying can be performed through the standard anterior rotator-interval cannula.

The presence of anteroinferior glenoid bone loss or residual suture anchors may make insertion of new suture anchors challenging. In the revision setting, it is common that the anteroinferior glenoid has inadequate "real estate" for insertion of multiple suture anchors. In this situation, the authors' preference is to place one double-loaded anchor at the 5 o'clock position with knot fixation (2.4- or 3-mm double-loaded). When using knot fixation, the first step is to position the drill sleeve onto the anteroinferior glenoid using a sharp trochar introduced through a percutaneous trans-subscapularis 5 o'clock portal without the need for a cannula. When piercing through the subscapularis with the pointed trochar and drill sleeve, it is safer to aim toward the axillary pouch to avoid iatrogenic injury to the glenoid articular surface. Once through the subscapularis, the sharp trochar is removed and the drill is used through the drill sleeve placed onto the desired 5 o'clock glenoid position. After the glenoid is drilled, the double-loaded anchor is placed through the drill sleeve and the mallet is used to fully seat the anchor into position. The suture tails from the anchor are left in their percutaneous position. The 90-degree curved suture passer is introduced through the anterior rotator interval cannula and passed under the capsule and labrum inferior to the anchor at the 5:30 position so that knot tying will shift and reduce the inferiorly displaced labrum up to the 5 o'clock anchor position. The PDS is retrieved out of the 7 o'clock portal. One limb of one of the sutures is retrieved out of the 7 o'clock portal, where it is tied to the PDS. The PDS is then retrograded through the anterior cannula, passing the suture under the labrum. The other end of the same suture is retrieved through the anterior cannula, creating a simple suture pattern. An arthroscopic knot is tied using a knot pusher, choosing the limb that passed through the labrum as the post to prevent the knot from abrading the articular surface. This knot is then cut with the suture-cutting device. The second suture is typically passed at the 4:30 position, just superior to the anchor and tied in a similar fashion. It is important to pass and tie the inferior (5:30) suture before the superior (4:30) suture in order to adequately reduce the inferiorly displaced Bankart lesion to the glenoid.

Step 6: Additional Anterior Anchor Placement

In a revision setting, it is important to use at least 3 anchors for the Bankart repair. Once the anteroinferior anchors have been placed, the surgeon can progress up the glenoid face toward the 3 o'clock position, depending on the extent of the Bankart lesion. Typically, the most superior anchor is at the 3 o'clock position, but about 5% to 10% of Bankart lesions can extend superiorly to involve the superior labrum and bicep insertion. The surgeon must be aware of anatomic variations of the anterosuperior labrum such as a sublabral foramen or Buford complex, which should not be "repaired." The authors' preference is for knotless fixation at the 3 o'clock position. The curved suture passer is introduced through the anterior cannula and the PDS suture is passed under the labrum at the 3:30 or 4 o'clock position and retrieved out of the 7 o'clock portal. The broad low-profile suture is tied to the PDS and pulled back under the labrum and out the anterior cannula. A suture retriever is used to pull the other limb of the labral tape out of the anterior cannula, creating a simple suture pattern. The drill sleeve is inserted up onto the glenoid articular cartilage at the 3 o'clock position by the surgeon while the assistant drills through the drill sleeve. The labral tape is passed through the suture anchor (2.9 mm) islet and the anchor is seated into the drilled glenoid site with a mallet. The labral tape ends are cut flush with the glenoid articular surface. This process is repeated if further superior labral stabilization is needed. At the end of the procedure, a load and shift test can be repeated and documented. The complete revision Bankart repair with augmentation can be seen in Figure 4-5.

POSTOPERATIVE PROTOCOL

▶ Weeks 1 through 4: Sling for 4 weeks, with motion restricted to 90 degrees of FF, 40 degrees of ER at side, internal rotation to stomach, and 45 degrees of abduction. Passive ROM exercises are started first, followed by active-assist ROM and, ultimately, active ROM as tolerated.

▶ Weeks 4 through 8: Discontinue sling at 4 weeks. Increase active ROM to 140 degrees of FF, 40 degrees of ER at side, internal rotation to posterior belt, and 60 degrees of abduction. Strengthening begins during this phase, including isometrics, light bands, and scapular stabilizers.

▶ Weeks 8 through 12: If ROM is lacking, increase to full with gentle passive stretching at end ranges. Advance strengthening as tolerated. Isometrics are first, bands second, and light weights third.

▶ Months 3 through 12: Strengthening continues 3 times per week, as well as closed chain exercises. Sports-specific rehab begins at 3 months. Return to throwing begins at 4.5 months and throw from mound at 6 months. Full recovery is expected by 1 year.

POTENTIAL COMPLICATIONS

Recurrent instability is the most common complication following revision arthroscopic shoulder stabilization. A systematic review of 16 articles and 349 patients undergoing revision arthroscopic Bankart repair found an overall recurrence rate of 12.7%.[11] Other complications may include loss of motion, deep infection, or neurologic injury.

TOP TECHNICAL PEARLS FOR THE PROCEDURE

1. Elevate all of the labrum and capsule as one large sleeve until it can be adequately reduced up onto the glenoid surface.

2. Augment the revision Bankart repair with an inferior and posteroinferior capsulolabral plication through a 7 o'clock portal.

3. Using a trans-subscapularis 5 o'clock portal is helpful to place the anteroinferior anchor in an optimal trajectory, especially in revision cases in which the glenoid may be compromised.

4. Use a double-loaded anchor in the anteroinferior position when bone loss and previous anchors prohibit placement of multiple anchors.

5. Pass the suture under the labrum inferior to the anchor position so the suture will shift and reduce the displaced labrum superiorly to the anchor.

REFERENCES

1. Voos JE, Livermore RW, Feeley BT, et al. Prospective evaluation of arthroscopic Bankart repairs for anterior instability. *Am J Sports Med.* 2010;38(2):302-307.
2. Porcellini G, Campi F, Pegreffi F, Castagna A, Paladini P. Predisposing factors for recurrent shoulder dislocation after arthroscopic treatment. *J Bone Joint Surg.* 2009;91(11):2537-2542.
3. Owens BD, DeBerardino TM, Nelson BJ, et al. Long-term follow-up of acute arthroscopic Bankart repair for initial anterior shoulder dislocations in young athletes. *Am J Sports Med.* 2009;37(4):669-673.
4. Balg F, Boileau P. The instability severity index score. A simple pre-operative score to select patients for arthroscopic or open shoulder stabilisation. *J Bone Joint Surg Br.* 2007;89(11):1470-1477.
5. Ahmed I, Ashton F, Robinson CM. Arthroscopic Bankart repair and capsular shift for recurrent anterior shoulder instability. *J Bone Joint Surg Am.* 2012;94(14):1308.
6. Mologne TS, Provencher MT, Menzel KA, Vachon TA, Dewing CB. Arthroscopic stabilization in patients with an inverted pear glenoid: results in patients with bone loss of the anterior glenoid. *Am J Sports Med.* 2007;35(8):1276-1283.
7. Arce G, Arcuri F, Ferro D, Pereira E. Is selective arthroscopic revision beneficial for treating recurrent anterior shoulder instability? *Clin Orthop Relat Res.* 2011;470(4):965-971.
8. Nho SJ, Frank RM, Van Thiel GS, et al. A biomechanical analysis of anterior Bankart repair using suture anchors. *Am J Sports Med.* 2010;38(7):1405-1412.
9. Burkhart SS, Debeer JF, Tehrany AM, Parten PM. Quantifying glenoid bone loss arthroscopically in shoulder instability. *Arthroscopy.* 2002;18(5):488-491.
10. Lo IK, Lind CC, Burkhart SS. Glenohumeral arthroscopy portals established using an outside-in technique: neurovascular anatomy at risk. *Arthroscopy.* 2004;20(6):596-602.
11. Abouali JAK, Hatzantoni K, Holtby R, et al. Revision arthroscopic Bankart repair. *Arthroscopy.* 2013;29(9):1572-1578.

Please see videos on the accompanying website at

www.ArthroscopicTechniques.com

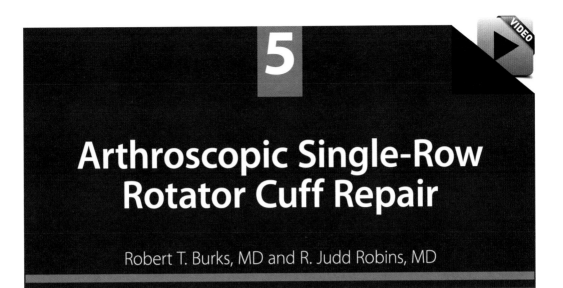

Arthroscopic Single-Row Rotator Cuff Repair

Robert T. Burks, MD and R. Judd Robins, MD

INTRODUCTION

Rotator cuff injury is a common problem for patients as they age but attempt to remain active. Injury to the rotator cuff occurs from acute trauma, such as falls, axial-load injuries to the shoulder, grabbing objects to break a fall, shoulder dislocations, and attempting to lift or move heavy objects. In addition, degenerative changes in the cuff tendon tissue and changes in vascularity to this tissue as patients age can lead to rotator cuff tears. Reasons for these age-related changes are not completely understood, but they can create a significant challenge for surgeons attempting to diagnose and treat acute, acute-on-chronic, and degenerative rotator cuff tears. Using arthroscopically assisted techniques for rotator cuff repair has become the preferred approach for addressing rotator cuff pathology due to improved techniques, arthroscopic instrumentation, and implant design. When adequate, acceptable healthy tissue remains, forms of rotator cuff tear patterns can now successfully be addressed arthroscopically, including partial bursal- or articular-side tears, full thickness tendon disruptions, and multi-tendon "massive cuff tears" with or without retraction. Debate remains, however, regarding how to optimize repair to improve healing rates as surgeons deal with loss of rotator cuff tendon length and continuous decline in biological and biomechanical properties of the muscle and cuff tissue.[1-4] Techniques have focused on attempting better coverage of the insertion "footprint" with more rotator cuff tendon tissue, improving compression of that tissue over the footprint, and increasing the stiffness and strength of the fixation construct to withstand physiologic loads during the healing phases following surgery.[3-5] The ultimate goal of treating rotator cuff tears is to reduce pain and restore strength and shoulder function. While rotator cuff repair has demonstrated reliable results in reducing pain and improving outcomes scores, recurrent tears can be problematic, with some studies reporting re-tear rates in large rotator cuff tears greater than 50% to 90%.[6,7] Despite the creation of improved biomechanical constructs and tendon-to-bone healing observed with imaging, no statistically significant improvements in functional outcomes comparing types of rotator cuff repair have been demonstrated.[8-16]

The single-row rotator cuff repair approach does not necessarily attempt to optimize footprint coverage with native rotator cuff tissue. The philosophy behind this approach recognizes and

Ryu RKN, Angelo RL, Abrams JS, eds. *The Shoulder: AANA Advanced Arthroscopic Surgical Techniques* (pp 49-60). © 2016 AANA.

addresses the loss of native tendon length, which can result in various tear patterns of the rotator cuff.[1] The goal of single-row repair focuses on the following principles:

- ▶ Optimize healing of degenerative cuff tissue by avoiding overtensioning the remnant cuff tendon-muscle unit[1,17]

- ▶ Improve biomechanical strength of the repair construct by optimizing (medializing as needed) suture anchor placement within the rotator cuff footprint[9]

- ▶ Maximize number of sutures per anchor (2 to 3) and arthroscopic knot strength[9,18]

- ▶ Limit the number of implants and subsequent "defects" in the bony footprint needed for repair

Based on these principles, single-row rotator cuff repair has been found to be a cost-effective method for treating rotator cuff tears.[19]

INDICATIONS

- ▶ Injury (ie, fall with axial load, dislocation, etc) to the shoulder resulting in a symptomatic acute disruption of the rotator cuff

- ▶ A tear of any size with minimal tendon loss that can be reduced to its insertion on the greater tuberosity in patients with persistent symptoms despite conservative measures, which include a trial of physical therapy, oral nonsteroidal anti-inflammatory medications, and possibly a subacromial corticosteroid injection

- ▶ Symptomatic partial thickness bursal- or articular-sided rotator cuff tear

- ▶ Loss of rotator cuff tendon length/degenerative tear[1]

- ▶ Retracted rotator cuff tendon tears requiring mobilization

Controversial Indications

- ▶ Chronic tear with higher degree of fatty infiltration (> Goutallier Stage II)

- ▶ Elderly patients (> 65 years)[20,21]

- ▶ Patients with chronic and persistent tobacco exposure

- ▶ Patients with medical comorbidities affecting tendon healing (renal disease, diabetes, immune disorders)

- ▶ Small partial thickness rotator cuff tear in patients with little or no pain and/or mild weakness[22,23]

- ▶ Young, active individuals with an incidental finding of rotator cuff tear without symptoms[21-23]

PERTINENT PHYSICAL FINDINGS

- ▶ Notable loss of active motion secondary to pain and weakness, but preservation of passive motion when compared to the contralateral side

- ▶ Subacromial crepitus with range of motion (ROM) of the shoulder

- ▶ Tenderness to palpation over the anterosuperior and/or posterosuperior shoulder region

- ▶ Associated tenderness of the acromioclavicular joint and bicipital sheath/proximal biceps tendon

- ▶ Loss of strength, especially in resisted forward flexion, abduction, and external rotation (Jobe test)

- Inability to actively lower arm in the plane of the scapula (positive drop sign/drop arm test)
- Inability to maintain external rotation (external rotation lag sign, hornblower's sign)
- Positive tests for impingement (Neer impingement sign, Hawkins sign)
- Continued weakness despite improvement in pain with subacromial lidocaine injection (Neer impingement test)
- Rarely, relative atrophy in the supraspinatus/infraspinatus fossae compared to the contralateral side

PERTINENT IMAGING

- Radiographs of the affected shoulder (anteroposterior, true anteroposterior [Grashey view], axillary, scapular Y, possibly Zanca view)
- Magnetic resonance imaging with sagittal, coronal, and axial views
- Ultrasound of the affected shoulder (can be performed during clinic appointment)
- Computed tomography arthrogram in patients who cannot undergo magnetic resonance imaging

EQUIPMENT

Standard arthroscopic pump and equipment for shoulder arthroscopy is required. This typically includes use of a 30-degree arthroscope, 4- or 5-mm shaver, arthroscopic burr, and an arthroscopic electrocautery wand. The use of cannulas is recommended to provide access to the subacromial space, instrument passage, and fluid management. Specialized arthroscopic graspers including a looped variety greatly facilitate suture management in particular, and in performing various tasks of the procedure overall. Use of both antegrade and retrograde suture-passing and shuttling devices are integral to creating different arthroscopic rotator cuff repair constructs. In addition, an arthroscopic knot pusher and arthroscopic suture cutters aid in managing arthroscopic knots. It is also helpful to have an assortment of arthroscopic rasps, angled tendon elevators, and a 2-mm punch for biologic preparation of the insertion site.

POSITIONING AND PORTALS

Rotator cuff repair surgery can be performed with the patient in the lateral decubitus or the beach chair position, though beach chair positioning facilitates placement of the upper extremity in various positions of abduction, adduction, internal rotation, and external rotation to optimize both exposure of the rotator cuff tendon tear as well as to facilitate reduction and repair of the cuff tissue to the footprint. Use of a mechanical or pneumatic "arm holder" attached to the bed greatly facilitates arm positioning and eliminates the need for an additional assistant in the operating room. General anesthesia with supplemental interscalene block or catheter is recommended to aid with postoperative pain management.[24,25] During patient positioning, attention is needed to avoid "pressure injury" at all bony prominences, ears, eyes, and vulnerable nerves (ulnar, median, common peroneal nerves, etc). The knees and hips should be flexed to avoid traction on the sciatic nerve, and the patient's head and neck region needs to be firmly held in place to avoid shifting during surgery with resultant traction on the brachial plexus. Care should be taken to orient the operative table to allow easy visualization of the video screen. Adequate length and slack in cords and tubing must permit the freedom of movement of the instruments and avoid contamination of the sterile field. The anesthetist should be provided easy access to the head for airway management.

STEP-BY-STEP DESCRIPTION OF THE PROCEDURE

Step 1: Diagnostic Arthroscopy

After prepping and draping the operative extremity, standard posterior and anterior portals are established to perform a complete intra-articular arthroscopic exam. Any intra-articular pathology is addressed at this time. Biceps tenotomy can be performed as indicated and tenodesis can be accomplished later in the procedure according to the patient's lifestyle demands and preferences. A thorough inspection of the subscapularis is a vital and necessary step to rule out partial or complete tear and possible retraction of the tendon. If encountered, the subscapularis tear is typically repaired at this time with use of 1 or 2 suture anchors. Techniques for this are discussed in another chapter.

Step 2: Subacromial Bursectomy

After completing intra-articular procedures, the arthroscope is placed into the subacromial space via the posterior portal, and a lateral portal is established under direct visualization by placing an 18-gauge spinal needle in line with the anterior edge of the acromion. A skin nick is made at that site and a cannula is used to establish the portal. Next, a 5-mm shaver with the aperture facing the undersurface of the acromion is introduced into the subacromial space while viewing with the arthroscope. A bursectomy is then performed to aid visualization of the rotator cuff and to expose the configuration and extent of the tear. Once a space is formed in the subacromial bursa with the shaver and the undersurface of the acromion is identified, a bipolar electrocautery is helpful for expediting removal of bursal tissue, including the posterior and lateral gutters of the subacromial space. A full-radius 5-mm shaver is useful to distinguish bursal and degenerative tissue from healthy rotator cuff tendon and to determine the configuration of the tear. Typically, midanterior and posterolateral portals are established as needed to help with visualization and exposure of the rotator cuff tear (Figure 5-1). An acromioplasty, while not routine, can be performed at this time for the removal of spurs and osteophytes in order to create space as needed.[26] The inclusion of a posterolateral portal has been shown to improve visualization and help the surgeon better define areas of delamination, retraction, and other aspects of the tear that will influence approach for repair.[27]

Step 3: Rotator Cuff Repair Preparation

The footprint on the greater tuberosity is exposed and prepared by clearing soft tissue and using a shaver or burr to create bleeding of the cortical bone. Care should be taken, however, not to remove all of the cortical bone as this affects both anchor pullout strength and healing integrity of the rotator cuff to the bone.

Mobilization of the rotator cuff tissue can then be assessed with use of a cuff grasper by pulling the tendon predominantly in an anterior and somewhat lateral vector. The length of the remnant tendon from the muscle-tendon junction should be noted. The goal is to identify the pattern and nature of the tear (L- vs U-shaped, "reverse L," delaminated, remnant tendon length, etc). If the rotator cuff is retracted medially, then mobilization of the muscle tendon unit can be accomplished as indicated. In some cases, release of the rotator interval, coracohumeral ligament, and coracoid attachments are necessary in chronic retracted tears to mobilize the supraspinatus tendon. Additional releases of the tendon can be performed as necessary to restore appropriate

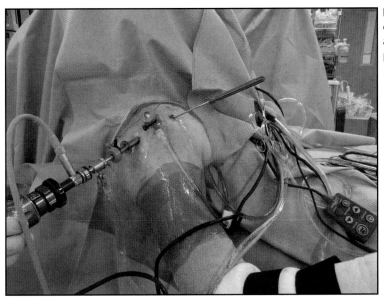

Figure 5-1. Demonstration of anterolateral, midlateral, and posterolateral portal placement.

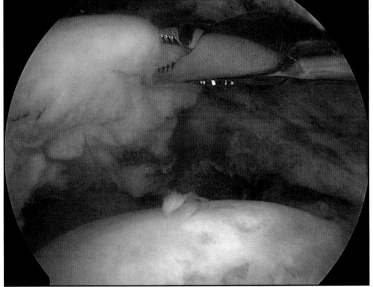

Figure 5-2. Visualization of the rotator cuff tear from the posterolateral portal.

tension to the muscle-tendon unit. A capsular release on the articular side as well as posterior interval slide between the supraspinatus and infraspinatus can be considered (see Chapter 6 for further explanation).

After mobilizing the rotator cuff, the site of anchor placement can then be determined by "rehearsing" reduction of the tendon to the footprint (Figures 5-2 and 5-3). Repairs that result in nonphysiologic tension (high tension) to cover the footprint are to be avoided at all costs as early failure of the repair is likely to occur. Anchors are placed as medial as necessary to minimize tension on the repaired tendon. In cases in which most of the tendon length remains, such as an acute rupture associated with shoulder dislocation, the anchors can be placed more centrally in the footprint to restore normal physiologic tension on the rotator cuff. Again, the goal is restoration of normal physiological tension of the rotator cuff muscles and avoidance of overtensioning.[17]

Figure 5-3. Mobilization of the rotator cuff tear and "rehearsing" of repair for anchor placement.

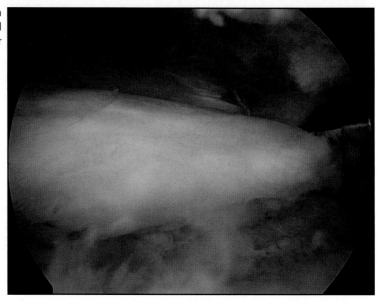

Figure 5-4. Placement of suture anchors within the footprint of the rotator cuff.

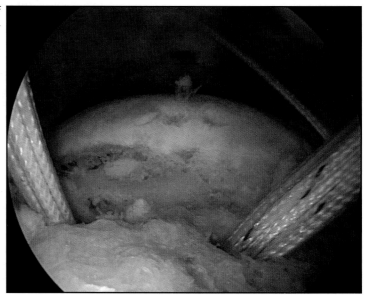

Seven- to 8-mm cannulas are used as necessary to facilitate visualization and passage of instruments. The camera can and should be moved between the anterolateral, midlateral, and posterior portals to improve visualization and recognition of the tear. In addition to the lateral portals, cannulas can also be placed in the anterior and posterior portals as desired to maintain fluid pressure, allow for nontraumatic passage of instruments including the camera, and facilitate suture management. Cannulas can be either hard or soft but should meet the needs listed previously.

Step 4: Rotator Cuff Repair

Typically, anchors are placed 5 to 10 mm apart (Figure 5-4). The number of anchors will vary based on tear size and character of each tear. Many anchors are typically loaded with two #2 braided sutures, but triple-loaded anchors are preferred. Anchors can be metallic, PEEK

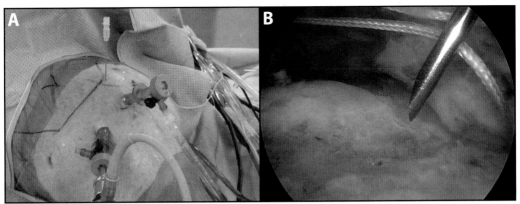

Figure 5-5. Use of a spinal needle to locate the superior lateral "poke-hole" incisions for optimal suture anchor placement.

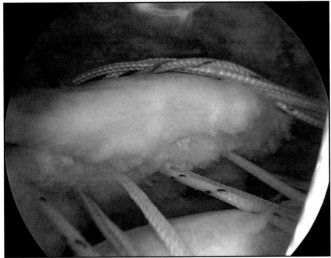

Figure 5-6. Passing of suture through cuff tendon tissue; sutures "parked" in anterior portal.

(polyetheretherketone), or biocomposite, though purely bioabsorbable anchors are not generally recommended. Anchors designed for cancellous bone should be selected, usually with a diameter of 3.5 to 5.5 mm. "All-suture" anchors are also becoming readily available. For patients with osteoporotic bone, 6.5-mm anchors are selected to decrease the risk of pullout. To aid in anchor placement, position the arm in adduction. Anchors are passed through supplemental "poke-hole" superolateral portals that are immediately adjacent to the lateral border of the acromion. This approach allows for optimal placement of the anchor and at an insertion angle that will not risk penetration of the chondral surface (Figure 5-5). Anchors are placed within the footprint based on the extent and location of tendon mobilization rehearsed earlier and in a pattern that allows for reduction of the tendon. A traction stitch can be passed to determine tension and hold the rotator cuff in a reduced position. This can facilitate the proper suture placement for each anchor. Sutures are then passed into the tendon, beginning anterior and progressing posterior, or whichever pattern allows for the best tissue reduction and secure purchase of the tendon. This is accomplished by passing the suture through the cuff tendon tissue using an antegrade suture passer, retrograde retriever, or other penetrating or suture-shuttling instrument. Instruments are typically introduced through the lateral portals and the suture delivered and subsequently "parked" in the anterior portal, posterior portal, or superolateral "poke-hole" portal (Figure 5-6). Once passed, sutures are clamped outside of the subacromial space to keep them separated and organized (Figure 5-7).

Figure 5-7. Clamping and separating of sutures optimizing suture management.

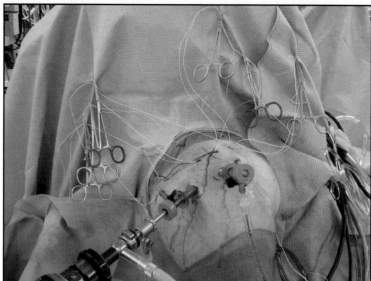

Figures 5-8. Tied and reduced rotator cuff tendon with triple-loaded suture anchors.

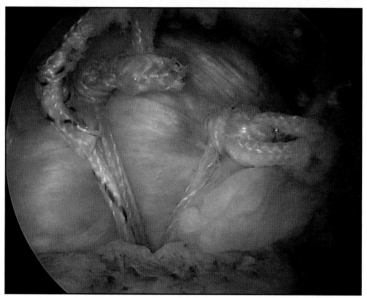

Care is taken to ensure that a bite of tissue 10 to 15 mm from the edge of the tear is accomplished, especially for a simple suture pattern. After all sutures have been passed, the arm is placed in a more abducted position prior to knot tying to reduce tension on the sutures. Begin tying pairs of sutures in the smallest gap or lowest tension point of the repair construct (eg, posterior sutures for posteromedial retracted tears). Each pair of sutures is retrieved separately and isolated in one of the lateral portals, where a sliding, locking knot is tied, delivered, and backed up with reversed half-hitches on alternating posts (Figure 5-8). In larger cuff defects, 3 simple sutures per anchor or a modified Mason-Allen "massive cuff tear" suture technique using 1 horizontal mattress and 1 or 2 simple sutures per anchor can be used to help optimize the biomechanical properties of the repair and prevent tendon-suture pull-out.[28,29] The arm is then taken through ROM to ensure the repair is secure and to determine if additional restrictions on postoperative ROM are needed. Visualization of the articular surface of the repaired rotator cuff from the glenohumeral joint can also be obtained at this time to confirm reduction and integrity of the repair.

Step 5: *Biological Augmentation*

For all types of repairs, the tuberosity can be trephinated with a 2-mm punch to create access to pluripotent mesenchymal bone marrow cells to enhance the reparative quality and volume of tissue at the repair site.[30]

POSTOPERATIVE PROTOCOL

Following wound closure and application of the dressing, the patient is placed into an abduction sling. The rehabilitation protocol is modified based on the age and comorbidities of the patient, quality of the tissue and the repair, and size of the tear. Under supervision, pendulums are started during the first week, and elbow, wrist, and finger motion is encouraged. Active supine motion is typically delayed for 6 weeks, or it can be initiated at 4 weeks depending on the repair qualities. Full active motion along with scapular stabilization exercises are initiated 6 to 8 weeks after surgery. Once full motion is obtained, rotator cuff strengthening exercises can begin 12 weeks from surgery. Patients should be counseled that full recovery takes at least 6 months with most functional outcome scores, ROM, and strength not reaching a plateau until 12 months from surgery.[31,32]

POTENTIAL COMPLICATIONS

The most common complication following rotator cuff repair is a re-tear, with rates reported from 12% to 94% depending on condition of the rotator cuff tissues, chronicity of the tear, patient age, and medical comorbidities.[6] A 2% to 7% incidence of postoperative stiffness has been reported, with risk factors including a single tendon repair, partial articular-sided tendon avulsions repair, calcific tendinitis, concomitant labral repair, and adhesive capsulitis prior to surgery.[32,33] Some degree of stiffness is probably more prevalent than reported in the literature. Also, failure to address other pathological conditions in the shoulder can lead to postoperative stiffness and adhesions. Additional complications can include injury to the axillary, musculocutaneous, and suprascapular nerves as well as injury to branches of the brachial plexus if portal sites are placed medial and inferior to the coracoid process. Risk of infection after arthroscopic rotator cuff repair is low and has been reported at 0.2% to 0.3%.[34] Finally, a rare risk of upper extremity venous thromboembolism or pulmonary embolism has been reported to occur at rates of less than 0.1%.[35]

TOP TECHNICAL PEARLS FOR THE PROCEDURE

1. Visualization is greatly aided by the use of a fluid inflow pump with or without "dual flow" or outflow control. Eight-millimeter hard or soft cannulas should be placed in each of the portal sites to maintain fluid pressure. In addition, a thorough bursectomy performed primarily with electrocautery for bursal tissue, and shaver on cuff tissue, allows for exposure of the rotator cuff tendon, tear site, and musculotendinous junction. This greatly aids performance for the remainder of the procedure and reduces the amount of time required to perform the sequence of steps during surgery. This, in turn, decreases the secondary soft-tissue swelling and edema that can develop, which will impair the ability to visualize important structures and anatomic landmarks for repair.

(continued)

2. "Rehearsal" prior to suture anchor placement or suture passage is vital to ensure that appropriate tension of the torn tendon is determined. This also helps the associated repair construct and design are implemented and individualized to the tear pattern being addressed. This step will allow the surgeon to determine remaining length of the tendon stump and the appropriate anchor placement location, clarify tear pattern (L-shaped, U-shaped, intrasubstance tear, musculotendinous tear, etc), determine whether any delamination exists, and identify whether additional releases are needed for mobilization of torn tendons. In addition, the arm should be repositioned liberally to aid in exposing the tear as well as to help determine anchor placement and appropriate reduction of the rotator cuff. Rehearsal reduces the risk of overtensioning, minimizes the risk of early re-tear, and avoids inadequate or inappropriate reduction of the tendon.

3. Judicious and careful use of portals, order and orientation of suture anchor placement, and sequential knot tying greatly assist with suture management. "Parking" and clamping sutures is often necessary to avoid entanglement and the creation of soft tissue bridges. Lining up sutures outside the shoulder and clamping them to the sterile drapes in the same order they were passed through the tissue can help in visualizing the repair pattern. The guiding principle is to be systematic with managing sutures.

4. The surgeon should be facile with both sliding and nonsliding knot-tying techniques. Understanding the intricacies of both methods will allow for appropriate tissue tensioning as well as appropriate knot and loop security that will withstand cyclic loading. Occasionally, sutures will not slide after being passed through the tendon, so readily transitioning between sliding and nonsliding suture knot techniques will allow for continued progression of the case while accomplishing the goal of secure fixation of the repaired tendon.[29] In addition, the surgeon should be facile with the multiple suture-passing devices necessary to handle different tear patterns.

5. When L-type and large U-type patterns are identified, use of a traction stitch aids in reducing the cuff to the foot print, as well as maintaining reduction during placement of side-to-side sutures. These side-to-side sutures can aid in lining up and reducing the number of suture anchors needed for a more low-tension repair. Side-to-side sutures can be passed independently or as horizontal mattress sutures coming from suture anchors (Figure 5-9).

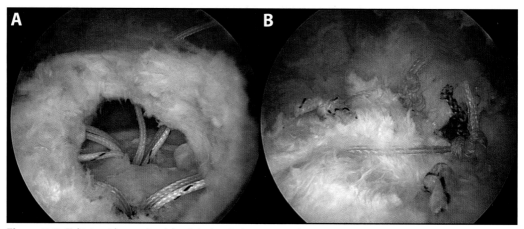

Figure 5-9. Side-to-side repair with triple-loaded suture anchors.

REFERENCES

1. Kim YK, Moon SH, Cho SH. Treatment outcomes of single- versus double-row repair for larger than medium-sized rotator cuff tears: the effect of preoperative remnant tendon length. *Am J Sports Med.* 2013;41(10):2270-2277.

2. Denard PJ, Burkhart SS. Techniques for managing poor quality tissue and bone during arthroscopic rotator cuff repair. *Arthroscopy.* 2011;27(10):1409-1421.

3. Ma CB, Comerford L, Wilson J, Puttlitz CM. Biomechanical evaluation of arthroscopic rotator cuff repairs: double-row compared with single-row fixation. *J Bone Joint Surg Am.* 2006;88(2):403-410.

4. Domb BG, Glousman RE, Brooks A, Hansen M, Lee TQ, ElAttrache NS. High-tension double-row footprint repair compared with reduced-tension single-row repair for massive rotator cuff tears. *J Bone Joint Surg Am.* 2008;90(Suppl 4):35-39.

5. Lo IK, Burkhart SS. Double-row arthroscopic rotator cuff repair: re-establishing the footprint of the rotator cuff. *Arthroscopy.* 2003;19(9):1035-1042.

6. Galatz LM, Ball CM, Teefey SA, Middleton WD, Yamaguchi K. The outcome and repair integrity of completely arthroscopically repaired large and massive rotator cuff tears. *J Bone Joint Surg Am.* 2004;86-A(2):219-224.

7. Sugaya H, Maeda K, Matsuki K, Moriishi J. Functional and structural outcome after arthroscopic full-thickness rotator cuff repair: single-row versus dual-row fixation. *Arthroscopy.* 2005;21(11):1307-1316.

8. Lapner PL, Sabri E, Rakhra K, et al. A multicenter randomized controlled trial comparing single-row with double-row fixation in arthroscopic rotator cuff repair. *J Bone Joint Surg Am.* 2012;94(14):1249-1257.

9. Burks RT, Crim J, Brown N, Fink B, Greis PE. A prospective randomized clinical trial comparing arthroscopic single- and double-row rotator cuff repair: magnetic resonance imaging and early clinical evaluation. *Am J Sports Med.* 2009;37(4):674-682.

10. Franceschi F, Ruzzini L, Longo UG, et al. Equivalent clinical results of arthroscopic single-row and double-row suture anchor repair for rotator cuff tears: a randomized controlled trial. *Am J Sports Med.* 2007;35(8):1254-1260.

11. DeHaan AM, Axelrad TW, Kaye E, Silvestri L, Puskas B, Foster TE. Does double-row rotator cuff repair improve functional outcome of patients compared with single-row technique? A systematic review. *Am J Sports Med.* 2012;40(5):1176-1185.

12. Duquin TR, Buyea C, Bisson LJ. Which method of rotator cuff repair leads to the highest rate of structural healing? A systematic review. *Am J Sports Med.* 2010;38(4):835-841.

13. Ma HL, Chiang ER, Wu HT, et al. Clinical outcome and imaging of arthroscopic single-row and double-row rotator cuff repair: a prospective randomized trial. *Arthroscopy.* 2012;28(1):16-24.

14. Mihata T, Watanabe C, Fukunishi K, et al. Functional and structural outcomes of single-row versus double-row versus combined double-row and suture-bridge repair for rotator cuff tears. *Am J Sports Med.* 2011;39(10):2091-2098.

15. Nho SJ, Slabaugh MA, Seroyer ST, et al. Does the literature support double-row suture anchor fixation for arthroscopic rotator cuff repair? A systematic review comparing double-row and single-row suture anchor configuration. *Arthroscopy.* 2009;25(11):1319-1328.

16. Saridakis P, Jones G. Outcomes of single-row and double-row arthroscopic rotator cuff repair: a systematic review. *J Bone Joint Surg Am.* 2010;92(3):732-742.

17. Davidson PA, Rivenburgh DW. Rotator cuff repair tension as a determinant of functional outcome. *J Shoulder Elbow Surg.* 2000;9(6):502-506.

18. Jost PW, Khair MM, Chen DX, Wright TM, Kelly AM, Rodeo SA. Suture number determines strength of rotator cuff repair. *J Bone Joint Surg Am.* 2012;94(14):e100.

19. Genuario JW, Donegan RP, Hamman D, et al. The cost-effectiveness of single-row compared with double-row arthroscopic rotator cuff repair. *J Bone Joint Surg Am.* 2012;94(15):1369-1377.

20. Namdari S, Donegan RP, Chamberlain AM, Galatz LM, Yamaguchi K, Keener JD. Factors affecting outcome after structural failure of repaired rotator cuff tears. *J Bone Joint Surg Am.* 2014;96(2):99-105.

21. Kukkonen J, Joukainen A, Lehtinen J, et al. Treatment of non-traumatic rotator cuff tears: a randomised controlled trial with one-year clinical results. *Bone Joint J.* 2014;96(1):75-81.

22. Moosmayer S, Tariq R, Stiris M, Smith HJ. The natural history of asymptomatic rotator cuff tears: a three-year follow-up of fifty cases. *J Bone Joint Surg Am.* 2013;95(14):1249-1255.

23. Yamaguchi K, Tetro AM, Blam O, Evanoff BA, Teefey SA, Middleton WD. Natural history of asymptomatic rotator cuff tears: a longitudinal analysis of asymptomatic tears detected sonographically. *J Shoulder Elbow Surg.* 2001;10(3):199-203.

24. Bryan NA, Swenson JD, Greis PE, Burks RT. Indwelling interscalene catheter use in an outpatient setting for shoulder surgery: technique, efficacy, and complications. *J Shoulder Elbow Surg.* 2007;16(4):388-395.

25. Davis JJ, Swenson JD, Greis PE, Burks RT, Tashjian RZ. Interscalene block for postoperative analgesia using only ultrasound guidance: the outcome in 200 patients. *J Clin Anesth.* 2009;21(4):272-277.

26. Chahal J, Mall N, MacDonald PB, et al. The role of subacromial decompression in patients undergoing arthroscopic repair of full-thickness tears of the rotator cuff: a systematic review and meta-analysis. *Arthroscopy.* 2012;28(5):720-727.

27. Han Y, Shin JH, Seok CW, Lee CH, Kim SH. Is posterior delamination in arthroscopic rotator cuff repair hidden to the posterior viewing portal? *Arthroscopy.* 2013;29(11):1740-1747.

28. Gerhardt C, Hug K, Pauly S, Marnitz T, Scheibel M. Arthroscopic single-row modified mason-allen repair versus double-row suture bridge reconstruction for supraspinatus tendon tears: a matched-pair analysis. *Am J Sports Med.* 2012;40(12):2777-2785.

29. Ponce BA, Hosemann CD, Raghava P, Tate JP, Sheppard ED, Eberhardt AW. A biomechanical analysis of controllable intraoperative variables affecting the strength of rotator cuff repairs at the suture-tendon interface. *Am J Sports Med.* 2013;41(10):2256-2261.

30. Jo CH, Shin JS, Park IW, Kim H, Lee SY. Multiple channeling improves the structural integrity of rotator cuff repair. *Am J Sports Med.* 2013;41(11):2650-2657.

31. Keener JD, Galatz LM, Stobbs-Cucchi G, Patton R, Yamaguchi K. Rehabilitation following arthroscopic rotator cuff repair: a prospective randomized trial of immobilization compared with early motion. *J Bone Joint Surg Am.* 2014;96(1):11-19.

32. Koo SS, Parsley BK, Burkhart SS, Schoolfield JD. Reduction of postoperative stiffness after arthroscopic rotator cuff repair: results of a customized physical therapy regimen based on risk factors for stiffness. *Arthroscopy.* 2011;27(2):155-160.

33. Denard PJ, Ladermann A, Burkhart SS. Prevention and management of stiffness after arthroscopic rotator cuff repair: systematic review and implications for rotator cuff healing. *Arthroscopy.* 2011;27(6):842-848.

34. Yeranosian MG, Arshi A, Terrell RD, Wang JC, McAllister DR, Petrigliano FA. Incidence of acute postoperative infections requiring reoperation after arthroscopic shoulder surgery. *Am J Sports Med.* 2014;42(2):437-441.

35. Martin CT, Gao Y, Pugely AJ, Wolf BR. 30-day morbidity and mortality after elective shoulder arthroscopy: a review of 9410 cases. *J Shoulder Elbow Surg.* 2013;22(12):1667-1675 e1661.

Please see videos on the accompanying website at

www.ArthroscopicTechniques.com

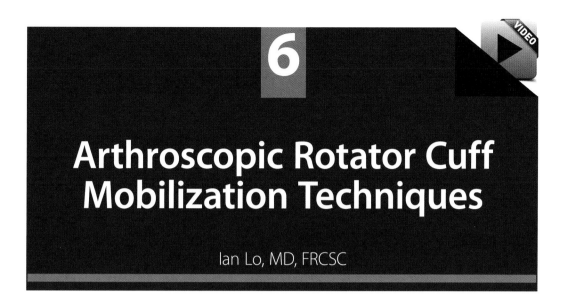

6

Arthroscopic Rotator Cuff Mobilization Techniques

Ian Lo, MD, FRCSC

INTRODUCTION

The majority of rotator cuff tears may be repaired without advanced releases (eg, interval slides) as long as the natural mobility of the tendon tear is understood, which therefore dictates the repair strategy. However, almost all rotator cuff tears will require at least some basic releases to delineate the tear margins and improve mobility. These basic releases (eg, bursal release) are performed routinely in conjunction with rotator cuff repair.

Classically, tears of the rotator cuff may be categorized according to their configuration of crescent shaped, U-shaped, L-shaped, reverse L-shaped, and massive contracted immobile rotator cuff tears.[1] Massive, contracted, immobile tears represent approximately 5% of massive tears and have minimal mobility from a medial-to-lateral and an anterior-to-posterior direction. These tears, which have previously been considered irreparable, may be reparable using advanced releases including interval slides.[2]

INDICATIONS

▶ Rotator cuff releases may be performed to improve the mobility during any rotator cuff repair.

▶ Basic bursal releases are performed routinely during any rotator cuff repair.

▶ Intra-articular releases are commonly performed in crescent-shaped tears with moderate tension, selective L-shaped or reverse L-shaped tears, and rotator cuff repair performed in the presence of adhesive capsulitis.

▶ Excavation of the rotator cuff is indicated when the scarring of the rotator cuff is severe enough to obscure tendon margins (eg, revision rotator cuff repair).

▶ Interval slides are performed in patients with massive contracted immobile tears, which are irreparable despite previous releases (ie, bursal release, intra-articular release). The decision to proceed with interval slides is based on the patient's age, the quality of the tissue (ie, both tendon and muscle quality), and the patient's symptoms (ie, pain vs weakness).

Ryu RKN, Angelo RL, Abrams JS, eds. *The Shoulder: AANA Advanced Arthroscopic Surgical Techniques* (pp 61-69).

Controversial Indications

▶ While there has been a recent trend toward the utilization of reverse shoulder arthroplasty in patients with large or massive rotator cuff tears, advanced releases and a rotator cuff repair are performed in the majority of patients under age 65 years who desire improvements in pain and function. In most cases, a partial or even complete repair can be performed and can lead to significant improvements in pain and function.[3]

▶ In patients with severe chronic proximal humeral migration with acetabularization of the acromion and femoralization of the humerus, rotator cuff repair is usually not achievable even with advanced releases, and arthroscopic debridement may be alternatively performed.

PERTINENT PHYSICAL FINDINGS

▶ Similar to any rotator cuff tear, but may present with findings consistent with a massive tear including impingement findings, active motion loss, external rotation lag signs in adduction and 90 degrees of abduction, and positive subscapularis signs (eg, positive lift-off, positive belly press signs).

▶ Massive tears requiring release will commonly present with atrophy of the supraspinatus and infraspinatus muscles and weakness.

▶ Beware of stiffness, which may indicate the presence of adhesive capsulitis and the necessity for an intra-articular release.

PERTINENT IMAGING

▶ Similar to preoperative planning for a standard rotator cuff repair, including standard radiographs and magnetic resonance imaging (MRI).

▶ Standard radiographs (anteroposterior, trans-scapular lateral, axillary views) are utilized to assess for chronic proximal humeral migration, acetabularization of the acromion, and femoralization of the humeral head. These findings indicate chronic cuff tear arthropathy and an irreparable rotator cuff tear despite advanced releases.

▶ MRI or MR arthrogram is desirable for an accurate assessment of retraction, muscle atrophy, and fatty infiltration. Care is taken to obtain sagittal oblique images medial to the scapular spine to ensure adequate assessment of muscular atrophy and fatty infiltration. In patients with severe muscular atrophy or stage III fatty infiltration or more, the decision to proceed with advanced releases including interval slides is made with caution and appropriate preoperative patient counselling. These patients are less likely to have significant benefit following arthroscopic repair with advanced release in particular related to strength.

EQUIPMENT

The instruments used to complete an arthroscopic release of the rotator cuff are similar to instruments used to perform any rotator cuff repair, including the following:

▶ Switching stick, probe, and grasper

▶ 15-degree Bankart knife or elevator

▶ Traction sutures (#2 Fiberwire [Arthrex, Inc])

▶ Multiple suture passers (antegrade suture passer [Scorpion Suture Passer, Arthrex], shuttle device [Spectrum II Suture Passer, Conmed-Linvatec], retrograde suture passer [0-degree, 22.5-degree, and 45-degree BirdBeak Suture Passer, Arthrex])

▶ Arthroscopic scissors (straight, right curved, and left curved)

▶ Shaver (5.5-mm Gator [Conmed-Linvatec])

▶ Electrocautery instrument, radiofrequency device

▶ 70-degree arthroscope

▶ Cannulae (8.25 mm x 7 cm Twist-In cannula [Arthrex])

Positioning and Portals

Shoulder arthroscopy is routinely performed in the lateral decubitus position. However, patient positioning for rotator cuff releases may be performed in either the lateral decubitus or beach chair position for arthroscopic rotator cuff repair. Standard arthroscopic subacromial portals are created including a posterior portal, lateral portal, and anterior portal. In addition, certain releases may require accessory lateral or anterosuperolateral portals (see next).

Step-by-Step Description of the Procedure

Basic Rotator Cuff Releases

Step 1: Bursal Release (Video 6-1)

Prior to rotator cuff repair, the tendon must be exposed and separated from the bursa, overlying acromion, and inner deltoid fascia. In the majority of cases, the bursal release is performed in conjunction with a subacromial decompression. This involves performing a partial subacromial bursectomy to delineate and expose the margins of the rotator cuff tear. A clear view of the interval between the rotator cuff and the surrounding deltoid should be created anteriorly, laterally, and posteriorly.

Standard anterior and lateral subacromial portals are established and the subacromial space is cleared of overlying bursa using a power shaver (and electrocautery device or radiofrequency device). While viewing through a lateral subacromial portal, instruments are introduced through the posterior portal (ie, shaver, electrocautery) to expose the scapular spine. The scapular spine will appear as a "keel"-shaped structure at the posterior medial portion of the acromion (Figure 6-1). This bony landmark is routinely exposed during rotator cuff repair and is helpful for determining the interval between the supraspinatus and infraspinatus tendons. Once the margins of the tendon tear are delineated, the mobility of the tear may be determined.

Step 2: Excavating the Rotator Cuff (Video 6-2)

In some cases of massive tearing, the margins of the rotator cuff tendon will become obscured due to scarring and adhesions between the rotator cuff and the undersurface of the acromion and inner deltoid fascia. This may occur during revision rotator cuff repair where scar tissue can obliterate tissue planes and anatomic landmarks.[4] This can make rotator cuff repair extremely difficult and tedious. In these cases, the rotator cuff must first be separated from the overlying acromion and the inner deltoid fascia. Then, the margins are secondarily identified and delineated.

To perform this technique, the subacromial space is viewed through a lateral subacromial portal. Instruments are then introduced through the posterior portal in the fibrofatty interval between

Figure 6-1. Arthroscopic view of a right shoulder from the lateral subacromial portal, demonstrating the keel-like structure of the scapular spine.

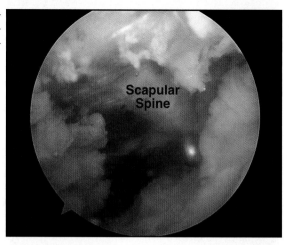

Figure 6-2. Arthroscopic view of a left shoulder from the lateral subacromial portal, demonstrating "blind" instrument insertion from the posterior portal into the fibrofatty interval between the acromion and rotator cuff.

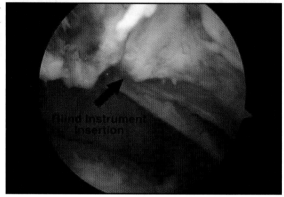

the undersurface of the acromion and the rotator cuff. Instruments are essentially inserted "blindly" into the interval by locating the posterior aspect of the acromion and then sliding just beneath it, palpating for the bony undersurface of the acromion (Figure 6-2). This interval is easiest to locate along the medial aspect of the acromion, and the tissue is followed laterally and posteriorly dissecting the tissue away from the undersurface of the acromion and inner deltoid. The dissection is continued anteriorly and laterally as well. It is critical that the dissection occur adjacent to the undersurface of the acromion to ensure that damage to the remaining cuff is avoided, especially in revision cases.

As the tissue planes are defined, the rotator cuff will be separated along with a large bursal leader, which will extend into the inner deltoid fascia (Figure 6-3). The true margins of the rotator cuff are then delineated by excising the bursal leader. Bursal leaders may be differentiated from the rotator cuff tendon as the tissue is usually thin and adventitial, not inserting into the humerus but extending into the inner deltoid fascia. Once the margins of the tendon are identified and exposed, the mobility of the tendon may be assessed.

Step 3: Intra-articular Release (Video 6-3)

Following assessment of mobility (and classification of the tear), an intra-articular or capsular release may be performed in select cases. This release is most valuable in tears that have moderate tension but are still reducible to the bone bed. This release will provide approximately 1 to 1.5 cm of excursion and therefore may decrease repair tension, but it rarely allows an "irreparable tear" to be repairable.

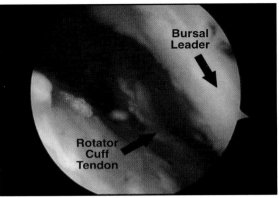

Figure 6-3. Arthroscopic view of a left shoulder from the lateral subacromial portal, demonstrating the bursal "leader" and the rotator cuff tendon. The bursal leader must be excised to delineate the true margins of the rotator cuff.

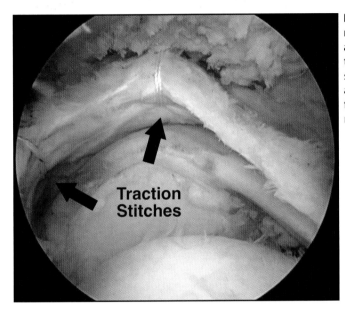

Figure 6-4. Arthroscopic view of a right shoulder from the lateral subacromial portal, demonstrating traction stitches placed in the supraspinatus and infraspinatus tendons and retrieved through the modified Neviaser and posterior portals, respectively.

An intra-articular release is most commonly performed in crescent-shaped tears but may be performed in select L-shaped or reverse L-shaped tears. In addition, because of the global capsular contracture present in most patients with adhesive capsulitis, this release is essential when repairing rotator cuff tears in the presence of significant stiffness.

To perform an intra-articular release, the arthroscope is placed in the lateral or posterior lateral subacromial portal. A traction stitch is placed along the margin of the supraspinatus and infraspinatus tendons and retrieved through the modified Neviaser and posterior portals, respectively (Figure 6-4). These stitches are used to provide superior and lateral traction of the tendon margin to improve exposure and excursion. In addition, a switching stick or hook probe may be used as well.

While viewing through the lateral or posterolateral portal, an electrocautery device and/or elevator is introduced through an accessory lateral portal. This portal is established approximately 1 to 2 cm posterior to the lateral portal to allow a direct approach to the capsule above the glenoid rim and beneath the supraspinatus and infraspinatus tendons. Needle localization is utilized to ensure the correct angle of approach.

The capsule is carefully incised just above the glenoid rim (Figure 6-5A). Care is taken to perform the release as lateral and away from the bony glenoid as possible because the suprascapular nerve lies approximately 1.5 to 2 cm medial to the glenoid rim. The release is complete when the

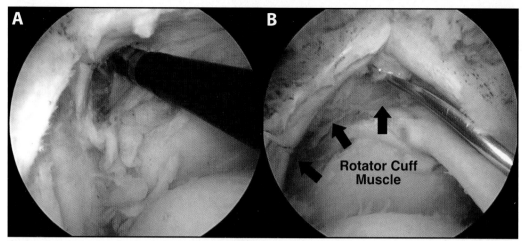

Figure 6-5. Arthroscopic view of a right shoulder from the lateral subacromial portal. (A) Instruments (eg, electrocautery, elevator) are introduced through an accessory lateral portal and the capsule is incised at about the glenoid. (B) The intra-articular release is complete when the underlying muscle of the rotator cuff is exposed.

muscle fibers deep to the capsule are visualized (Figure 6-5B). Tension on the traction sutures can help orient the release and improve exposure and visualization. In addition, by pulling the rotator cuff superiorly and laterally, the release may be performed safely away from the glenoid rim.

Advanced Releases

Step 4: Interval Slides (Video 6-4)

When faced with a rotator cuff tear with minimal mobility in the medial-to-lateral and anterior-to-posterior direction, interval slides may be performed to improve tendon excursion. Many of these tears have previously been considered irreparable but may be repaired using anterior and/or posterior interval slides.[3,4] The anterior interval slide releases the interval between the supraspinatus tendon and rotator interval while the posterior interval slide releases the interval between the supraspinatus and infraspinatus tendons.

In some cases, the inherent mobility of the rotator cuff tear may direct which slide should be performed. However, in the author's experience, a posterior interval slide is more commonly performed and will provide sufficient mobility. An anterior interval slide is only performed when necessary.

The posterior interval slide releases the interval between the supraspinatus and infraspinatus tendons and therefore can improve excursion of both tendons. In general, the posterior interval slide is performed as an initial release, and improved excursion of 3 to 4 cm may be obtained.

The key anatomic landmark for the posterior interval slide is the scapular spine, which directs and orients the release between the supraspinatus and infraspinatus tendons (Figure 6-6).[5] The rotator cuff is viewed through a lateral or accessory lateral portal and traction stitches are again placed through the supraspinatus and infraspinatus tendons. The traction stitches are retrieved through the anterior and posterior portals, respectively.

An accessory lateral portal is established in line with the direction of the posterior interval. An arthroscopic scissor is then introduced through the accessory lateral portal and the posterior interval is incised toward the scapular spine (Figure 6-7A). Tension is applied to the traction stitches, which will help direct the rotator cuff and separate the tendons as the release is performed. This

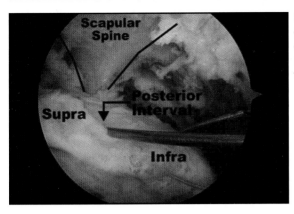

Figure 6-6. Arthroscopic view of a left shoulder through an accessory lateral portal, demonstrating the spine of the scapula, which is used as a landmark to direct the orientation of the posterior interval slide.

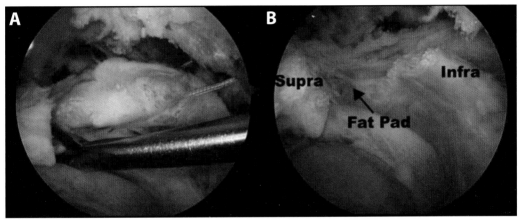

Figure 6-7. Arthroscopic view of a left shoulder through an accessory lateral portal. (A) An arthroscopic scissor is introduced through a lateral portal and incises the tissue between the supraspinatus and infraspinatus tendons. (B) The posterior interval slide is complete when the fibrofatty tissue is encountered lateral to the scapular spine, which heralds the presence of the suprascapular nerve.

creates an apex at the interval between released and unreleased tissue, improving visualization of the tips of the scissors and ensuring a precise and safe posterior interval slide.

Care is taken to lift the tips of the scissors away from the bony glenoid to protect the suprascapular nerve. The release is continued until the fibrofatty tissue, which heralds the presence of the suprascapular nerve, is exposed (Figure 6-7B). If not previously performed, the capsule in now released under the supraspinatus and infraspinatus tendons, connecting the intra-articular release to the posterior interval slide.

Excursion of the supraspinatus tendon and the infraspinatus tendons is then evaluated. If sufficient mobility is obtained to allow tendon repair to bone, then definitive fixation may proceed with standard suture anchor repair to bone. If there is still insufficient excursion, then further mobility may be obtained with an anterior interval slide.

Step 5: The Anterior Interval Slide

The anterior interval slide involves the release of the leading edge of the supraspinatus tendon from the rotator interval, coracohumeral ligament, and coracoid and subscapularis.[3,5] The key anatomic landmark for performing an anterior interval slide is the base of the coracoid, which lies anterior and medial to the base of the long head of the biceps tendon (Figure 6-8).

Figure 6-8. Arthroscopic view of a left shoulder through the lateral portal, demonstrating the orientation of the anterior interval slide. The anterior slide is performed toward the base of the coracoid, which can be palpated anterior and medial to the root of the biceps tendon.

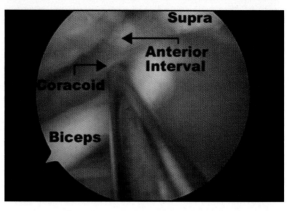

To perform this release, the rotator cuff is viewed from a lateral or accessory lateral subacromial portal. A traction stitch is placed in the supraspinatus tendon and retrieved through the posterior or posterolateral portal. The base of the coracoid may be palpated as a bony prominence anterior and medial to the base of biceps root.

An accessory lateral portal is established in line with the anterior interval toward the base of the coracoid. An arthroscopic scissor is introduced through the accessory lateral portal and the release is performed in line and toward the base of the coracoid. Tension on the traction stitch again will facilitate release and enhance visualization. The anterior release is complete when the bony prominence of the base of the coracoid is encountered. The intra-articular release may then be completed to connect with the anterior interval release. With the anterior interval release, increased excursion of 1 to 2 cm of the supraspinatus is anticipated.

POSTOPERATIVE PROTOCOL

The postoperative protocol following rotator cuff repair is individualized and based on the size of the tear and the security of the repair. A more conservative rehabilitation approach is used in massive tears, which require extensive mobilization and releases. Alternatively, a more aggressive rehabilitation program may be utilized in smaller tears treated in the presence of adhesive capsulitis, where the risk of postoperative stiffness is significant. The authors' general postoperative protocol utilizes sling immobilization for 6 weeks with immediate active range of motion of the hand, wrist, and elbow as tolerated. Passive external rotation with the arm at the side is permitted immediately postoperatively and as tolerated. Forward elevation is initiated approximately 6 weeks postoperatively, progressing from passive to active assisted to active forward elevation. Strengthening begins 12 to 14 weeks postoperatively, progressing to functional activities and sport-specific activities 6 to 8 months postoperatively.

POTENTIAL COMPLICATIONS

Complications related to releases are essentially similar to complications related to arthroscopic rotator cuff repair. However, specifically related to mobilization techniques, the suprascapular nerve is at risk, particularly when performing intra-articular releases or interval slides (ie, posterior interval slide). Therefore, extreme care is taken to ensure that the instruments do not penetrate beyond 1.5 cm medial to the glenoid, the release is performed away from the bony glenoid, and the releases are discontinued prior to potentially injuring the suprascapular nerve (eg, when the fibrofatty layer around the scapular spine is identified).

TOP TECHNICAL PEARLS FOR THE PROCEDURE

1. Expose the scapular spine. This will improve your orientation in the subacromial space and serve as a landmark for the interval between supraspinatus and infraspinatus tendons.

2. Remember that most tears do not require advanced releases. After delineating the tear margins, take time to assess the natural mobility of the rotator cuff tendon to determine whether a tension-free repair may be obtained to bone.

3. Use traction stitches. Traction stitches are routinely used when performing releases. Traction stitches will improve the ease of performing the release, improve visualization, and help orient the direction of the release.

4. If you perform only one advanced release, perform the posterior interval slide. The posterior interval slide provides the most mobility of all of the individual releases and improves mobility of both the supraspinatus and infraspinatus tendons.

5. Protect the suprascapular nerve. The suprascapular nerve may be at risk when performing the posterior interval slide or intra-articular release. Care is taken when performing these slides to ensure instruments are kept as lateral and superior as possible to the bony glenoid. Releases are immediately stopped when the fibrofatty tissue (in the case of the posterior interval slide) or the muscle belly (in the case of the intra-articular release) is identified.

REFERENCES

1. Burkhart SS, Lo IK. Arthroscopic rotator cuff repair. *Arthroscopy.* 2007;14(6):333-346.
2. Lo IK, Burkhart SS. Arthroscopic repair of massive, contracted, immobile rotator cuff tears using single and double interval slides: technique and preliminary results. *Arthroscopy.* 2004;20(1):22-33.
3. Berdusco R, Trantalis JN, Nelson AA, et al. Arthroscopic repair of massive, contracted, immobile tears using interval slides: clinical and MRI structural follow-up. *Knee Surg Sports Trauma Arthro.* 2015;23(2):502-507. doi: 10.1007/s00167-013-2683-9. Epub 2013 Sep 22.
4. Lo IK, Burkhart SS. Arthroscopic revision of failed rotator cuff repairs: technique and results. *Arthroscopy.* 2004;20(3):250-267.
5. Klein JR, Burkhart SS. Identification of essential anatomic landmarks in performing arthroscopic single- and double-interval slides. *Arthroscopy.* 2004;20(7):765-770.

Please see videos on the accompanying website at

www.ArthroscopicTechniques.com

7

Arthroscopic Acromioclavicular Joint Repair for Acute Injury

Craig R. Bottoni, MD and Kevin P. Krul, MD

INTRODUCTION

Although acromioclavicular joint (ACJ) repair for chronic injuries can be controversial, operative treatment of an acute high-grade ACJ injury is recommended to restore normal anatomy and to return the patient back to manual work or the athlete back to sport more reliably. Injuries to the ACJ constitute approximately 3.2% of shoulder injuries.[1] Overall rates of ACJ injuries are higher in men and contact athletes, specifically those who participate in rugby, wrestling, and hockey.[2] The mechanism of injury has been described as an inferiorly directed force on the acromion, displacing the scapula down and medially.[3] This typically occurs when an athlete falls or is tackled with an adducted arm. The shoulder—specifically the acromion—strikes the ground first and is driven inferiorly, separating the distal clavicle from its scapular connections. This may be the origin of the lay term, *a separated shoulder*, for this injury. The AC ligament fails first, followed by the 2 components of the coracoclavicular (CC) ligaments, the more anterolateral trapezoid, and the posteromedial conoid. The clinical manifestation of the acute injury is pain, limited shoulder function, and a prominence over the lateral shoulder representing the superiorly displace distal clavicle.

Originally, AC dislocations were classified by Tossy et al into types 1, 2, and 3.[3] AC dislocations were later classified into 6 types by the Rockwood system, defining more severe injuries. A type I and II injury represents an incomplete tear of the AC and CC ligaments, while a type III through VI injury represents a complete disruption of both the AC and CC ligaments. A type III or higher injury indicates complete disruption of the CC ligaments and may be indicated for acute operative intervention.[4-8]

Myriad surgical techniques have been described to repair and hold the reduction of the displaced type V AC separation. Most of the procedures entail transfixing the distal clavicle to either the acromion or the coracoid. Plates, screws, wires, sutures, and tape have all been proposed to stabilize this injury. ACJ reduction with acute CC fixation reapproximates the ruptured CC ligaments by securing the clavicle to the coracoid. The need for reconstruction in an acute injury is debated; however, postoperative MRI has demonstrated ligament healing in reduced ACJs without primary repair.[9] While motion at the ACJ contributes to less than 10 degrees of motion with

Ryu RKN, Angelo RL, Abrams JS, eds. *The Shoulder: AANA Advanced Arthroscopic Surgical Techniques* (pp 71-80). © 2016 AANA.

Figure 7-1. A CT scan of a coracoid nonunion in a patient who presented for CC ligament reconstruction. This would be a contraindication to arthroscopically assisted acute ACJ reconstruction.

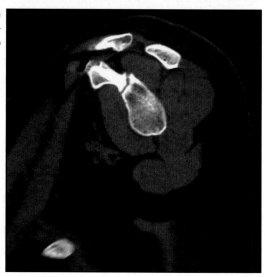

elevation of the arm, rigid fixation of the joint can lead to early hardware failure.[1] The advantages of an arthroscopically assisted acute ACJ repair are smaller incisions, the ability to evaluate for concomitant glenohumeral pathology, strong yet nonrigid fixation, and the ability to achieve direct visualization of the base of the coracoid while stabilizing the clavicle.

The authors present an arthroscopically assisted technique for CC fixation with strong suture tape that allows for maintenance of the AC reduction and healing of the ruptured conoid and trapezoid ligaments in the acute setting. Standard shoulder arthroscopic equipment is utilized in conjunction with commercially available fixation buttons that allows for fixation of the displaced clavicle to the coracoid.

INDICATIONS

▶ Rockwood type V ACJ dislocations The optimal timing is debated; however, the earlier the injuries are treated, the better. The acute operative stabilization defined for this technique is within 2 weeks from injury.[6,8,10-12]

Controversial Indications

▶ Acute Rockwood type III ACJ dislocation in the dominant arm of a laborer or athlete[8,11,12]

▶ Patients who are not medically fit for surgery or who cannot maintain postoperative protocols. The lone publication that reports on nonoperative treatment of type V AC injuries demonstrates that patients may have fair results being treated nonoperatively.[13]

Contraindications

▶ A concomitant coracoid fracture, nonunion, or any previous surgery involving the transfer of the coracoid (ie, Bristow-Latarjet) would be an absolute contraindication. If any question exists regarding coracoid integrity, a computed tomography (CT) scan should be obtained, which will clearly delineate the fracture or nonunion (Figure 7-1).

▶ Conditions that may preclude any surgery (ie, bleeding disorders, irreversible blood thinning agents such as Plavix [clopidogrel], and any systemic condition precluding any operation)

▶ Patients not able to tolerate general anesthesia as it is typically utilized for this operation. Although this procedure can be performed under a regional interscalene block alone, the superior shoulder and clavicle are poorly covered with a regional block and would have to be supplemented with local anesthesia.

▶ The open injury, posteriorly displaced (type IV), inferiorly displaced (type VI), and those with combined clavicular and/or scapular fractures are typically treated operatively but are not the subject of this chapter. The focus of this technique is the closed, type V AC injury.

▶ Delayed presentation: It is paramount that this procedure be performed acutely and as soon after the injury as is feasible. Past 10 to 14 days from injury, additional graft augmentation is recommended. (See Chapter 8 on arthroscopic ACJ reconstruction with allograft or autograft.)

PERTINENT PHYSICAL FINDINGS

▶ Best test: To differentiate between a type III or a type V ACJ injury, have the patient stand with adducted arms and then perform a shrug of both shoulders. A type V injury will not reduce with a shrug, while a type III injury will. Alternatively, an ACJ that is irreducible by the examiner also indicates an injury higher than type III.

▶ The classic presentation is severe pain localized to the top of the shoulder following a fall or athletic injury.

▶ Skin integrity is important to first ascertain whether the injury is open, and second to assess for abrasions, which are common given the mechanism of injury. Abrasions and lacerations over the area of expected skin incisions may necessitate a delay in operative treatment.

▶ The differentiation between types III and V ACJ injuries can be difficult. The interobserver reliability is poor.[14,15] An intrarticular injection of 0.25% bupivacaine into the ACJ may provide significant relief and better allow the shoulder examination.

▶ Tenting of the skin may indicate disruption of the trapezial fascia and further support the diagnosis of a type V injury.[16]

▶ Neurological evaluation is necessary. The brachial plexus traverses just inferomedial to the coracoid. Traction or direct injury may manifest as neurological deficit in the ipsilateral upper extremity.

▶ The entire clavicle should be palpated as associated sternoclavicular joint injuries have been described with concomitant ACJ injuries.[17]

PERTINENT IMAGING

▶ A standard radiographic series of the injured shoulder, including anteroposterior, scapular Y, and axillary views[18]

▶ An anteroposterior view of the contralateral side or whole chest view including both ACJs allows for comparison of the CC interval. While the normal CC distance has been described as 1.1 to 1.3 cm, this is quite variable.[4,19] On radiographs, the CC distance is measured from the superior portion of the coracoid directly to the inferior border of the clavicle. A type I injury has no radiographic abnormality. A type II injury has a < 25% increase in the CC distance. A type III injury has a 25% to 100% increase in the CC distance. A type V injury has a > 100% increase. Alternatively, a type V injury has also been defined as greater than 2 cm of absolute superior displacement of the clavicle.[4,11,13] A type IV injury will be displaced

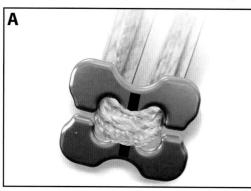

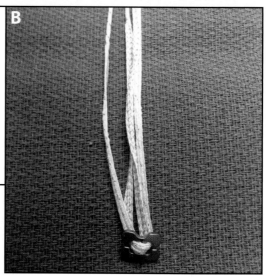

Figure 7-2. (A) The assembled construct consisting of a metal button called a Dogbone because of the shape resembling a bone. The open sides allow for sutures to be easily threaded into the button. (B) The Dogbone and FiberTape construct ready for insertion into joint.

posteriorly on the axillary or scapula-Y view. A type VI injury demonstrates an inferiorly displaced distal clavicle seen radiographically lying beneath the coracoid.[4]

▶ As noted in the previous section, the coracoid should be inspected for any abnormalities or evidence of previous surgery. If in doubt, a CT scan should be obtained to better visualize the coracoid and other related bony structures.

EQUIPMENT

The arthroscopically assisted ACJ reconstruction depends on the availability of and familiarity with specialized equipment. The surgeon should be familiar with routine shoulder arthroscopy, instrumentation, and labral repair.

▶ Standard 30- and 70-degree arthroscope

▶ Standard arthroscopic instruments including graspers, probes, shavers, electrocautery, and cannulas

▶ Anterior cruciate ligament (ACL) tibial guide

▶ 2.4-mm tibial guide pin

▶ Small-sized (3 to 4.5 mm) cannulated reamer

▶ Reinforced suture or tape, such as FiberWire or FiberTape (Arthrex)

▶ Fixation buttons, such as the Dogbone button (Arthrex)

▶ A large enough cannula to pass the instruments, such as the PassPort (Arthrex)

▶ A flexible suture passing device similar to the 1.1-mm nitinol wire with a looped end (SutureLasso SD Wire Loop [Arthrex])

POSITIONING AND PORTALS

The arthroscopically assisted technique entails reducing the ACJ then securing the clavicle to the coracoid, with a construct consisting of 2 metal buttons and 2 strong sutures (FiberWire or FiberTape; Figure 7-2). The patient can be positioned in either the beach chair or lateral decubitus

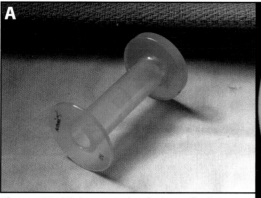

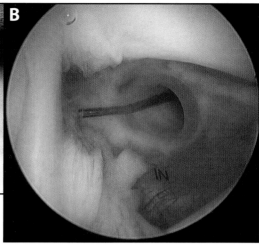

Figure 7-3. (A) An example of a large flexible cannula preferred for this procedure. (B) The cannula after properly inserted into the rotator interval.

position. Standard arthroscopy is first performed, but both the posterior entry portal and the anterior portals should be made slightly more lateral than usual to visualize and to allow easier access to the base of the coracoid. The anterior cannula should be large enough to allow instrumentation including the ACL tibial guide to pass through the cannula. The authors prefer a flexible plastic cannula (Passport [Arthrex]; Figure 7-3) inserted into the rotator interval. It allows passage of multiple instruments simultaneously and easily accommodates the ACL guide. The shoulder joint should first be examined arthroscopically for concomitant pathology. Although the ACJ dislocation is usually found in isolation, superior labral anteroposterior tears, rotator cuff injuries, and chondral defects have been encountered and should be addressed prior to ACJ stabilization.

STEP-BY-STEP DESCRIPTION OF THE PROCEDURE

The patient is positioned in either a beach chair or lateral decubitus position. The authors prefer a commercially available beach chair positioner that allows easy access to the posterior shoulder for arthroscopy. While draping, the anterior shoulder and clavicle are left exposed. From the anteroinferior portal, an electrocautery (Surface Energy [Stryker Endoscopy]) is used to create a capsulotomy through the rotator interval just anterior to the glenoid between the superior and middle glenohumeral ligaments. Occasionally, an anatomical variant—the sublabral hole—is present, which allows easy access to the base of the coracoid with minimal capsular ablation. At this point, the standard 30-degree arthroscope is switched for a 70-degree arthroscope. Although the procedure can be performed without the 70-degree scope, it facilitates visualization around the anterosuperior labrum and is strongly recommended. The arthroscope follows the cautery approximately 1.5 to 2 cm medial to the glenoid to identify the base of the coracoid. It is important to identify the base of the coracoid and not the tip that often projects well anterolateral from the base. It is also imperative to use the cautery judiciously medial to the base of the coracoid as the brachial plexus is passing inferiorly several centimeters from the base of the coracoid. Once identified, the base of the coracoid is cleared of soft tissue to expose the medial and lateral margins.

Next, a 3-cm incision is made over the superior clavicle and the periosteum incised longitudinally from the center of the clavicle. The periosteum is carefully reflected with electrocautery to expose the anterior and posterior margins of the distal clavicle. These periosteal flaps will be closed over the top of the clavicle to reinforce the repair and to mitigate the complaint of symptomatic hardware over the clavicle. A standard ACL tibial aiming guide is inserted though the anterior arthroscopy portal. The tip of the aiming guide is placed at the base of the coracoid,

Figure 7-4. The drill tip guide pin is passed using an ACL tibial guide from the clavicle through the middle of the base of the coracoid.

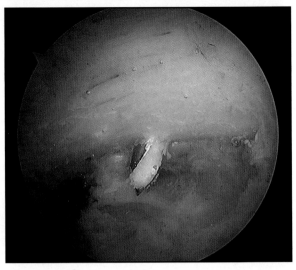

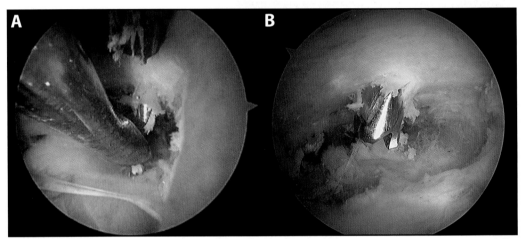

Figure 7-5. (A) A small arthroscopic curette is used to prevent advancement of the guide pin during drilling of the clavicle and coracoid. (B) The cannulated reamer with the guide pin removed. It is left projecting 1 to 2 mm from the inferior coracoid to facilitate nitinol wire passage.

centered between the medial and lateral bone edges. Although a procedure-specific guide is available that has a solid receiving end to prevent inferior penetration of the guide pin, the authors have not found this necessary if good visualization is maintained and care is taken in advancing the guide pin through the coracoid. The drill sleeve is secured on the superior surface of the clavicle between the anterior and middle third of the bone. The drill guide and subsequent pin should be directed perpendicular to the clavicle at approximately 2.5 to 3 cm from the distal end of the clavicle. The metal 2.4-mm drill tip ACL tibial guide pin is drilled through the clavicle and then the coracoid while observing arthroscopically beneath the coracoid to avoid overpenetration (Figure 7-4). The pin should only exit the base of the coracoid by 1 to 2 mm. It is imperative that the pin is as close to the middle of the coracoid base as possible. Since the coracoid is a cylindrical structure, this can be difficult to ascertain. However, if the pin is too far medial or lateral, the subsequent hole can fracture the coracoid and fixation will be lost.

While securing the pin tip with a small curette, the pin is overdrilled with a 4-mm cannulated drill (Figure 7-5A). After penetration of the inferior coracoid, the drill is left in place and the guide pin is removed (Figure 7-5B). Through the drill, a flexible 1.1-mm nitinol wire with

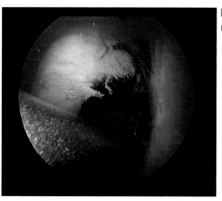

Figure 7-6. An arthroscopic grasper is used to retrieve the nitinol wire, after which the reamer is removed.

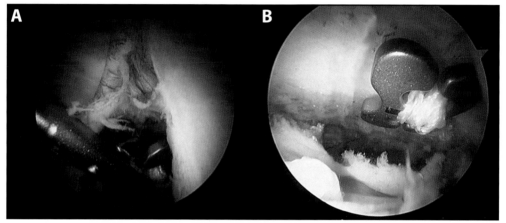

Figure 7-7. (A) The button is passed into the joint and under the coracoid using an arthroscopic grasper. (B) The Dogbone button in proper position with the laser line parallel to the long axis of the coracoid.

a looped end (SutureLasso SD Wire Loop) is passed down the cannulated drill with the looped end leading. The wire is secured and pulled out of the anterior portal with an arthroscopic grasper (Figure 7-6). The cannulated drill is now removed. The wire loop on the nitinol wire is used to pass the lead sutures or tape for the suture button construct. The free ends of 2 stands of FiberTape are pulled through the coracoid and out of the clavicular hole while visualizing arthroscopically. The button (Dogbone) is attached to the 2 tapes outside of the anterior cannula and then secured with a locking arthroscopic grasper. It is pushed into the joint and then under the coracoid while the tapes are pulled taut above the clavicle (Figure 7-7A). The optimal suture button orientation is confirmed by a laser line, which should be directed with its long axis running anterior to posterior (Figure 7-7B). The button can be manipulated with a probe or grasper if necessary. The 4 free ends of the FiberTape are now passed through a second metal fixation button (Dogbone) and cinched down to the top of the clavicle.

The ACJ is reduced with manual pressure on the superior clavicle while applying an upward force on the flexed elbow. While holding the ACJ reduced, the first 2 sutures are tied over the metal button on top of the clavicle. Intraoperative fluoroscopy should be used to ensure adequate reduction. If satisfactory ACJ reduction is confirmed, the remaining 2 sutures are tied over the clavicle button and then cut at the knots. If reduction cannot be obtained, rarely, a distal clavicle resection may need to be performed. The periosteal flaps are now closed over the clavicle with absorbable suture and routine skin closure performed.

Figure 7-8. An example of a potential complication: a fracture after minimal trauma due to eccentric placement of the clavicular tunnel and button.

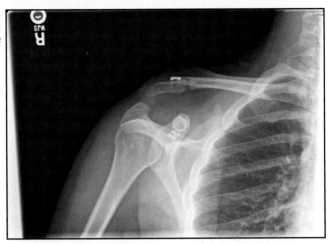

POSTOPERATIVE PROTOCOL

The clavicle serves as the only strut between the axial and appendicular skeleton. The medial end (the scapulothoracic articulation) serves as a relatively fixed point on the manubrium. With shoulder motion, the scapula rotates, protracts, and retracts. Since the clavicle is fixed at the ACJ, the clavicle too moves in conjunction with the scapula. It rotates and elevates with glenohumeral forward flexion. Therefore, high forces are transmitted to the coracoid through the intact CC ligaments during shoulder motion. Because of this, shoulder motion must be minimized during the first 6 weeks postoperatively. Most importantly, the arm must not be used to push up the body as occurs when one rises from a chair and pushes to a standing position. The force involved in this or a similar maneuver is enough to disrupt the repair in the early stages.

The recommended rehabilitation protocol is as follows:

▶ Maintain the arm in a sling for 6 weeks. No active forward flexion or abduction is allowed and no passive motion beyond 90 degrees.

▶ Pendulum exercises may be performed immediately. No formal physical therapy is required during this period. Shoulder stiffness is typically not a problem as minimal intra-articular work is done.

▶ At 6 weeks, the patient may remove the sling and use the upper extremity for activities of daily living. Physical therapy is begun to restore full motion before allowing gradual strengthening at 3 months postoperatively.

▶ Resumption of full sporting activities is not allowed until 4 to 6 months postoperatively.[20]

POTENTIAL COMPLICATIONS

Loss of reduction and recurrence of the deformity are the most common complications. This may occur through button pullout, fracture, or suture breakage.[21] Intraoperative complications or technical errors that can lead to failure include eccentric drilling of the clavicle or, more commonly, the coracoid. Coracoid fracture can occur with eccentric drilling or trauma postoperatively. Clavicular fracture can also occur but usually requires a fall or trauma postoperatively (Figure 7-8). Pain at the superior clavicle is another potential problem that rarely may require hardware removal once healing is ensured, but it should wait a minimum of 8 to 10 months postoperatively.

Top Technical Pearls for the Procedure

1. Ensure you have adequate exposure of both the posterior shoulder (for the arthroscopy) and the anterior chest (to access the clavicle) when draping the patient.

2. Portal placement that is slightly lateral and a 70-degree arthroscope will assist in visualization of the inferior coracoid. Adequate visualization of the coracoid is essential to ensure proper pin placement in the center of the base of the base of the coracoid. Incorrect pin placement and eccentric drilling may lead to coracoid fracture and loss of reduction.

3. Use a large cannula in the anterior portal, preferably the flexible Passport, to allow instrument and ACL guide passage.

4. Before tying the second set of sutures, ensure the ACJ is reduced. Fluoroscopic confirmation is recommended as palpation alone may not allow confirmation of reduction.

5. Strict compliance with rehabilitation restrictions is imperative to avoid early loading and failure of the surgery (Figure 7-9).

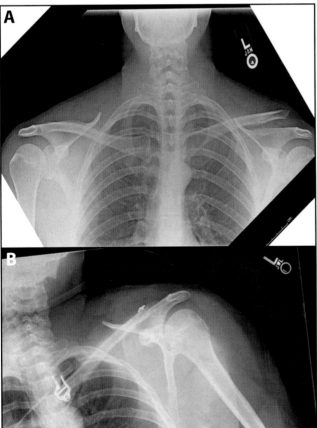

Figure 7-9. (A) Preoperative radiograph of a 27-year-old male with a Rockwood grade 5 injury. (B) 3 months postoperative radiograph of the same patient demonstrating anatomic reduction. Note the low profile of the implant.

REFERENCES

1. Mazzocca AD, Arciero RA, Bicos J. Evaluation and treatment of acromioclavicular joint injuries. *Am J Sports Med.* 2007;35(2):316-329.
2. Pallis M, Cameron KL, Svoboda SJ, Owens BD. Epidemiology of acromioclavicular joint injury in young athletes. *Am J Sports Med.* 2012;40(9):2072-2077.
3. Tossy JD, Mead NC, Sigmond HM. Acromioclavicular separations: useful and practical classification for treatment. *Clin Orthop Relat Res.* 1963;28:111-119.
4. Williams G, Nguyen V, Rockwood C. Classification and radiographic analysis of acromioclavicular dislocations. *Appl Radiol.* 1989;18:29-34.
5. Smith TO, Chester R, Pearse EO, Hing CB. Operative versus non-operative management following Rockwood grade III acromioclavicular separation: a meta-analysis of the current evidence base. *J Orthop Traumatol.* 2011;12(1):19-27.
6. Phillips AM, Smart C, Groom AF. Acromioclavicular dislocation. Conservative or surgical therapy. *Clin Orthop Relat Res.* 1998(353):10-17.
7. Reid D, Polson K, Johnson L. Acromioclavicular joint separations grades I-III: a review of the literature and development of best practice guidelines. *Sports Med.* 2012;42(8):681-696.
8. Tamaoki MJ, Belloti JC, Lenza M, Matsumoto MH, Gomes Dos Santos JB, Faloppa F. Surgical versus conservative interventions for treating acromioclavicular dislocation of the shoulder in adults. *Cochrane Database Syst Rev.* 2010(8):CD007429.
9. Di Francesco A, Zoccali C, Colafarina O, Pizzoferrato R, Flamini S. The use of hook plate in type III and V acromio-clavicular Rockwood dislocations: clinical and radiological midterm results and MRI evaluation in 42 patients. *Injury.* 2012;43(2):147-152.
10. Simovitch R, Sanders B, Ozbaydar M, Lavery K, Warner JJ. Acromioclavicular joint injuries: diagnosis and management. *J Am Acad Orthop Surg.* 2009;17(4):207-219.
11. Johansen JA, Grutter PW, McFarland EG, Petersen SA. Acromioclavicular joint injuries: indications for treatment and treatment options. *J Shoulder Elbow Surg.* 2011;20(2 Suppl):S70-82.
12. Flint JH, Wade AM, Giuliani J, Rue JP. Defining the terms acute and chronic in orthopaedic sports injuries: a systematic review. *Am J Sports Med.* 2014;42(1):235-241.
13. Bannister GC, Wallace WA, Stableforth PG, Hutson MA. The management of acute acromioclavicular dislocation. A randomised prospective controlled trial. *J Bone Joint Surg Br.* 1989;71(5):848-850.
14. Kraeutler MJ, Williams GR, Jr, Cohen SB, et al. Inter- and intraobserver reliability of the radiographic diagnosis and treatment of acromioclavicular joint separations. *Orthopedics.* 2012;35(10):e1483-1487.
15. Cho CH, Hwang I, Seo JS, et al. Reliability of the classification and treatment of dislocations of the acromioclavicular joint. *J Shoulder Elbow Surg.* 2014;23(5):665-670.
16. Green DP, Rockwood CA, Bucholz RW, Heckman JD, Tornetta P. *Rockwood and Green's Fractures in Adults.* Vol 1. Philadelphia, PA: Lippincott Williams & Wilkins; 2010.
17. Echo BS, Donati RB, Powell CE. Bipolar clavicular dislocation treated surgically. A case report. *J Bone Joint Surg Am.* 1988;70(8):1251-1253.
18. Vaisman A, Villalon Montenegro IE, Tuca De Diego MJ, Valderrama Ronco J. A novel radiographic index for the diagnosis of posterior acromioclavicular joint dislocations. *Am J Sports Med.* 2014;42(1):112-116.
19. Bearden JM, Hughston JC, Whatley GS. Acromioclavicular dislocation: method of treatment. *J Sports Med.* 1973;1(4):5-17.
20. Cote MP, Wojcik KE, Gomlinski G, Mazzocca AD. Rehabilitation of acromioclavicular joint separations: operative and nonoperative considerations. *Clin Sports Med.* 2010;29(2):213-228, vii.
21. Geaney LE, Miller MD, Ticker JB, et al. Management of the failed AC joint reconstruction: causation and treatment. *Sports Med Arthrosc.* 2010;18(3):167-172.

Please see videos on the accompanying website at

www.ArthroscopicTechniques.com

8

Arthroscopic Acromioclavicular Joint Reconstruction With Allograft/Autograft

Lane N. Rush, MD; Michael J. O'Brien, MD; and Felix H. Savoie III, MD

INTRODUCTION

Anatomy of the Native Acromioclavicular Joint

The acromioclavicular (AC) joint is a diarthrodial joint between the medial margin of the acromial process of the scapula and the lateral aspect of the clavicle. Interposed within the AC ligaments is a meniscus-like disc of fibrocartilage. The exact function of the disk is unknown, but it has shown to have a tremendous variation in size and shape.[1]

Stability in the anteroposterior plane is provided by the AC ligaments, which are thickenings of the capsule that envelop the joint. They consist of the superior, inferior, anterior, and posterior ligaments, with the superior ligaments being the strongest.[2] The superior AC ligament merges with the attachments of the deltoid and trapezius muscles along the superior aspect of the clavicle and acromial process, thereby strengthening the ligament complex and adding stability to the AC joint.

The coracoclavicular (CC) ligament complex is composed of 2 ligaments: the medial conoid ligament and the more laterally located trapezoid ligament. The conoid has a broad origin on the inferior clavicle and tapers from superior to inferior as it courses to the posterior aspect of the coracoid. The conoid provides optimal stabilization in the vertical as well horizontal plane during shoulder motion.[3] The distance from the lateral edge of the clavicle to the medial edge of the conoid is approximately 47 mm.

The trapezoid ligament attaches more laterally to the undersurface of the clavicle. It is located an average of 25 mm from the lateral end of the clavicle, and its attachment to the clavicle forms a linear, ribbon-like form in the anteroposterior plane.

AC joint stability is maintained by the CC ligaments, the stout AC capsule, and the AC ligaments. Studies have shown that the trapezoid ligament has a greater role in resistance to posterior displacement of the clavicle and the conoid, a greater role in anterior displacement.[4]

Ryu RKN, Angelo RL, Abrams JS, eds. *The Shoulder: AANA Advanced Arthroscopic Surgical Techniques* (pp 81-93). © 2016 AANA.

Figure 8-1. An anatomic illustration of the normal AC joint and CC ligaments.

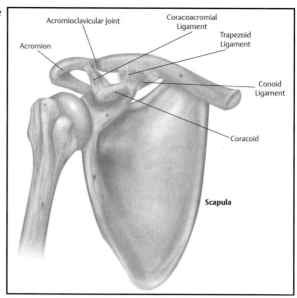

The role of the AC joint capsule and ligaments has been studied extensively with respect to distal clavicle resection. Posterior abutment of the clavicle against the acromion is avoided with only 5 mm of bone removal. This preserves the capsule and ligaments, maintaining anteroposterior stability of the AC joint. Larger resections have been shown to result in excessive posterior translation.[5]

These experiments have led to the following general conclusions: horizontal stability is controlled by the AC ligaments, and vertical stability is controlled by the CC ligaments (Figure 8-1).

Biomechanics of the Acromioclavicular Joint

AC joint biomechanics involve static stability, dynamic stability, and AC joint motion. Fixation methods for stabilization of the AC instability vary widely, and recently, more sophisticated techniques in biomechanical research have shed light on the roles of various structures about the joint. These studies have also shown that well-known and popular fixation methods, such as the Weaver-Dunn procedure, a transfer of the acromial attachment of the coracoacromial (CA) ligament to the resected end of the distal clavicle, do not replicate the normal AC biomechanics and lack the stability of more anatomic techniques.

Recent studies by Grutter and Peterson indicate a load to failure of the native AC and CC ligament complex to be 815 N.[6] The transferred CA ligament provides only 25% of the strength of the intact AC joint complex, with a load to failure of 145 N. Lee et al found that anatomic reconstruction of the CC ligaments with a tendon graft was biomechanically superior to CA ligament transfer.[7] The use of a free tendon graft can aid in the initial stability of the construct and provide strength equivalent to the native ligaments, representing a tremendous advantage over previous nonanatomic reconstruction methods. These biomechanical findings have prompted the recent popularity in the techniques described next, including the anatomic CC reconstruction (ACCR).

Mechanism and Classification of Acromioclavicular Joint Separations

A dislocation of the AC joint is almost always the result of a direct trauma. This is classically produced by the patient falling onto the lateral aspect of the shoulder with the arm in an adducted

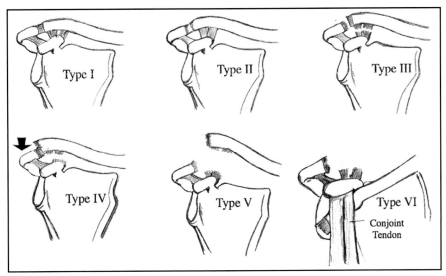

Figure 8-2. The Rockwood classification of AC joint injuries.

position.[8] The acromion is forced inferiorly and medially, and the entire shoulder girdle is displaced inferiorly. A sufficient downward force will result in either a fracture of the clavicle or a sprain of the AC ligaments. An increase in force will sequentially result in an AC ligament tear, followed by a sprain of the CC ligaments, and, ultimately, a complete rupture of the CC ligaments and deltoid and trapezius muscle attachments. As a consequence, the affected upper extremity has lost its suspensory support from the clavicle, and the entire forequarter displaces inferiorly. This, combined with the slight upward pull of the trapezius on the clavicle, results in the characteristic inferior displacement of the shoulder seen in complete AC dislocations.

The Rockwood Classification, proposed by Rockwood and colleagues, subclassifies AC joint disruption into 6 grades. This has become the universally accepted classification system (Figure 8-2).

INDICATIONS

- ► Medically stable patients with type IV, type V, and type VI injuries
- ► Open injuries

Controversial Indications

- ► Acute type III separations in high-demand athletes, heavy manual laborers
- ► Chronic type III separations that have failed nonoperative management, resulting in persistent pain, significant tenting of the skin, and shoulder dysfunction

PERTINENT PHYSICAL FINDINGS

- ► Point tenderness at AC joint
- ► Pain with cross body adduction test
- ► Must rule out associated sternoclavicular injury and dislocation

- Skin tenting in grade II or higher injuries
- Reducibility of the AC joint

Most patients with an acute AC injury will present with the injured upper extremity in an adducted and supported position to limit pain. Pain, point tenderness, and swelling around the AC joint can all be expected in the acute period. Inspection of the affected shoulder and comparison with the contralateral side may reveal gross deformity. Pain accentuated with abducted and cross body adduction of the arm is consistent with AC injury. Tenting of the skin along the distal aspect of the clavicle may be seen in type III or type V injuries. Vascular compromise has not been documented in acute AC injury, but transient paresthesias of the injured limb has been described with type VI AC injury.[2]

The AC joint should be tested for ease of reduction. An irreducible joint indicates the presence of interposed tissue that will have to be removed intraoperatively.

PERTINENT IMAGING

- Anteroposterior, scapular Y, and axillary radiographs
- Zanca view
- Magnetic resonance imaging (MRI) to confirm or exclude concomitant pathology

Initial radiographs of the injured AC joint should include standard anteroposterior, axillary, and scapular Y views. Anteroposterior radiographs will show the degree of superior displacement of the clavicle relative to the acromion, and the axillary view is of paramount importance in detecting type IV AC separations, in which the clavicle is displaced posteriorly.

The most accurate radiograph to visualize the AC joint is the Zanca view, in which the x-ray beam is directed from anterior to posterior with a 10- to 15-degree cephalic tilt.[9] The normal width of the AC joint is 1 to 3 mm. A joint space of 7 mm or greater in men and 6 mm or greater in women is considered pathologic.[8]

The Zanca view can also be used to assess the CC distance.[9] The average distance between the superior aspect of the coracoid process and the inferior aspect of the clavicle varies between 13 to 15 mm. Bearden et al reported that a 40% to 50% increase of the CC distance compared to the contralateral side is indicative of complete CC disruption, while Rockwood and Young found a 25% side-to-side CC difference to be indicative of disruption.[2,9,10]

MRI has become an important aspect of preoperative planning for AC joint injuries, and MRI is routinely recommended in all of these patients prior to considering surgical intervention. MRI is not routinely recommend for patients in whom nonoperative management is selected. While radiographs rely on osseous relationships to determine ligamentous damage, MRI has the advantage of directly visualizing AC and CC ligament disruptions, as well as identifying associated glenohumeral pathology. Concomitant glenohumeral pathology can occur in up to 18.2% of patients with grade III to grade V AC joint separations.[11]

EQUIPMENT

- Semitendinosus allograft/autograft
- Braided PDS (polydioxanone) suture (Johnson & Johnson, Ethicon)
- PEEK Bio-Tenodesis interference screw (Arthrex)

Treatment Options

Conservative Treatment

Rockwood type I and II separations are typically treated nonoperatively. Although most authors recommend simple sling immobilization, the authors prefer scapular retraction bracing to attempt to bring the arm back up to the clavicle. The time of immobilization varies with the degree of injury. One week of immobilization is usually all that is needed for type I injuries, while type II injuries may require up to 2 to 3 weeks. Once the patient is asymptomatic, the sling may be discontinued and physical therapy initiated, focusing on passive and active shoulder range of motion. Return to full activity should not be allowed until the patient demonstrates a painless full range of motion. For type I injuries, return typically requires 1 to 2 weeks, whereas type II injuries can take as long as 6 to 8 weeks to heal.

Other treatment modalities include ice therapy, anti-inflammatory medications, activity modification, and complete rest. Corticosteroid and/or anesthetic injections into the AC joint are also used in high-level athletes to allow quicker return to play.

Grade III AC Injuries

The management of type III AC injury remains controversial. Nonsurgical management has traditionally been advocated for all but the most high-level athletes. Most patients treated nonoperatively can expect a good functional outcome and a return to previous levels of activity. However, some authors recommend early surgical intervention in high-demand athletes and heavy manual laborers.[12]

Based on the current literature, the consensus is that no functional difference is demonstrated between the nonsurgical and surgical management of type III AC joint injuries. However, there is a trend toward higher overall complications and longer time before return to previous level of sport or work in the surgical group.

It is the authors' opinion that most acute type III AC injuries be managed nonoperatively with scapular retraction bracing for 3 to 4 weeks, followed by gentle range of motion exercises and strengthening. The normal healing time for nonoperative treatment is 3 to 4 months. Although some patients still have a distal clavicle prominence, most will do well with nonoperative management. Those patients with persistent horizontal instability, diagnosed primarily by crepitation and horizontal (anteroposterior) movement of the clavicle on the acromion with resisted cross chest adduction and abduction, will usually experience a poor result and will most likely desire surgical reconstruction. Patients who fail conservative care, defined by the persistence of symptoms or inability to return to their desired level of activity or sport, are considered potential candidates for AC joint reconstruction.

STEP-BY-STEP DESCRIPTION OF THE PROCEDURE

Several variations of the arthroscopically assisted ACCR have been described, yet 3 key components remain essential to a successful result:

1. Anatomic reduction of the AC joint

2. Repair or reconstruction of the CC and AC ligaments

3. Supplementation of the repair with a synthetic material or implant to maintain stability during the acute phase of healing[2]

Each construct consists of a stent and a biologic component. The stent is a synthetic material or rigid implant designed to maintain AC joint stability during the acute phases of healing. The stent is often a suture, cortical fixation button, screw, or synthetic tape.

The use of the biologic component may differ with the timing of the surgery and the severity of the injury. In acute cases, it may be possible to repair the native AC and CC ligaments. In chronic cases, an autograft or allograft tendon is used to reconstruct the AC and CC ligaments. Semitendinosus tendon is the most common graft used.

Described next are 2 techniques for arthroscopic-assisted ACCR. The first technique describes ACCR with a single, looped allograft, and the second describes a combined allograft and cortical fixation button technique. The third technique employs an open approach to introduce an AC hook plate supplemented with allograft semitendinosus. This latter method is the authors' preferred method for revision AC joint reconstruction.

Arthroscopic-Assisted Anatomic Coracoclavicular Ligament Reconstruction With Looped Allograft

Positioning

The patient is placed in the lateral decubitus position, rolled back 30 degrees. The neck is directed 10 to 15 degrees laterally away from the operative site to allow for better access and to avoid interference with laterally directed drill approaches during the case. The patient is draped to expose the entire clavicle. The clavicle, acromion, and coracoid are palpated and marked as a guide for portal placement.

Portal Placement and Initial Arthroscopic Approach

An arthroscope is then introduced through a standard posterior portal into the glenohumeral joint for diagnostic arthroscopy. Concomitant pathologies are identified and addressed at that time. Once diagnostic arthroscopy and concomitant procedures are complete, the arthroscope is removed from the glenohumeral joint and placed into the subacromial space through the same posterior skin portal. A lateral portal 3 cm distal to the anterolateral corner of the acromion is then established using an outside-in technique with a spinal needle while visualizing from the posterior portal. The correct placement of the portal is confirmed by arthroscopic visualization. The arthroscope is transferred to the lateral viewing portal. The CA ligament is identified but not taken down. The posterior border of the CA ligament is used as a guide down to the tip of the coracoid.

An anterior portal is made directly anterior and slightly inferior to the medial coracoid by use of an outside-in technique with a spinal needle. The needle must be positioned to allow for easy access above and below the coracoid (Figures 8-3 and 8-4).

An 8-mm cannula is then inserted into this portal. An electrocautery device is used to remove soft tissue from the anterior, inferior, and superior aspect of the coracoid (Figure 8-5). Damage to the nearby neurovascular structures is avoided by keeping the electrocautery in close contact with bone at all times. It may be necessary to release the pectoralis minor tendon from the medial surface of the coracoid at this time, especially in cases of chronic contracture refractory to preoperative stretching, or in cases where visualization of the coracoid is unsatisfactory.

The undersurface of the clavicle is identified and exposed with an electrocautery device and a shaver to improve visualization. Remnants of the CC ligaments are preserved (Figure 8-6). A superior AC portal is established, and the AC joint is inspected. A distal clavicle excision is then performed with the arthroscope in the lateral portal and the shaver in the anterior portal in all chronic cases, resecting at least 5 mm of distal clavicle to allow for adequate reduction and to reduce the risk of painful AC arthrosis.

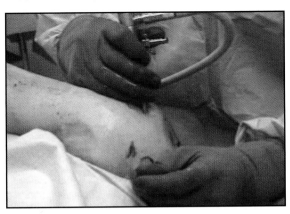

Figure 8-3. Portal placement in the lateral decubitus position. A lateral viewing portal is used to confirm outside-in placement of the anterior portal.

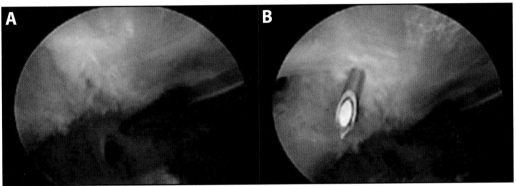

Figure 8-4. Anterior portal set up. (A) The spinal needle is visualized inferior to the coracoid. (B) The spinal needle is visualized superior to the coracoid. (Reprinted with permission from Felix H. Savoie III, MD.)

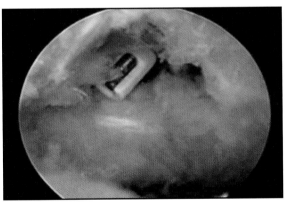

Figure 8-5. The superior and inferior surfaces of the coracoid are debrided using electrocautery. The active surface is always kept in contact with the bone of the coracoid to avoid neurologic injury. (Reprinted with permission from Felix H. Savoie III, MD.)

Mini-Open Procedure and Tunnel Placement

Attention is once again returned to the marked skin incision over the clavicle. An incision is made 2 to 4.5 cm medial to the lateral edge of the clavicle to approximate the insertion site of the CC ligaments. Dissection with a needle-tip electrocautery is completed to the level of the deltotrapezial fascia. Full thickness skin flaps are created using Metzenbaum scissors. The fascia and the AC capsule are incised in one layer parallel to the long axis of the clavicle using electrocautery. Homan retractors are placed anterior and posterior to the clavicle to visualize the distal clavicle.

Figure 8-6. The undersurface of the clavicle is evaluated and debrided in the area of the origin of the CC ligaments. This is usually performed with a cautery to prevent inadvertent bleeding. The surface of the cautery is kept in contact with the bone of the displaced clavicle. The CC ligament remnants are preserved as a landmark for clavicular tunnel placement. (Reprinted with permission from Felix H. Savoie III, MD.)

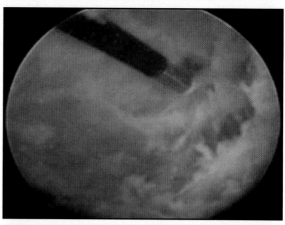

Figure 8-7. View from the lateral portal. Kirschner wires are inserted through the clavicle at the sites of origin of the CC ligaments. The insertion points are confirmed arthroscopically, and the wires are over-reamed with a 5-mm reamer. (Reprinted with permission from Felix H. Savoie III, MD.)

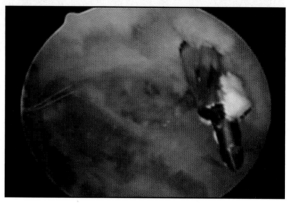

Two Kirschner wires are then placed through the clavicle and directed toward the coracoid. They will serve as the medial and lateral clavicular tunnels. These are inserted at the site of the origin of the CC ligaments. This step is visualized arthroscopically from the lateral portal, and the retained edges of the CC ligaments serve as a landmark for Kirschner wire placement (see Figures 8-6 and 8-7).

The conoid ligament tunnel (the medial tunnel) is placed 45-mm medial to the AC joint and at the posterosuperior aspect of the clavicle. The trapezoid ligament tunnel is placed 2.5 cm medial to the AC joint at the direct superior aspect of the clavicle. The Kirschner wires are over-reamed with a cannulated reamer of 4.5 to 6 mm based on the size of the graft. The holes are then tapped to accommodate screw insertion.

Graft Passage

Visualization continues via the anterolateral portal and a passing suture is inserted through the anterior portal, directed under the coracoid, and retrieved out of the medial clavicular tunnel. A second passing suture is then placed through the anterior cannula, retrieved superior to the coracoid, and pulled out the lateral clavicular tunnel.

The medial suture is used to pull the graft from the anterior portal, under the coracoid, and through the medial clavicular tunnel, thus exiting the incision. The lateral suture is used to retrieve the opposite end of the graft with a previously prepared braided PDS suture stent. The other end of the stent is then placed under the coracoid and retrieved out of the AC joint portal. (Figure 8-8).

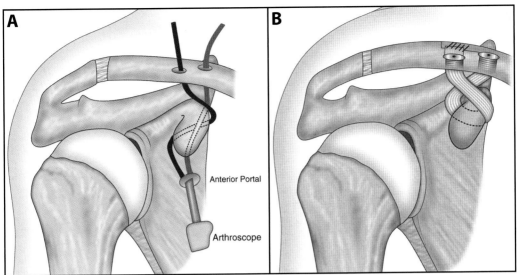

Figure 8-8. (A) 1. The passing suture is placed through the anterior portal, retrieved inferior to the coracoid, and pulled out of the medial clavicular tunnel. 2. A second passing suture (purple) is passed through the anterior portal, retrieved superior to the coracoid, and transferred out of the lateral clavicular tunnel. (B) 3. The green passing suture is used to lead the semitendinosus graft inferior to the coracoid and out of the medial clavicular tunnel. 4. Viewing from the lateral portal, the graft is followed as it moves up and into the medial clavicular tunnel. 5. The second passing suture pulls the opposite end of the graft through the cannula, over the coracoid, and into the lateral clavicular tunnel. 6. The graft is in place and tensioned to eliminate soft tissue constraints or laxity, and satisfactory positioning is confirmed. Note the 2 limbs of the graft cross in the space between the coracoid and clavicle. (Reprinted with permission from Felix H. Savoie III, MD.)

Graft Tensioning and Interference Screw Placement

A nitinol pin is placed through the medial and lateral clavicular tunnels and the graft is then tensioned appropriately. The medial interference screw is placed and tightened first until it is flush against the superior cortex of the clavicle. The screwdriver is left in the screw and used to over-reduce the clavicle toward the coracoid while continuing to visualize the entire AC joint arthroscopically. The suture stent runs around the base of the clavicle with the graft and through the drill holes in the clavicle with the knot between the clavicle and coracoid, not on top of the clavicle, to prevent skin irritation The graft is then retensioned to confirm proper restoration of the CC anatomy, and the lateral interference screw is inserted.

The 2 limbs of the graft are sutured to each other and the excess graft is tunneled under the skin to the acromion and fixed to the acromion or lateral AC capsule using percutaneous suture to reconstruct the anterior and posterior AC ligaments. Surgical C-arm images may be obtained throughout the case to confirm reduction.

Anatomic Coracoclavicular Reconstruction With Tendon Graft and Cortical Fixation Button

The arthroscope is introduced into the glenohumeral joint utilizing the standard posterior portal. Some authors prefer to keep the arthroscope in the joint, excise the rotator interval, and continue to view from this portal during the procedure. The authors prefer to use the same anterior and lateral portals described previously. Diagnostic arthroscopy is performed and concomitant pathology is addressed. The initial stages of coracoid exposure are as previously detailed in the graft technique. The pectoralis minor attachment to the coracoid is kept intact.

Figure 8-9. The semitendinosus allograft is looped through the hook plate and around the coracoid.

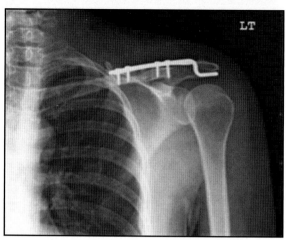

A 5-cm incision is then made longitudinally over the clavicle. Dissection to the level of the deltotrapezial fascia is carried out with electrocautery. With the clavicle adequately visualized, the clavicular drill holes are made with the same technique as described previously.

A 4.5-mm hole is created in the coracoid and must be placed as close to the coracoid base as possible to avoid an iatrogenic fracture. The fixation button is then passed through the conoid hole in the clavicle and inferiorly through the coracoid, and the button is flipped beneath the coracoid. It is important to obtain direct visualization of the cortical fixation button as it is flipped. A passing suture is placed around the coracoid in a medial-to-lateral fashion and posterior to the conjoined tendon. The graft is passed around the coracoid and through the corresponding clavicle hole.

The AC joint is reduced anatomically and the cortical fixation stent is tensioned and tied. Having reduced and secured the AC joint, each end of the graft is then tensioned and secured with a bicortical interference screw.

Hook Plate Fixation (Nonarthroscopic Technique)

For cases in which more rigid fixation is desired, a hook plate may be used as the "stent." Utilizing this device commits the patient to a second surgery at 4 months to remove the plate, but it does have the advantage of requiring less immobilization in the early postoperative phase.

The patient is placed in the beach chair position. General anesthesia is administered. A 7-cm–long skin incision is made in line with the lateral clavicle and AC joint. The AC joint is exposed and inspected for scar tissue and signs of arthrosis. The AC joint is reduced and a hook plate is positioned with the hook inferiorly beneath the acromion and fixed to the clavicle with screws. Once the plate is properly positioned and this is confirmed under fluoroscopy, a semitendinosus allograft is placed through an empty hole in the hook plate (Figures 8-9 and 8-10).

The graft is looped posteriorly and anteriorly beneath the clavicle and around the coracoid, providing an allograft reconstruction of the CC ligaments. Excess graft is brought onto the posterior and superior portion of the AC ligaments and sutured in place to reinforce the AC joint.

POSTOPERATIVE PROTOCOL

Arthroscopic

Postoperatively, the shoulder is supported with a shoulder immobilizer and abduction pad full-time for 6 weeks. Elbow, wrist, and hand motion exercises are allowed during this time.

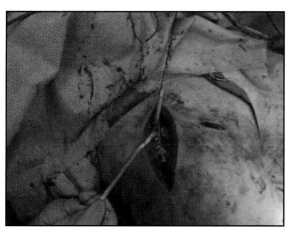

Figure 8-10. Anterior portal radiographs of acromial hook plate. The hook plate is subsequently removed at 3 to 6 months.

Radiographs are obtained at the first postoperative visit. Passive range of motion exercises are initiated at 2 weeks. A dynamic scapular retraction brace is worn beginning at 4 weeks following surgery for use during daytime activities, and the abduction sling is gradually discontinued. Active range of motion is also started at that time, but cross chest adduction is avoided until 8 weeks postoperatively. At 6 to 8 weeks, aggressive rehabilitation is started with a return to normal activities, usually by 12 to 16 weeks following repair.

Hook Plate

The patient is placed in a pillow sling for 1 week. One week postoperatively, the sling is discontinued except at night and physical therapy is then initiated. The patient is encouraged to return to normal activity. After 4 months, the plate is removed and the patient is followed radiographically at monthly intervals to monitor for any erosion into the scapular spine.

POTENTIAL COMPLICATIONS

Although arthroscopic AC joint reconstruction procedures were designed to minimize surgical complications associated with a large, open procedure, they are not without their risks. Common complications of arthroscopically assisted ACCR procedures include loss of reduction, soft tissue irritation/infection, and distal clavicle osteoarthritis.

A multitude of factors can lead to loss of reduction, including graft failure, button slippage, button pullout, hardware failure, osteolysis of the clavicular tunnel, coracoid fractures, and clavicle fractures. Loss of reduction has been reported to occur in 30% to 89% of cases, but this is usually asymptomatic and associated with a good functional outcome.[3,13] Schliemann et al reported that a loss of reduction equal to a Rockwood II to III lesion may be asymptomatic and associated with a good functional outcome, but patients with a loss of reduction equivalent to a Rockwood V lesion were clinically symptomatic and required revision.[14]

Soft tissue complications are often related to PDS suture granulomas that result in pain, irritation, and, occasionally, erosion through the skin overlying the superior clavicle. This complication is caused by suture knots that sit too prominently on the superior surface of the clavicle. These cases often require oral antibiotic suppression and local wound care until 12 weeks postoperatively, at which time the suture knot can be removed under local anesthesia.[15]

AC joint arthrosis is believed to be a common cause of persistent postoperative pain. Presently, there is little evidence to support or refute routinely performing a concomitant distal clavicle excision.[16] Some studies have shown that the retained distal clavicle is a pain generator that leads to symptomatic arthritis requiring further treatment.[17] In their series of 16 patients undergoing ACCR, Carofino and Mazzocca reported no instances of AC joint symptoms in 14/16 patients with a retained distal clavicle.[16]

CONCLUSION

Arthroscopic AC joint reconstruction combines the desirable features of an open anatomic reconstruction of the CC ligaments with the benefits of a less invasive surgery. The new generation of AC reconstructions, based on sound biomechanical and anatomic data, have ushered forth hybrid reconstructive techniques that afford a stable and secure construct utilizing minimally invasive techniques.

The arthroscopic technique for reconstruction of the injured AC joint is still evolving but shows much promise for the future management of these challenging injuries.

TOP TECHNICAL PEARLS FOR THE PROCEDURE

1. Proper portal placement is key.
2. Adequate circumferential access to the coracoid process is essential.
3. Clavicle tunnels must be spaced 20 to 25 mm to prevent iatrogenic fracture. The lateral tunnel must not be closer than 15 to 20 mm from the lateral edge of the clavicle.
4. Avoid prominent suture knots or fixation devices on the superior surface of the clavicle as they may erode through the skin and cause infection.
5. Synthetic or metal fixation stents, especially those placed through a drill hole in the coracoid, have a high rate of complications and, if used, must be observed carefully for potential loosening or fracture.

REFERENCES

1. DePalma AF. The role of the disks of the sternoclavicular and the acromioclavicular joints. *Clin Orthop.* 1959;13:222-233.
2. Li X, Ma R, Bedi A, Dines DM, Altchek DW, Dines JS. Management of acromioclavicular joint injuries. *J Bone Joint Surg Am.* 2014;96(1):73-84.
3. Urist, MR. Complete dislocations of the acroioclavicular joint:the nature of the traumatic lsion and effective methods of treatment with an analysis of forty-one cases. *J Bone Joint Surg.* 1946;28(4):813-837.
4. Salzmann GM, Walz L, Buchmann S, Glabgly P, Venjakob A, Imhoff AB. Arthroscopically assisted 2-bundle anatomical reduction of acute acromioclavicular joint separations. *Am J Sports Med.* 2010;38(6):1179-1187.
5. Blazar PE, Iannotti JP, Williams GR. Anteroposterior instability of the distal clavicle after distal clavicle resection. *Clin Orthop.* 1998;(348):114-120.
6. Grutter PW, Petersen SA. Anatomical acromioclavicular ligament reconstruction: a biomechanical comparison of reconstructive techniques of the acromioclavicular joint. *Am J Sports Med.* 2005;33(11):1723-1728.
7. Lee SJ, Nicholas SJ, Akizuki KH, McHugh MP, Kremenic IJ. Reconstruction of the coracoclavicular ligaments with tendon grafts: a comparative biomechanical study. *Am J Sports Med.* 2003;31(5):648-655.

8. Rockwood CA, Williams GR, Young CD. Injuries to the acromioclavicular joint. In: Rockwood CA, Green DP, Bucholz RW, Heckman JD, eds. *Fractures in Adults*. Vol 2, 4th ed. Philadelphia, PA: Lippincott-Raven, 1996:1341-1414.

9. Zanca P. Shoulder pain: involvement of the acromioclavicular joint. (Analysis of 1,000 cases). *Am J Roetgenol Radium Ther Nucl Med.* 1971;112(3):493-506.

10. Bearden JM, Hughston JC, Whatley GS. Acromioclavicular dislocation: method of treatment. *J Sports Med.* 1973;1:5-17.

11. Tischer T, Salzmann GM, El-Azab H, Vogt S, Imhoff AB. Incidence of associated injuries with acute acromioclavicular joint dislocations type III through V. *Am J Sports Med.* 2009;37(1):136-139.

12. Bannister GC, Wallace WA, Stableforth PG, et al. The management of acute acromioclavicular dislocation. A randomised prospective controlled trial. *J Bone Joint Surg Br.* 1989;71:848-850.

13. Scheibel M, Droschel S, Gerhardt C, Kraus N. Arthroscopically assisted stablization of acute high-grade acromioclavicular joint separations. *Am J Sports Med.* 2011;39(7):1507-1516.

14. Schliemann B, Roblenbroich SB, Schneider KN, et al. Why does minimally invasive coracoclavicular ligament reconstruction using a flip button repair technique fail? An analysis of risk factors and complications. *Knee Surg Sports Traumatol Arthrosc.* 2015;23(5):1419-1425.

15. VanSice W, Savoie FH. Arthroscopic reconstruction of the acromioclavicular joint using semitendinosus allograft: technique and preliminary results. *Tech Shoulder Elbow Surg.* 2008;9(3):109-113.

16. Carofino B, Mazzocca A. The anatomic coracoclavicular ligament reconstruction: Surgical technique and indications. *J Bone Joint Surg.* 2010;19(2 Suppl):37-46.

17. Park JP, Arnold JA, Coker TP. Treatment of acromioclavicular separations. A retrospective study. *Am J Sports Med.* 1980;8(4):251-256.

9

Arthroscopic Extracellular Matrix Rotator Cuff Replacement/Augmentation

Nolan R. May, MD and Stephen J. Snyder, MD

INTRODUCTION

Rotator cuff injuries continue to be a common clinical problem. The incidence of full thickness rotator cuff tears is related to increasing age, with an estimated incidence between 28% and 40% in patients over age 60 years.[1] The reported re-tear rate of surgically repaired full thickness rotator cuff tears ranges from 15% to 60%, with large or massive cuff tears having failure rates reported as high as 94%.[2] Patient age, tear size, fatty infiltration, smoking, muscle atrophy, and the chronic nature of the tear are all factors that can lead to repair failure.[2-14]

Asymptomatic or minimally symptomatic patients with irreparable tears or re-tears should be treated conservatively or with the minimal surgery needed to relieve symptoms resulting from loose bodies, biceps disease, acromioclavicular (AC) joint pathology, and impingement. When conservative treatment fails, surgeons look to alternate options. Reverse total shoulder arthroplasty is a useful surgical option that can be utilized more in the elderly or lower-demand patient population with significant arthritis, but should not be considered when a repairable cuff tear is present or an adequate cuff stump is available for performing an allograft augmentation or replacement.

For the younger or higher-demand patient with a large or massive cuff tear, biologic repair is preferred to eliminate the restrictions associated with reverse arthroplasty. Newer techniques are being utilized that involve supplemental scaffolds to enhance the rotator cuff repair constructs by replacing or reinforcing the damaged cuff tendon. Numerous types of scaffolds exist, including synthetic nonbiologic scaffold material, dermal xenografts, dermal allografts, and other collagen products. The new biologic materials are often referred to as *extracellular matrix (ECM) grafts*. The ECM grafts can assist in the healing of the damaged rotator cuff by augmenting a weak tendon after direct repair of the tendon to the bone (augmentation technique). For those cases where the tendon is unable to be directly repaired to the bone because of poor tissue quality or excess tissue tension, the ECM graft can be used to bridge the defect (bridge technique).

Regardless of whether the graft is used for augmenting or bridging, the aim of the ECM graft is to increase the initial repair strength and assist in cell recruitment and adherence[15,16] and thus facilitate cuff-like tissue tendon regrowth. Acellular dermal grafts have successfully

Ryu RKN, Angelo RL, Abrams JS, eds. *The Shoulder: AANA Advanced Arthroscopic Surgical Techniques* (pp 95-105). © 2016 AANA.

restored deficient rotator cuff tendons in numerous animal laboratory studies.[17,18] Human studies with midterm follow-up utilizing ECM grafts have also been promising.[15,19-22] Similar to using allograft tissue to reconstruct other areas of the body, the biologic activity, the source and preparation of the tissue, and the strength of the graft are all characteristics that must be considered by the surgeon prior to use.

INDICATIONS

- ► Patients with large, degenerative tears (greater than 2 cm) and those at risk for re-tear are ideal candidates for allograft augmentation or allograft bridge techniques.
- ► Those patients considered high risk for re-tear include prior failed repairs, evidence of significant retraction, fatty infiltration or atrophy on preoperative magnetic resonance imaging (MRI), or patients who failed to heal a repair on the contralateral shoulder.
- ► Ideally, patients should have minimal glenohumeral chondromalacia, only mild or moderate pain, active forward flexion greater than 130 degrees, and evidence of some power with external rotation strength testing.
- ► Patients with poor motion, severe pain, failed prior repairs, and early cartilage wear are still considered candidates, but results are likely to be inferior to the "ideal" candidate description, and preoperative clinic visits must focus on patient expectations.

Contraindications

While the indications and contraindications for allograft rotator cuff reconstruction are still evolving, the only true contraindications are as follows:
- ► Active infection
- ► Severe stiffness
- ► An incompetent deltoid
- ► Severe glenohumeral arthritis
- ► Lack of a medial rotator cuff tendon stump
- ► Medical comorbidities that would pose a substantial risk during the perioperative period must also be considered.
- ► Relative contraindications are cost, surgeon's skill and experience, and additional operative time.

PERTINENT PHYSICAL FINDINGS

A standard shoulder-focused exam is essential, including the following:
- ► Evaluation of neck motion
- ► Skin inspection for muscle atrophy
- ► Localized tenderness to palpation
- ► Active and passive shoulder motion, as well as muscle strength, should be assessed and documented. Patients with massive rotator cuff tears frequently have pronounced weakness of supraspinatus and infraspinatus testing.

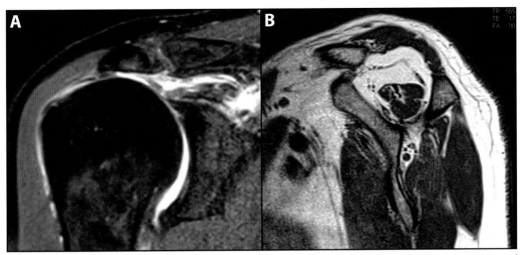

Figure 9-1. Coronal T2 and sagittal T1 images of a right shoulder demonstrating a large, retracted tear of the supraspinatus tendon and significant fatty infiltration, respectively.

Pertinent Imaging

Patients should have recent good-quality radiographs. This preoperative series should include the following:

- Four standard radiographs: anteroposterior, Zanca AC, axillary lateral, and scapular outlet views. The degree of glenohumeral or AC arthritis, acromial arch shape and thickness, cystic tuberosity changes, humeral head elevation, and the presence of previously used anchors can all be appreciated from this 4-view series.

- MRI scans are also necessary to allow the surgeon to further assess for potential articular surface defects, cystic changes of the tuberosity, and prior anchor placement. Likewise, the MRI will reveal the degree of tendon retraction and confirm that an adequate tendon stump is present for graft fixation. The status of the subscapularis, biceps tendon, and remaining cuff tissue should also be reviewed prior to the case. Frequently, coronal (Figure 9-1A) and sagittal (Figure 9-1B) images demonstrate significant fatty infiltration and a large, retracted tear of the supraspinatus tendon.

Equipment

- Acellular dermal allograft (> 1.8 mm thick)
- Suture shuttling system
- Four cannulas: three 7 mm and one 8 to 10 mm (depending on graft size)
- Knotted measuring suture with knots at 1-cm increments
- #2 braided sutures for short-tailed interference knot (STIK) knots (#10 to 12)
- Anchors: triple-loaded suture anchors, preferably titanium, to easily identify on postoperative radiographs.

Figure 9-2. External view of a right shoulder demonstrating standard anterior and posterior portals, as well as a larger lateral subacromial portal for passage of the graft. The 2 triple-loaded suture anchors placed at the anterior and posterior margins of the rotator cuff tear are clamped tightly against the skin creating the 2 "suture stacks." All sutures from the graft must be shuttled between the "stacks" to avoid crossing the sutures and tangling of the graft. One suture from each anchor is passed and tied through the borders of the rotator cuff tear to stabilize the lateral margin.

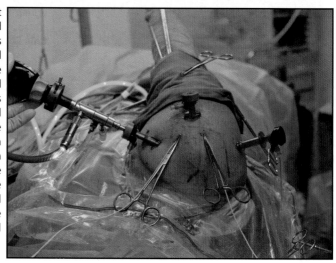

POSITIONING AND PORTALS

The procedure is performed with the patient in the lateral decubitus position with all bony prominences well-padded and an axillary roll in good position. The glenohumeral joint work is performed with the arm in 70 degrees of abduction and 5 degrees of forward flexion, which is achieved with 10 to 15 lbs of balanced arm traction, depending on patient size. The bursal surgery is performed with the arm in 15 degrees of abduction. The arm in "midposition" (45 degrees of abduction) is necessary for evaluating the lateral aspect of the greater tuberosity and for lateral row anchor placement if they are used.

The initial portals created are the standard posterior mid-glenoid and anterior mid-glenoid portals. Either 1 (Figure 9-2) or 2 lateral portals are also established. If 2 lateral portals are utilized, an anterolateral working cannula will be used for graft passage and anchor placement, while a posterolateral portal will be used for viewing and should be positioned just posterior to the middle of the tear. It is also very helpful to create a suprascapular notch portal as described in the next section.

STEP-BY-STEP DESCRIPTION OF THE PROCEDURE

Initial Arthroscopic Exam

A complete 15-point arthroscopic evaluation of the glenohumeral joint is performed, viewing from both the posterior and anterior portals. Any intra-articular surgery that is needed is performed at this time, including labral debridement, subscapularis repair, and preparation of the articular side of the rotator cuff. The superior capsule is released from the glenoid to mobilize the retracted stump of the rotator cuff. The arm is adjusted to 15 degrees of abduction and the bursal space is entered. A lateral portal for viewing is established in addition to the standard anterior and posterior portals. To aid in visualization, bursal tissue is debrided and a subacromial decompression and distal clavicle resection is performed as needed.

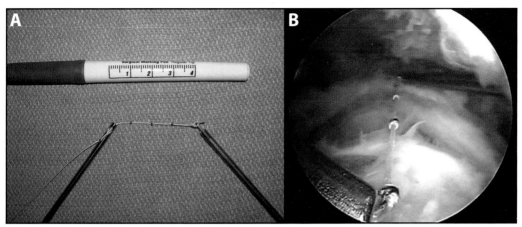

Figure 9-3. (A) A measuring suture is created with knots placed at 1-cm increments and marked with a pen. (B) The measuring suture is drawn across the tear with a knot pusher to estimate graft size.

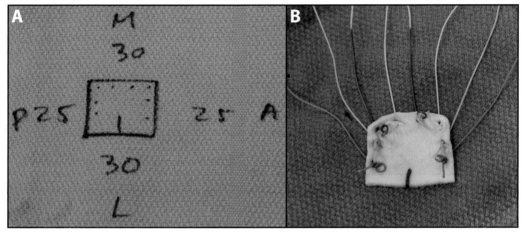

Figure 9-4. (A) A preliminary template of the graft is created after measurement. (B) After cutting the graft, STIK sutures are passed along the posterior, medial, and anterior border of the graft at premarked (usually 8 mm) intervals from a bursal-to-articular direction. Ensure that the shiny (epidermal) side of the graft is positioned up toward the acromion.

Graft Preparation

The frayed edges of the rotator cuff tear are debrided and the tear size is measured in anterior-to-posterior and medial-to-lateral dimensions using a knotted suture (Figure 9-3) as a measuring device. The knotted suture measuring device is created by tying a loop STIK on one end in a #1 suture and placing simple half-hitch knots in exact 1-cm increments. The allograft patch is hydrated if necessary and cut to size on the back operating room table after creating a measurement template (Figure 9-4A). It is important to intentionally oversize the graft by 3 mm on each side to allow for placement of the STIK sutures 3 mm away from the edge. A loop-STIK suture consists of a bulky interference knot (mulberry-type knot) tied on the end of a #2 suture after looping it over a 1-mm metal rod. A mark is placed using a surgical marking pencil at the midline on the lateral aspect of the graft and blue dots are placed to indicate the location of all perimeter STIKs. The authors recommend placing 3 to 5 STIK sutures circumferentially around

Figure 9-5. Right shoulder. Staging the graft on the lateral arm with passage of the middle suture of the posterior suture stack. After passage of this suture through the posterolateral corner of the graft, another STIK is tied to provide traction and remaining slack in the suture is removed. Subsequently, the remaining STIK sutures already passed through the graft are sequentially shuttled through the RCT in a posterior-to-medial-to-anterior sequence. Again, it is imperative to always pass the suture hooks posterior or anterior to the suture stack and retrieve the shuttle between the stacks and anterior and parallel to the previous stitch to prevent twisting.

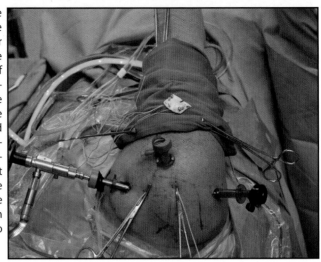

the posterior, medial, and anterior aspects of the graft, approximately 3 mm from the graft edge (Figure 9-4B). Two #2 sutures are placed laterally if a lateral row of suture anchors is being used.

Initial Cuff Repair

An arthroscopic rotator cuff repair is performed in standard fashion as the majority of tears can be completely repaired back to bone. The authors prefer to use the Southern California Orthopedic Institute (SCOI) row technique: a single row of 2 or 3 medially based, triple-loaded suture anchors located just lateral to the articular margin. One suture from each anchor is not used to repair the cuff. Rather, these sutures are stored outside of the cannula for later lateral graft fixation. Five to 7 bone marrow vents are punched in the prepared lateral tuberosity bone to facilitate creation of the crimson duvet, the red velvety bone marrow clot that extends from the tuberosity over the cuff and allograft and supplies the fibrin matrix containing mesenchymal stem cells, platelets with growth factors, and a permanent neovascular blood supply.

Suture Passage

An 8.5- to 10-mm cannula is utilized in the midlateral portal. The graft is positioned on the lateral arm in the correct orientation (Figure 9-5). A suture hook is inserted through the posterior cannula and penetrates the most posterior and lateral cuff tissue, creating a small full-thickness "pinch." A suture shuttle device is passed through the suture needle and retrieved out of the lateral cannula. The free end of the corresponding STIK suture is loaded in the shuttle and then carried through the cuff tendon and back out of the posterior cannula. This shuttling technique is repeated, progressing along the posterior cuff, then medially, and finally anteriorly, shuttling all of the STIK sutures. It is critical that the STIK sutures are not tangled during these steps. This is accomplished by keeping the path of each subsequent shuttle, grasper, and STIK suture anterior and parallel to the previously passed sutures as they are retrieved into the lateral cannula.

Graft Insertion

The slack must first be pulled out of the STIK sutures, thus positioning the graft at the lateral cannula aperture. The graft is then folded on and advanced down the cannula (Figure 9-6) using a

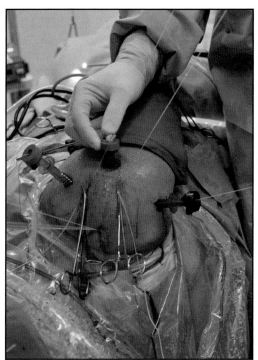

Figure 9-6. Graft insertion, right shoulder. The graft sutures are uniformly tensioned by pulling the slack out, thereby delivering the graft to the mouth of the cannula. The graft is rolled onto itself to facilitate passage through the cannula diaphragm. A "push-pull" technique is used; as the sutures are tensioned, the graft is pushed down the cannula with a closed blunt tool. The free end of the STIK sutures are pulled from their respective cannulae, keeping the sutures uniformly taut. It is important not to allow slack in any of the sutures since the loops formed may tangle with the STIK knots.

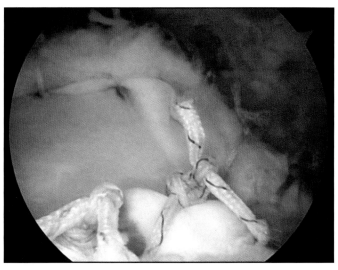

Figure 9-7. Right shoulder. Arthroscopic view from the lateral subacromial portal after rotator cuff reconstruction using acellular human dermal allograft tissue.

push-pull technique (the STIK suture ends are pulled from their respective posterior and anterior cannulas, while the graft is pushed with a grasper). Once the graft is entirely through the cannula, each suture end is pulled to unfold the graft. The free end and the knot of each STIK is retrieved into the lateral cannula and sequentially tied (Figure 9-7). The remaining anchor sutures, which were stored outside of the cannula, are passed through the graft using standard suture shuttle technique to fix the lateral margin of the graft to the tuberosity. These are passed and tied similar to a routine rotator cuff repair.

STEP-BY STEP DESCRIPTION OF THE PROCEDURE: BRIDGE TECHNIQUE

Initial Arthroscopic Exam

The initial 15-point glenohumeral exam and bursal exam utilize the same techniques as the augmentation method described earlier. The greater tuberosity and the frayed cuff edges are debrided.

Placement of Anterior and Posterior Anchors

A triple-loaded suture anchor is inserted into the posterior aspect of the footprint just lateral to the articular margin. The most posterior suture in the anchor is passed through the posterior cuff using standard shuttle technique and tied using a sliding, locking knot to establish a stable posterior edge of the tear for measurement purposes. A second anchor is then inserted into the anterior aspect of the footprint, again just lateral to the articular margin and slightly posterior to the biceps tendon or groove. The most anterior suture from this anchor is passed through the interval tissue and tied to establish the anterior edge of the tear.

Graft Preparation

The dimensions of the tear, both anteroposterior and mediolateral, are measured using a knotted measuring suture as described previously (see Figure 9-3). The graft is prepared on the back table in a similar fashion as the augmentation technique after a sample template is created (see Figure 9-4A). STIK sutures (described earlier) are placed 3 mm from the graft edge and spaced every 5 to 7 mm circumferentially around the anterior, medial, and posterior aspect of the graft (see Figure 9-4B). The anterolateral corner and the posterolateral corner of the graft do not need STIKs because limbs from the previously placed anchors will be utilized in these areas. To aid in suture identification within the shoulder, it is easier to use alternating colored sutures.

Suture Passage

The arthroscope is maintained in an anterior viewing portal and an 8.5- to 10-mm lateral cannula is used for suture shuttling and graft passage. The graft is positioned on the lateral arm in the correct orientation to aid in suture management (see Figure 9-5). The most posterior, medial limb from the posterior anchor is retrieved out of the midlateral cannula. A straight Keith needle is used to pass this suture through the posterolateral corner of the graft from its undersurface to the upper surface. A bulky STIK knot is tied so the knot rests on the upper surface of the graft. A crescent-shaped suture hook is inserted through the posterior cannula and used to penetrate the most posterior and lateral cuff tissue and exit under the edge of the cuff. A suture shuttle is retrieved out of the lateral cannula with a grasper. The free end of the corresponding posterior STIK suture is then loaded in the shuttle and carried through the cuff tendon and back out of the posterior cannula. The stitching and shuttling technique is repeated for all of the STIK sutures. The anterior stitches are passed with the suture hook in the anterior cannula. To keep the sutures from becoming tangled, the paths of each subsequent suture hook, shuttling suture, grasper, and STIK suture must all be kept anterior and parallel to the previously passed sutures. After all sutures are passed through the cuff, a small suprascapular notch portal is created and all of the sutures from the medial portion of the graft are retrieved out of this portal. Positioning the medial sutures in this portal facilitates the task of pulling the graft into the shoulder. The most anterior medial limb of the anterior anchor is retrieved out of the lateral operating cannula and is passed through the anterolateral corner of the graft using a straight Keith needle. A STIK knot is tied, which rests upon the upper side of the graft.

Graft Seating

The slack is pulled out of all the free ends of the STIK sutures, docking the graft at the aperture of the lateral cannula. The graft is rolled onto itself to aid in passage through the diaphragm of the cannula (see Figure 9-6) and the push-pull technique described earlier is used. The STIK suture ends stored in the supraclavicular notch portal are pulled first as leader sutures for graft passage. Once the graft passes through the cannula, each suture end is sequentially tightened to unfold the graft. Clamps are placed on the medial and lateral STIKs adjacent to the skin to hold the graft taut. The sutures are then retrieved and tied through any convenient cannula, but the authors often prefer to tie via the lateral cannula while viewing through the posterior or anterior cannula.

Lateral Fixation

The final suture from the posterior anchor is then passed through the posterior portion of the lateral edge of the graft using a shuttle technique. This process is repeated for the remaining suture in the anterior anchor. These sutures are stored outside of the posterior and anterior cannula, respectively, using plastic suture covers if desired. One or 2 additional double-loaded sutures anchors are placed just lateral to the graft. These anchors are positioned halfway anterior and posterior to the midline mark on the lateral edge of the graft. The 4 sutures from the anchors are then passed through the lateral edge of the graft from posterior to anterior using standard shuttle technique. Each suture pair is retrieved and stored outside of the posterior cannula. The lateral sutures are then tied via the lateral cannula from anterior to posterior using a sliding locking knot (see Figure 9-7).

POSTOPERATIVE PROTOCOL

In the authors' experience, the therapy program does not differ between patients who undergo augmentation or interposition/bridge reconstruction. A sling with a 15-degree abduction pillow is worn for 6 weeks. Gentle pendulum, elbow, wrist, and hand motion exercises are initiated on postoperative day 1 and performed 3 times per day. Formal physical therapy, which is focused on passive motion with progression to active as tolerated, is begun around 6 weeks postoperatively. Strengthening is only allowed once full painless active elevation has been achieved by the patient.

POTENTIAL COMPLICATIONS

The complications typically arise with suture management and graft entanglement. To facilitate graft preparation, an orientation line is placed using a surgical marking pencil at the midline on the lateral aspect of the graft, and blue dots are placed to indicate the location of all perimeter STIKs. A suture hook and suture shuttling technique are used to pass the posterior and medial STIK sutures through the posterior cannula, while the anterior stitches are passed with the suture hook in the anterior cannula. To keep the sutures from becoming tangled, the paths of each subsequent suture hook, shuttling suture, grasper, and STIK suture must all be kept anterior and parallel to the previously passed sutures. Undersizing the graft is another complication, which can be eliminated with the use of an exact measuring suture.

TOP TECHNICAL PEARLS FOR THE PROCEDURE

1. Start the shoulder arthroscopy with a standard 15-point glenohumeral exam, viewing from both the anterior and posterior portals.

2. Thorough debridement of the subacromial bursa is necessary to aid in visualization throughout the entire case.

3. Make the knotted measuring suture with simple half-hitch knots at exactly 1-cm increments to measure the anteroposterior distance, as well as the mediolateral distance of the desired graft size. Oversize the graft by 3 mm on each side to allow for the STIK sutures. Alternate the color of the STIK sutures to assist in suture management.

4. Use a suture hook and suture shuttling technique to pass the corresponding posterior and medial STIK sutures through the posterior cannula, while the anterior stitches are passed with the suture hook in the anterior cannula. To keep the sutures from becoming tangled, the paths of each subsequent suture hook, shuttling suture, grasper, and STIK suture must all be kept anterior and parallel to the previously passed sutures.

5. Postoperatively, a sling with a 15-degree abduction pillow is worn for 5 to 6 weeks, while gentle pendulum, elbow, wrist, and hand motion exercises are initiated on postoperative day 1. Formal therapy is not started until 6 weeks postoperatively.

REFERENCES

1. Sher JS, Uribe JW, Posada A, Murphy BJ, Zlatkin MB. Abnormal findings on magnetic resonance images of asymptomatic shoulders. *J Bone Joint Surg Am.* 1995;77:10-15.
2. Galatz LM, Ball CM, Teefey SA, Middleton WD, Yamaguchi K. The outcome and repair integrity of completely arthroscopically repaired large and massive rotator cuff tears. *J Bone Joint Surg Am.* 2004;86:219-224.
3. Boileau P, Brassart N, Watkinson DJ, Carles M, Hatzidakis AM, Krishnan SG. Arthroscopic repair of full-thickness tears of the supraspinatus: does the tendon really heal? *J Bone Joint Surg Am.* 2005;87:1229-1240.
4. Bishop J, Klepps S, Lo IK, Bird J, Gladstone JN, Flatow EL. Cuff integrity after arthroscopic versus open rotator cuff repair: a prospective study. *J Shoulder Elbow Surg.* 2006;15:290-299.
5. Cole BJ, McCarty LP III, Kang RW, Alford W, Lewis PB, Hayden JK. Arthroscopic rotator cuff repair: prospective functional outcome and repair integrity at minimum 2-year follow-up. *J Shoulder Elbow Surg.* 2007;16:579-585.
6. Verma NN, Dunn W, Adler RS, et al. All-arthroscopic versus mini-open rotator cuff repair: a retrospective review with minimum 2-year follow-up. *Arthroscopy.* 2006;22:587-594.
7. Nho SJ, Brown BS, Lyman S, Adler RS, Altchek DW, MacGillivray JD. Prospective analysis of arthroscopic rotator cuff repair: prognostic factors affecting clinical and ultrasound outcome. *J Shoulder Elbow Surg.* 2009;18:13-20.
8. Harryman DT II, Mack LA, Wang KY, Jackins SE, Richardson ML, Matsen FA III. Repairs of the rotator cuff. Correlation of functional results with integrity of the cuff. *J Bone Joint Surg Am.* 1991;73:982-989.
9. Anderson K, Boothby M, Aschenbrener D, van Holsbeeck M. Outcome and structural integrity after arthroscopic rotator cuff repair using 2 rows of fixation: minimum 2-year follow-up. *Am J Sports Med.* 2006;34:1899-1905.
10. Huijsmans PE, Pritchard MP, Berghs BM, van Rooyen KS, Wallace AL, de Beer JF. Arthroscopic rotator cuff repair with double-row fixation. *J Bone Joint Surg Am.* 2007;89:1248-1257.

11. Lafosse L, Brozska R, Toussaint B, Gobezie R. The outcome and structural integrity of arthroscopic rotator cuff repair with use of the double-row suture anchor technique. *J Bone Joint Surg Am.* 2007;89:1533-1541.

12. Sugaya H, Maeda K, Matsuki K, Moriishi J. Repair integrity and functional outcome after arthroscopic double-row rotator cuff repair. A prospective outcome study. *J Bone Joint Surg Am.* 2007;89:953-960.

13. Snyder SJ. Why I prefer the "SCOI" single row technique for all full thickness rotator cuff repairs. *Inside AANA Newsletter.* 2012;28(1):6-9.

14. Fuchs B, Weishaupt D, Zanetti M, Hodler J, Gerber C. Fatty degeneration of the muscles of the rotator cuff: assessment by computed tomography versus magnetic resonance imaging. *J Shoulder Elbow Surg.* 1999;8(6):599-605.

15. Snyder SJ, Arnoczky SP, Bond JL, Dopirak R. Histologic evaluation of a biopsy specimen obtained 3 months after rotator cuff augmentation with GraftJacket Matrix. *Arthroscopy.* 2009;25(3):329-333. Epub 2008 Jul 24.

16. Montgomery SR, Petrigliano FA, Gamradt SC. Biologic augmentation of rotator cuff repair. *Curr Rev Musculoskelet Med.* 2011;4:221-230.

17. Adams JE, Zobitz ME, Reach JS Jr, et al. Rotator cuff repair using an acellular dermal matrix graft: an in vivo study in a canine model. *Arthroscopy.* 2006;22:700-709.

18. Xu H, Wan H, SAndor M, et al. Host response to human acellular dermal matrix transplantation in a primate model of abdominal wall repair. *Tissue Eng Part A.* 2009;14:2009-2019.

19. Bond JL, Dopirak RM, Higgins J, et al. Arthroscopic replacement of massive, irreparable rotator cuff tears using a Graft-Jacket allograft: technique and preliminary results. *Arthroscopy.* 2008;24:403-409.

20. Burkhead WZ, Schiffern SC, Krishnan SG. Use of a Graft Jacket as an augmentation for massive rotator cuff tears. *Semin Arthroplasty.* 2007;18:11-18.

21. Wong I, Burns J, Snyder S. Arthroscopic GraftJacket repair of rotator cuff tears. *J Shoulder Elbow Surg.* 2010;19:104-109.

22. Barber FA, Burns JP, Deutsch A, Labbe MR, Litchfield RB. A prospective, randomized evaluation of acellular human dermal matrix augmentation for arthroscopic rotator cuff repair. *Arthroscopy.* 2012;28:8-15.

Please see videos on the accompanying website at

www.ArthroscopicTechniques.com

10

Arthroscopic Hill-Sachs Remplissage

Nathan D. Faulkner, MD; Matthew D. Driscoll, MD;
and Mark H. Getelman, MD

INTRODUCTION

A Hill-Sachs lesion (HSL) is an impaction fracture of the posterior superior humeral head that can result from traumatic anterior glenohumeral dislocation. This lesion was first identified by Flower in 1861,[1] but it is named after Hill and Sachs, who were the first to describe the mechanism by which it occurs.[2] HSLs are estimated to occur in up to 67% of first-time anterior glenohumeral dislocations and over 80% of patients with recurrent anterior instability.[3]

Remplissage is a French word meaning "to fill." The concept of filling the humeral head defect with an open transfer of the infraspinatus tendon and its greater tuberosity insertion was originally described by Connolly in 1972.[4] In 2004, Wolf and Pollack developed an arthroscopic, minimally invasive modification of the Connolly procedure that they termed the *Hill-Sachs remplissage*.[5] This technique involves an arthroscopic infraspinatus tenodesis and posterior capsulodesis, which fills the bed of the HSL and effectively renders the HSL extra-articular. As a result, the lesion can no longer engage the anterior inferior glenoid during range of motion (ROM). The posterior capsulodesis also results in decreased anterior translation of the humeral head, further reducing the likelihood of recurrent dislocation.[6]

HSLs vary in size, location, and orientation; therefore, not all HSLs contribute similarly to recurrent anterior glenohumeral instability. Most occur in conjunction with injury to the anterior labrum and glenohumeral ligaments as well as the anterior bony rim of the glenoid. As such, any evaluation of an HSL must also include an evaluation of the other static and dynamic stabilizers of the glenohumeral joint (Table 10-1). Several investigators have identified instability-related bone loss as a particularly strong predictor of recurrence following an isolated soft-tissue arthroscopic Bankart repair.[7-9] Burkhart and De Beer[7] retrospectively reviewed 197 patients who underwent arthroscopic Bankart repair for traumatic anterior glenohumeral instability to identify risk factors for recurrence. They determined that patients with significant bone loss were at a 10 times higher risk for recurrent instability (67% for patients with significant bone loss vs 6.5% for patients with no significant bone loss).[7] Significant bone loss, in this landmark study, was defined for both the glenoid and the Hill-Sachs involvement. Bone loss resulting in a loss of ≥25% of inferior glenoid

Ryu RKN, Angelo RL, Abrams JS, eds. *The Shoulder:*
AANA Advanced Arthroscopic Surgical Techniques (pp 107-121).
© 2016 AANA.

Table 10-1. Static and Dynamic Stabilizers of the Shoulder

STATIC	DYNAMIC
Coracohumeral ligament	Rotator cuff muscles
Glenohumeral ligaments	Biceps
Labrum	Deltoid
Joint contact	
Scapular inclination	
Intra-articular pressure	

diameter was deemed an *inverted-pear*, where the inferior half of the glenoid demonstrates a smaller anterior radius than the superior half. Similarly, an *engaging HSL* was defined as an HSL that becomes oriented parallel with the anterior glenoid in a position of function (abduction and external rotation), thus enabling it to engage or key on the anterior glenoid.[7]

A thorough history and physical exam are essential in the evaluation of patients with glenohumeral instability. It is important to distinguish subluxations from dislocations requiring reduction as well as voluntary vs involuntary instability episodes. The mechanism of injury and number of previous instability events should be determined because the likelihood of glenoid bone loss and HSLs increases in patients who experience multiple dislocations.[3] The patient's age, occupation, and participation in sports are important factors that impact the risk for recurrence, likelihood of associated injuries, and patient expectations following surgery.

A comprehensive physical exam should include evaluation of the cervical spine and brachial plexus along with an assessment for generalized ligamentous laxity. The shoulder exam begins with visual inspection from both the front and back of the patient, carefully evaluating for any atrophy or asymmetry. Passive and active ROM should be assessed, including both the glenohumeral joint and scapulothoracic contributions to shoulder motion. Patients with large HSLs will likely have positive anterior apprehension and apprehension suppression or relocation tests. Apprehension in lesser degrees of abduction and external rotation can indicate significant glenoid and/or humeral head bone loss. The load and shift test assesses glenohumeral translation and is valuable for determining engagement of the HSL as well as integrity of the anterior inferior glenohumeral ligament. Finally, posterior and inferior instability should be assessed with a jerk test and sulcus sign, respectively.

The radiographic work-up for all patients with a history of shoulder instability should include anteroposterior, scapular Y, and axillary lateral views. The Stryker notch view[10] and 45-degree internal rotation anteroposterior view[11] are particularly sensitive for detecting HSLs and should be considered in patients with suspected bone loss. A Bernageau profile view, on the other hand, is helpful for assessing glenoid bone loss and has been shown to correlate highly with computed tomography (CT) scan measurements.[12] The radiographs should be evaluated to determine the alignment of the glenohumeral joint as well as the presence and location of any fractures, bone fragments, glenoid bone loss, and HSLs. Any flattening of the posterior superior humeral head may signify an HSL; however, on occasion, the only sign of an HSL will be a subtle "line of condensation," which represents compression or compaction of the cancellous bone of the humeral head at the base of the lesion.[2]

A CT scan with 3D reconstruction is considered the gold standard for quantifying bony defects of the glenohumeral joint; however, they provide little information regarding the extent of the soft tissue injury. A magnetic resonance imaging (MRI) study with or without intra-articular contrast is superior for evaluating soft-tissue injury including Bankart or anterior labral periosteal sleeve avulsion lesions, superior labral anteroposterior tears, humeral avulsion of the glenohumeral ligaments, reverse humeral avulsion of the glenohumeral ligaments, cartilage lesions, and rotator cuff tears. In addition, an approximation of glenoid bone loss can be made using the sagittal oblique image tangential to the glenoid articular surface. The authors prefer MRI with intra-articular contrast as the primary imaging modality in any patient with suspected shoulder instability. CT scans should be considered if there are any bony defects requiring precise measurement and quantification of the location and size of the lesions. CT scans should include 3D reconstructions with humeral subtraction, which allow for an en fosse view of the glenoid and a more accurate measurement of bone loss. Measurement techniques for MRI are currently being developed and may soon eliminate the need for additional radiation associated with CT scans.

Several methods have been proposed for determining the size and grade of the HSL. Rowe et al developed one of the initial methods in 1984.[13] The Rowe classification grades the HSL as mild (2-cm long x 3-mm deep), moderate (4-cm long x 0.3- to 1-cm deep), or severe (4-cm long x ≥ 1-cm deep) based on intraoperative evaluation.[13] A few years later, Calandra et al proposed a grading scale based on the depth of penetration of the HSL, with grade 1 consisting of a defect in the articular surface down to subchondral bone, grade 2 including the subchondral bone, and grade 3 being a large defect extending deep to the subchondral bone.[14] Flatow and Warner proposed a separate classification system based on percent involvement of the humeral head: < 20% clinically insignificant; 20% to 40% variable significance; and > 40% clinically significant.[15] Other classification systems have been proposed, but none have yet been shown to guide or predict successful surgical treatment.

The concept of a glenoid track (GT), as described by Itoi and colleagues,[16] is likely the best method for determining the significance of an HSL and may be the optimal way to conceptualize the role of remplissage in reducing the risk of recurrent instability. In their initial investigation, Yamamoto et al performed a cadaveric study placing the glenohumeral joint in horizontal extension and maximum external rotation while increasing glenohumeral abduction from 0 to 30 and 60 degrees.[16] With increased abduction, the glenohumeral contact area was noted to shift from inferomedial to superolateral along the posterior aspect of the humeral head, creating a zone of contact called the GT. The GT extended, on average, 18.4 mm medial to the rotator cuff footprint, a distance equivalent to 84% of the inferior glenoid diameter.[16] In a similar study using 3D motion analysis with open MRI, Omori et al determined that the size of the GT represents 83% of the inferior glenoid diameter.[17] The size of the GT is directly affected by the amount of glenoid bone loss, with increasing glenoid bone loss resulting in proportional narrowing of the track. The significance of the HSL, on the other hand, is determined not only by its size, but also its location and orientation in relation to the GT.

These concepts may prove to be particularly useful in developing treatment algorithms for cases of combined glenoid and humeral bone loss. Di Giacomo et al recently described a method for calculating the size of the GT and determining whether an HSL will be "on-track" or "off-track."[18] In cases with glenoid bone loss, the GT is calculated as 83% of the normal inferior glenoid diameter (D) minus the defect width of glenoid bone loss (d) (GT = 0.83D − d; Figure 10-1). The Hill-Sachs interval (HSI), which is the distance from the rotator cuff attachment to the medial margin of the HSL, is calculated as the width of the HSL (HS) plus the width of the bony bridge (BB) between the HSL and the rotator cuff attachment (HSI = HS + BB; Figure 10-2). If the HSI > GT, the HSL is considered off-track and, therefore, likely to engage or lead to recurrent instability. If HSI < GT, the HSL is on-track, or nonengaging (Figure 10-3). These measurements can be made on a preoperative 3D CT with humeral subtraction or intraoperatively using a calibrated probe.[18] The relationship between the HSL and GT helps explain why even a small HSL can contribute to glenohumeral instability if associated with a significant amount of glenoid bone loss. Di Giacomo et al proposed a treatment algorithm based on both the amount of glenoid bone loss and whether the HSL is calculated to be on- or off-track (Table 10-2).[18]

Figure 10-1. Illustration of the glenoid showing how to calculate the GT. GT = 0.83D – d. D, normal inferior glenoid diameter; d, diameter of glenoid bone loss. A2-B2 is the long axis of the glenoid.

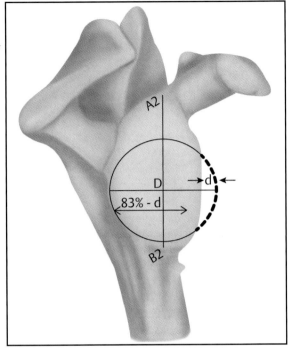

Figure 10-2. Illustration showing how to determine the HSI. HSI = HS + BB. BB, bony bridge between the HSL and the rotator cuff attachment; HS, width of HSL. L1 represents the medial margin of the rotator cuff footprint and L2 represents the medial margin of the HSL.

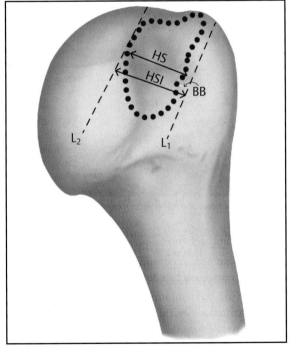

While the relationship of the bony defects is paramount, the tension of the inferior glenohumeral ligament and its influence on the GT must also be considered. Kurokawa et al defined a "true engaging HSL" as either a lesion that engages *after* Bankart repair or a lesion that extends over the GT.[19] They argue that determining engagement of the HSL during dynamic operative assessment *before* Bankart repair could potentially lead to overdiagnosis of an engaging HSL

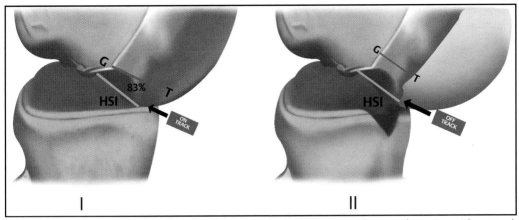

Figure 10-3. Illustration showing the glenohumeral joint in abduction and external rotation with on-track and off-track HSLs. If the HSI < GT, then the HSL is on-track or nonengaging (I). If the HSL extends medial to the medial margin of the GT (ie, HSI > GT), then the HSL is off-track or engaging (II).

Table 10-2. Treatment Algorithm for Anterior Glenohumeral Instability With Associated Glenoid and/or Humeral Head Bone Loss[18]

Group	Glenoid Defect	Hill-Sachs Lesion	Recommended Treatment
1	< 25%	On track	Arthroscopic Bankart repair
2	< 25%	Off track	Arthroscopic Bankart repair + remplissage
3	≥ 25%	On track	Latarjet procedure
4	≥ 25%	Off track	Laterjet procedure +/– humeral-sided procedure (humeral bone graft or remplissage) depending on engagement of HSL after remplissage

because ligamentous insufficiency could permit excessive anterior translation of the humeral head.[19] Indeed, studies that have evaluated the incidence of engaging HSLs following Bankart repair have noted much lower prevalence (7.1% to 7.4%)[19,20] compared to those that used dynamic arthroscopic assessment before Bankart repair (34% to 45%).[21,22]

In addition to the remplissage technique, several other options have been proposed for the treatment of HSLs, including rotational osteotomy, osteoarticular allograft transfer, disimpaction, and partial prosthetic resurfacing. Some authors believe that a Latarjet or other anterior glenoid bone grafting procedure should be the primary treatment for even large HSLs because it increases the length of the glenoid arc, which in most cases will make the HSL on track. Historically, humeral rotational osteotomy was used to retrovert the humeral head relative to the humeral shaft, thereby rotating the HSL posterolaterally and reducing the risk for engagement of the HSL. However, this technique has fallen out of favor due to high complication rates, including nonunion, delayed union, over-rotation, risk of fracture, and post-traumatic arthritis.[23] Osteoarticular allograft transfer to the humeral head defect can restore the anatomy and increase the articular arc, but this requires an open approach and can result in osteonecrosis with graft collapse and hardware complications.[24] Re et al have described a novel technique for disimpacting and grafting the compressed posterior humeral cancellous bone through a transhumeral bone tunnel adjacent to the lesser tuberosity.[25] While they were able to show clinical efficacy in their small series of 4 patients with greater than 1 year follow-up, this technique is relatively new with little biomechanical and clinical evidence to support its widespread use. Finally, partial and complete resurfacing of the humeral head has been described. Partial replacement eliminates the risk of disease transmission and resorption that can occur with allograft, but disadvantages include loss of fixation and eventual glenoid wear. Good results have been reported up to 2 years postoperatively with partial replacements, but current studies are limited to case reports with short-term follow-up.[26] Complete humeral head resurfacing vs total shoulder arthroplasty should be considered for older (>65 years), low-demand patients with lesions involving greater than 40% of the articular surface and/or significant cartilage degeneration.[23]

A recent systematic review of 7 studies (level II to IV) involving a total of 220 patients who underwent combined arthroscopic Bankart repair and remplissage (BRR) with mean follow-up of 26 months showed no clinically significant losses in ROM, 98% satisfaction rate, 5.3% recurrent dislocation/subluxation rate, and 72% return to presymptom activity level.[27] In one of the few studies to directly compare BRR to Bankart repair alone, Franceshi et al reported no difference in postoperative ROM between the 2 groups but a much lower recurrent instability rate in the BRR group (0% vs 12%).[28] Boileau et al evaluated 47 patients, including 9 who had previous instability surgery, and reported a mean deficit of 8 degrees for external rotation of the adducted arm.[6] This slight decrease in ROM did not significantly affect return to sport, including those involving overhead throwing activities.[6] This was also the first study to objectively evaluate healing of the remplissage with CT arthrogram or MRI, and it showed that soft tissues filled >75% of the HSL in most cases.[6] A separate study evaluated healing of the remplissage using MRI and showed that no defects were left unfilled, with 75% to 100% fill with granulation tissue (2/11), fibrous tissue (3/11), or both (6/11).[29]

In a series with one of the longest follow-up periods to date, Wolf and Arianjam published their results of BRR for 45 patients with anterior shoulder instability, significant HSL, and glenoid deficiency up to 25%.[30] Patients were followed for 2 to 10 years (average 58 months). Recurrent instability after traumatic dislocations occurred in only 4.4%, and patients reported high clinical outcome scores. There were no significant losses of ROM in any plane. Except for the traumatic dislocations, there were no reoperations or complications.

The majority of published studies evaluating recurrence rates following arthroscopic BRR, however, fail to precisely report the magnitude of glenoid and humeral bone loss. In the authors' series of 47 cases of combined BRR (submitted for publication), glenoid bone loss averaged 15% of anterior-to-posterior glenoid diameter (range 0% to 34%) and sagittal HSL width averaged 39% of axial humeral head diameter (range 16% to 61%).[31] The authors noted a trend toward higher recurrence rates among patients with >20% glenoid bone loss (21.4% [3/14]) compared to those with <20% glenoid bone loss (6.1% [2/33]) (p=0.059).[31] Thus, in patients with >20% glenoid bone loss, there is certainly a role for collective decision making with the patient in order to select the best surgical treatment for that individual (arthroscopic BRR vs open bone grafting procedure for the glenoid).

INDICATIONS

▶ Recurrent anterior shoulder instability with an HSL and mild glenoid bone loss
▶ Moderate-to-large HSL

Controversial Indications

▶ Associated glenoid bone loss (up to 25%)

PERTINENT PHYSICAL FINDINGS

▶ Anterior apprehension
  ▷ Apprehension in midrange abduction and lesser degrees of external rotation is a predictor of significant bone loss.
▶ Positive apprehension suppression or relocation test
▶ Increased translation with load and shift test
  ▷ During an exam under anesthesia, a clinically significant HSL can often be felt to engage the anterior glenoid with a palpable clunk.

PERTINENT IMAGING

▶ Pre- and postreduction radiographs to include anteroposterior, axillary lateral, and scapular Y views
▶ Internal rotation anteroposterior and Stryker notch views to best evaluate the HSL
▶ Bernageau profile view to evaluate glenoid bone loss
▶ MRI or MR arthrogram
▶ CT with 3D reconstruction and humeral subtraction can be considered

EQUIPMENT

▶ Arthroscope in the anterior superior viewing portal with a 5.5-mm cannula posteriorly and a 7-mm cannula anteriorly in the mid-glenoid portal
▶ Ringed and/or cupped curette
▶ 4.5-mm shaver
▶ Rasp
▶ Suture hooks or penetrating tissue grasper (ie, bird beak)
▶ Triple-loaded 4.5-mm or 5.5-mm suture anchors
▶ Crochet hook or looped grasper
▶ Knot pusher
▶ Suture savers

POSITIONING AND PORTALS

The preferred position is lateral decubitus with a beanbag and axillary roll. Once the patient is positioned appropriately, the arm is placed in 10 to 12 lbs of balanced suspension with a well-padded arm holder with a 3-point shoulder holder set initially at 70 degrees abduction and 10 to 15 degrees of forward flexion. A standard posterolateral portal is initially established, followed by an anterior superior portal (ASP) created high in the rotator interval just behind the long head of the biceps via an outside-in technique. An 18-gauge spinal needle is used to localize the optimal position before making the portal incision (Figure 10-4). Once the diagnosis of a Bankart and HSL is confirmed, a second anterior mid-glenoid (AMG) portal is established again via an

Figure 10-4. Arthroscopic view of an 18-gauge spinal needle being used to accurately determine the location of the ASP directly behind the biceps, high in the rotator interval.

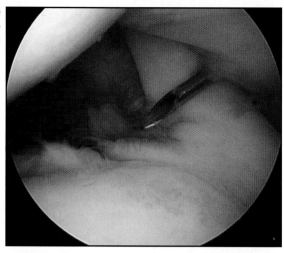

Figure 10-5. Arthroscopic view demonstrating the appropriate spread between the AMG and ASP.

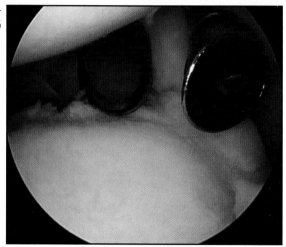

outside-in technique. It is important to determine that the 18-gauge needle can reach all essential areas of the glenoid for subsequent Bankart repair before making the portal. Care should also be taken to ensure that the portals are not too close together (Figure 10-5). The camera is switched to the ASP and the posterior portal becomes a working portal. Some authors advocate centering the posterior portal directly in line with the HSL,[30] but these authors typically make the posterolateral portal in the standard position. The AMG portal is the main working portal for the Bankart repair and is used to shuttle sutures for the remplissage. Both the AMP and standard posterior cannulas should be appropriately sized to accommodate suture shuttling instruments such as the spectrum suture hooks or penetrating graspers depending on the desired technique.

STEP-BY-STEP DESCRIPTION OF THE PROCEDURE

Each case of shoulder instability should begin with a thorough exam under anesthesia with a comparison to the opposite shoulder. ROM should be assessed in all planes, as well as a load shift exam in 90 degrees of abduction and neutral rotation, and then in external rotation to gauge the extent of glenohumeral translation. Posterior instability is assessed and sulcus testing is performed to evaluate for any rotator interval involvement.

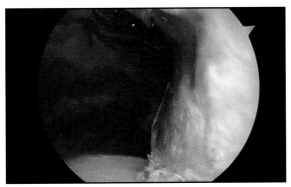

Figure 10-6. Arthroscopic image of a large HSL of a left shoulder viewed from the ASP.

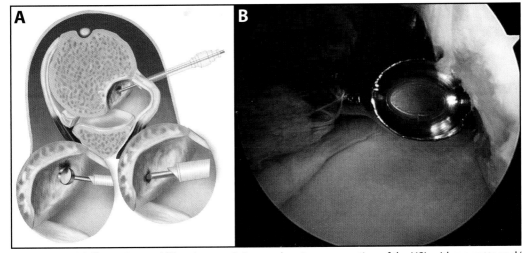

Figure 10-7. (A) Illustration and (B) arthroscopic image showing preparation of the HSL with a curette and/or shaver to create a bleeding bone bed.

After introducing the arthroscope, the authors begin with a standard 15-point diagnostic shoulder exam. The HSL is initially visualized with the arthroscope in the posterior portal. The arm is abducted and externally rotated to evaluate the ability of the HSL to engage the anterior/inferior glenoid. The arthroscope is then switched to the ASP, which is often the best position to evaluate the HSL of the humeral head relative to the glenoid (Figure 10-6). The next step is to fully mobilize the Bankart lesion. After mobilization of the anterior capsuloligamentous complex, the tissue is shifted superiorly and laterally to the anterior glenoid using a grasping clamp to simulate the position of the final labral advancement. The position of the HSL is re-evaluated with the labrum in this reduced position. Typically, the HSL will rotate out of the surgical viewing field once the anterior labrum and ligaments have been mobilized and reduced. This signifies that the HSL will not likely articulate with or engage the anterior/inferior glenoid through the glenoid arc. If, however, the HSL remains visible or approaches the anterior glenoid with humeral rotation, remplissage should be performed.

While timing of the remplissage is controversial, the authors believe that the best time to perform the remplissage is immediately after the completion of the anterior mobilization but before the labral repair because this is when the HSL is easiest to view. With the camera in the ASP, insert a ring curette and/or motorized shaver through the standard posterior portal to create a bleeding bed in the base of the HSL (Figure 10-7). If a shaver or burr is used, care should be taken to remove the smallest amount of bone possible to create a bleeding surface for healing. The posterior capsule should also be lightly abraded with a rasp or burr.

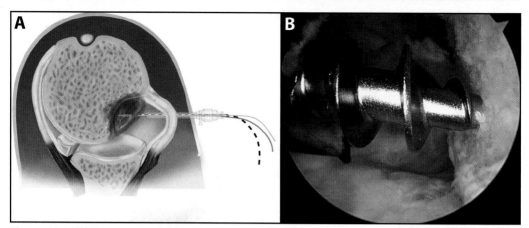

Figure 10-8. (A) Illustration and (B) arthroscopic image demonstrating the ideal inferior anchor position a few millimeters off the articular surface.

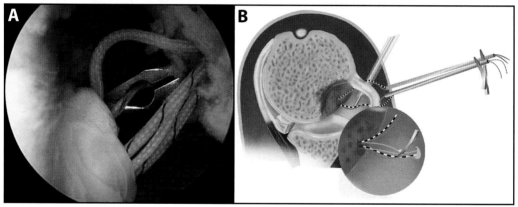

Figure 10-9. (A) Arthroscopic view of a penetrating grasper piercing the posterior capsule to retrieve one of the suture limbs from the anchor. (B) Illustration showing a penetrating grasper via an extra-articular cannula passed through the infraspinatus tendon/capsule laterally with the previously passed sutures stored in suture savers.

Once the base of the HSL is prepared, insert the most inferior anchor first. The authors recommend 4.5- or 5.5-mm triple-loaded suture anchors. The anchor should be close to the articular surface (Figure 10-8). The pilot hole for the anchor is created with a punch. The soft bone in this portion of the humeral head usually obviates the need for a tap. With the anchor seated, the sutures are tensioned to confirm that the anchor is securely fixed in the bone before removing the inserter. All of the sutures are taken outside of the posterior cannula using a switching stick. The posterior cannula is reinserted into the joint, then backed up to just outside of the capsule while visualizing from the ASP. The cannula is directed more laterally toward the infraspinatus tendon but inferior to the anchor. A penetrating tissue grasper pierces the infraspinatus tendon and posterior capsule laterally and enters the joint to retrieve the first limb of the most inferior suture pair (Figure 10-9). The suture is brought out of the posterior cannula and the penetrating grasper is then reinserted 3 to 4 mm away and more medially from the first pass, this time grasping the partner suture of the same color, creating a mattress suture configuration. It is essential to avoid incorporating the more medial capsular structures with the medial stitch. The sutures should be placed more laterally through the capsule and tendon of the infraspinatus to prevent limitation of postoperative ROM (Figure 10-10). A switching stick is inserted. The suture pair is brought

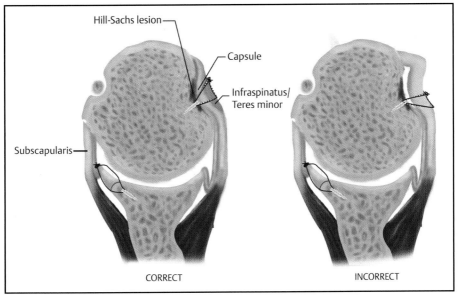

Figure 10-10. Illustration demonstrating correct suture position on the left side with all of the sutures passed through the infraspinatus tendon, whereas the image on the right demonstrates the incorrect position with sutures passed too far medially. This results in an overtensioned posterior capsule, which could significantly limit ROM and humeral rotation.

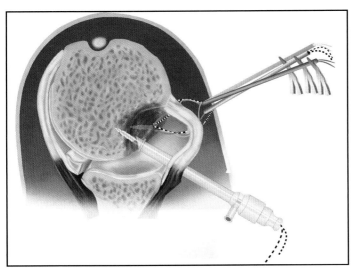

Figure 10-11. Illustration showing insertion of a second triple-loaded suture anchor more superiorly, again just off of the articular surface. The sutures from the more inferior anchor have all been passed and are stored in suture savers outside of the cannula.

outside of the posterior cannula and stored in a suture saver. The posterior cannula is reinserted over the switching stick. The process is repeated, moving more cephalad for each set of sutures until all suture pairs have been passed in a similar mattress fashion. One or 2 triple-loaded anchors are used depending on the size of the lesion (Figure 10-11).

Once all of the sutures are passed, attention is turned to completing the Bankart reconstruction. Tying the remplissage sutures before completing the anterior reconstruction can limit access inferiorly and compromise the repair. Once the Bankart reconstruction is complete, the remplissage sutures can be tied from inferior to superior. The posterior cannula is removed and a looped grasper is used to bring the suture saver into the cannula outside of the shoulder. The cannula is advanced over the suture saver through the deltoid but not through the infraspinatus or capsule.

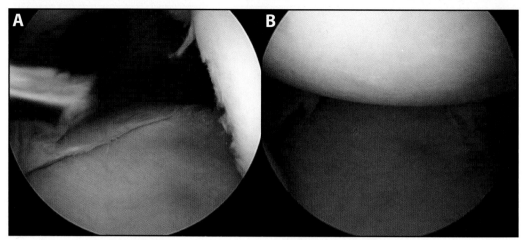

Figure 10-12. (A) Arthroscopic view of the humeral head–glenoid relationship. Note how the HSL is easily visualized and the humeral head is subluxed anteriorly relative to the bare spot on the glenoid. (B) Arthroscopic view after BRR. The HSL is rotated out of view and the head is now well-centered on the glenoid.

The knots are tied in a blind fashion using a sliding locking knot (eg, Seoul Medical Center [SMC] knot) with 3 reversed half-hitches on alternating posts. If preferred, the arthroscope can be placed in the subacromial space to view the knots as they are tied, but the sutures are often obscured by the posterior bursa. If suture savers are used, it is critical to slide the adjacent suture saver back a few millimeters before tying the knot to ensure that part of the adjacent suture saver does not become entrapped in the knot as it is tied.

Finally, the location and position of the humeral head relative to the center of the glenoid should be evaluated. The previously subluxated humeral head should be centered relative to the bare spot on the glenoid (Figure 10-12). (See accompanying video for demonstration.)

POSTOPERATIVE PROTOCOL

Following surgery, patients are immobilized in a neutral rotation sling for 4 weeks. They start immediate elbow, wrist, and hand exercises and are allowed to add gentle pendulums after the initial postoperative visit 1 week after surgery. Supervised physical therapy begins at 4 weeks when patients discontinue the sling. The emphasis is then on restoring ROM and scapular rhythm. Progressive strengthening begins after 3 months and anticipated return to sports and activity is typically at 6 months when full ROM and strength have been restored.

POTENTIAL COMPLICATIONS

Limitation of ROM is the primary concern after remplissage. Cadaveric studies have demonstrated significant limitations in adducted and abducted ROM as well as in horizontal extension ROM. Elkinson et al tested 8 cadaveric specimens following Bankart repair with and without remplissage for HSL involving either 15% or 30% of the humeral head diameter.[32] For both lesion sizes, BRR demonstrated significantly decreased internal-external arc of motion in adduction, but not abduction (15.1 degrees ± 11.1 degrees for the 15% HSL and 14.5 degrees ± 11.3 degrees for the 30% HSL).[32] A follow-up study by Omi et al simulated remplissage for small (50% glenoid width) and large (100% glenoid width) HSLs by placing suture anchors on the articular surface and tying down the infraspinatus at the medial edge of the would-be lesion site.[33] No decrease in ROM was observed for the smaller lesions, but remplissage for the large lesion resulted in significantly decreased adducted and abducted external rotation as well as horizontal extension at all abduction angles. Important limitations of this study are the use of older cadaveric specimens, lesser tuberosity osteotomy to perform the remplissage, and lack of pertinent injury conditions including creation of an HSL.

Despite the cadaveric data and a single case report showing significantly limited postoperative ROM following BRR,[34] the larger clinical series have not shown any clinically significant difference in ROM.[6] Boileau et al reported a mean deficit in external rotation of the adducted arm to be 8 degrees at the time of final follow-up, and 68% of patients were able to return to the same level of sport, including those involving overhead activities.[6] The recent systematic review by Leroux et al, described previously, showed no clinically significant losses in glenohumeral motion after arthroscopic BRR.[27] In order to prevent postoperative stiffness, it is imperative to place the sutures laterally in the tendon. If instead the sutures are passed more medially through the capsule and tendon, an excessive plication of the tissues may result and ROM may be significantly limited.

Other possible complications following remplissage are recurrent instability and degeneration of the infraspinatus tendon and muscle. Recurrent instability rates for BRR range from 0% to 10%,[27] but in one of the few studies by Franceschi et al directly comparing BRR to Bankart alone, remplissage lead to a significant decrease in postoperative instability (0% vs 12%).[28] A follow-up study by Park et al evaluated healing of remplissage with MRI in 11 patients with average follow-up of 18 months and showed the degree of atrophy to be minor (0% to 25%) for all patients studied.[29]

TOP TECHNICAL PEARLS FOR THE PROCEDURE

1. Completely mobilize the anterior capsulolabral structures before the remplissage.

2. Evaluate the location of the HSL and need for remplissage after the anterior capsulolabral structures have been mobilized and reduced with the arthroscope in the ASP.

3. Prepare a bleeding bone bed for the remplissage.

4. Place 1 to 2 anchors, depending on the size of the HSL, adjacent to the intact articular surface.

5. Make sure the sutures pass laterally through the infraspinatus tendon and not through the medial capsular structures to prevent limitation of ROM.

REFERENCES

1. Flower WH. On the pathological changes produced in the shoulder joint by traumatic dislocations, as derived from an examination of all specimens illustrating this injury in the museums of London. *Trans Pathol Soc London.* 1861;12:179-201.

2. Hill HA, Sachs MD. The grooved defect of the humeral head. A frequently unrecognized complication of dislocations of the shoulder joint. *Radiology.* 1940;35:690-700.

3. Spatschil A, Landsiedl F, Anderl W, et al. Posttraumatic anterior-inferior instability of the shoulder: Arthroscopic findings and clinical correlations. *Arch Orthop Trauma Surg.* 2006;12:217-222.

4. Connolly J. Humeral head defects associated with shoulder dislocations. *Instr Course Lect.* 1972;21:42-54.

5. Wolf EM, Pollack ME. Hill-Sachs "remplissage:" an arthroscopic solution for the engaging Hill-Sachs lesion. *Arthroscopy.* 2004;20(Suppl 1):e14-15.

6. Boileau P, Varga P, Pinedo M, Old J, Zumstein M. Anatomical and functional results after arthroscopic Hill-Sachs remplissage. *J Bone Joint Surg Am.* 2012;94:618-626.

7. Burkhart SS, De Beer JF. Traumatic glenohumeral bone defects and their relationship to failure of arthroscopic Bankart repairs: significance of the inverted-pear glenoid and the humeral engaging Hill-Sachs lesion. *Arthroscopy.* 2000;16:677-694.

8. Boileau P, Villalba M, Hery JY, Balg F, Ahrens P, Neyton L. Risk factors for recurrence of shoulder instability after arthroscopic Bankart repair. *J Bone Joint Surg Am.* 2006;88(8):1755-1763.

9. Ahmed I, Ashton F, Robinson CM. Arthroscopic Bankart repair and capsular shift for recurrent anterior shoulder instability: functional outcomes and identification of risk factors for recurrence. *J Bone Joint Surg Am.* 2012;94(14):1308-1315.

10. Rozing PM, de Bakker HM, Obermann WR. Radiographic views in recurrent anterior shoulder dislocation. Comparison of six methods for identification of typical lesions. *Acta Orthop Scand.* 1986;57(4):328-330.

11. Danzig LA, Greenway G, Resnick D. The Hill-Sachs lesion: an experimental study. *Am J Sports Med.* 1980;8(5):328-332.

12. Pansard E, Klouche S, Billot N, et al. Reliability and validity assessment of a glenoid bone loss measurement using the Bernageau profile view in chronic anterior shoulder instability. *J Shoulder Elbow Surg.* 2013;22(9):1193-1198.

13. Rowe CR, Zarins B, Ciullo JV. Recurrent anterior dislocation of the shoulder after surgical repair. *J Bone Joint Surg Am.* 1984;66-A(2):159-168.

14. Calandra JJ, Baker CL, Uribe J. The incidence of Hill-Sachs lesions in initial anterior shoulder dislocations. *Arthroscopy.* 1989;5(4):254-257.

15. Flatow EL, Warner JI. Instability of the shoulder: complex problems and failed repairs. Part I: relevant biomechanics, multidirectional instability, and severe glenoid loss. *Instr Course Lect.* 1998;47:97-112.

16. Yamamoto N, Itoi E, Abe H, et al. Contact between the glenoid and the humeral head in abduction, external rotation, and horizontal extension: a new concept of glenoid track. *J Shoulder Elbow Surg.* 2007;16:649-656.

17. Omori Y, Yamamoto N, Koishi H, et al. Measurement of the glenoid track in vivo, investigated by three-dimensional motion analysis using open MRI. Poster 502 presented at: 57th Annual Meeting of the Orthopedic Research Society; January 13-16, 2011; Long Beach, CA.

18. Di Giacomo G, Itoi E, Burkhart SS. Evolving concept of bipolar bone loss and the Hill-Sachs lesion: from "engaging/non-engaging" lesion to "on-track/off-track" lesion. *Arthroscopy.* 2014;30(1):90-98.

19. Kurokawa D, Yamamoto N, Nagamoto H, et al. The prevalence of a large Hill-Sachs lesion that needs to be treated. *J Shoulder Elbow Surg.* 2013;22:1285-1289.

20. Parke CS, Yoo JH, Cho NS, Rhee YG. Arthroscopic remplissage for humeral defect in anterior shoulder instability: is it needed? Paper presented at: 39th Annual Meeting of Japan Shoulder Society; October 5-6, 2012; Tokyo, Japan.

21. Cho SH, Cho NS, Rhee YG. Preoperative analysis of the Hill-Sachs lesion in anterior shoulder instability: how to predict engagement of the lesion. *Am J Sports Med.* 2011;39:2389-2395.

22. Zhu YM, Lu Y, Zhang J, Shen JW, Jian CY. Arthroscopic Bankart repair combined with remplissage technique for the treatment of anterior shoulder instability with engaging Hill-Sachs lesion: a report of 49 cases with a minimum 2-year follow-up. *Am J Sports Med.* 2011;39:1640-1647.

23. Provencher MT, Frank RM, LeClere LE, et al. The Hill-Sachs lesion: diagnosis, classification, and management. *J Am Acad Orthop Surg.* 2012;20(4):242-252.

24. Miniaci A, Gish MW. Management of anterior glenohumeral instability associated with large Hill-Sachs defects. *Tech Shoulder Elbow Surg.* 2004;5(3):170-175.

25. Re P, Gallo RA, Richmond JC. Transhumeral head plasty for large Hill-Sachs lesions. *Arthroscopy.* 2006;22:798.e1-798.e4.

26. Scalise J, Miniaci A, Iannotti J. Resurfacing arthroplasty of the humerus: indications, surgical technique, and clinical results. *Tech Shoulder Elbow Surg.* 2007;8:152-160.

27. Leroux T, Bhatti A, Khoshbin A, et al. Combined arthroscopic Bankart repair and remplissage for recurrent shoulder instability. *Arthroscopy.* 2013;29(10):1693-1701.

28. Franceshi F, Papalia R, Rizzello G, et al. Remplissage repair – new frontiers in the prevention of recurrent shoulder instability: a 2-year follow-up comparative study. *Am J Sports Med.* 2012;40(11):2462-2469.

29. Park MJ, Garcia G, Malhotra A, Major N, Tjoumakaris FP, Kelly JD IV. The evaluation of arthroscopic remplissage by high-resolution magnetic resonance imaging. *Am J Sports Med.* 2012;40:233-236.

30. Wolf EM, Arianjam A. Hill-Sachs remplissage, an arthroscopic solution for engaging Hill-Sachs lesion: 2- to 10-year follow-up and incidence of recurrence. *J Shoulder Elbow Surg.* 2013;1-7.

31. Driscoll MD, Snyder SJ, Burns JP. Arthroscopic Bankart repair and remplissage in patients with combined humeral and glenoid bone loss. *Arthroscopy.* In press.

32. Elkinson I, Giles JW, Faber KJ, et al. The effect of the remplissage procedure on shoulder stability and range of motion. *J Bone Joint Surg Am.* 2012;94:1003-1012.

33. Omi R, Hooke AW, Zhao KD, et al. The effect of the remplissage procedure on shoulder range of motion: a cadaveric study. *Arthroscopy.* 2014;30(2):178-187.

34. Deutsch AA, Kroll DG. Decreased range of motion following arthroscopic remplissage. *Orthopedics.* 2008;31(5):492.

Please see videos on the accompanying website at

www.ArthroscopicTechniques.com

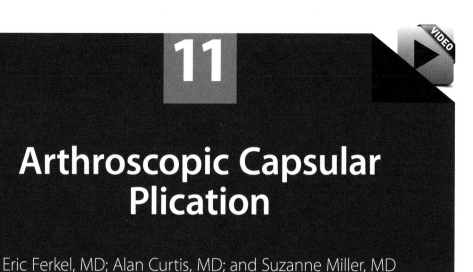

INTRODUCTION

Multidirectional instability (MDI) of the shoulder is a very complex problem to manage, representing anterior and posterior instability with inferior subluxation. The spectrum of MDI can range from chronic to acute, often presenting with variable pathology. MDI was originally described by Neer and Foster in 1980.[1] They introduced an open capsular shift to reduce the volume of the joint and reduce humeral head translation in the anterior, inferior, and posterior planes. The pathology was further classified by Matsen et al into TUBS (Traumatic etiology, Unidirectional instability, Bankart lesion, Surgery required) and AMBRI (Atraumatic: minor trauma, MDI may be present, Bilateral: asymptomatic shoulder is also loose, Rehabilitation is the treatment of choice, Inferior capsular shift is surgery required if conservative measures fail).[2]

The early surgical stabilization procedures used for MDI included the Putti-Platt, Magnuson-Stack, and Bristow; however, these often failed to provide improvement as they typically only addressed unidirectional instability. Over time, standard procedures further evolved to the Neer open capsular shift. These historic open procedures have progressed to arthroscopic options that have shown excellent results. Arthroscopic techniques have evolved from arthroscopic inferior capsular shift using a transglenoid technique[3-5] initially reported on by Duncan and Savoie[5] in 1993, to arthroscopic stabilization with bioabsorbable tacks. The arthroscopic, all-inside technique was described by Wichman and Synder in 1997.[6] Wichman and Snyder employed a rasp to excoriate the capsule and created a "bumper" with the labrum by tightening the loose ligamentous structures. This technique demonstrated improved tensioning of the capsule.

Anatomy and Pathology

In MDI, multiple episodes of instability cause recurrent stretching of the capsule, which eventually leads to the loss of proprioceptive feedback (in the capsule) and resulting disruption of the afferent system.[7] This loss leads to changes in the balance of the shoulder musculature and the force coupling that is responsible for maintaining humeral head centering. The imbalance that results can lead to impingement, periscapular dyskinesis, and rotator cuff pathology, all of which can be pain generators.[8]

Ryu RKN, Angelo RL, Abrams JS, eds. *The Shoulder:*
AANA Advanced Arthroscopic Surgical Techniques (pp 123-131).
© 2016 AANA.

INDICATIONS

- ▶ Traditional nonoperative management of MDI includes the following:
  - ▷ Rehabilitation of the static and dynamic stabilizers to improve and treat the scapulothoracic dyskinesis that has resulted from the instability
  - ▷ Rotator cuff strengthening and scapular stabilizers may also help improve humeral head centering
- ▶ After a patient has failed a well-supervised course of nonoperative management, surgical intervention is typically necessary to help the patient improve further.

Controversial Indications

- ▶ MDI in patients with Ehlers-Danlos syndrome has typically been managed nonsurgically with rehabilitation. Open inferior capsular shift has been used successfully in patients whom have failed nonoperative management.[1] Some authors choose tissue grafting due to failure with soft tissue procedures.

PERTINENT PHYSICAL FINDINGS

The diagnosis of MDI can be complex and difficult to elicit. Combining a thorough history with patient observation can often give a substantial amount of information.

- ▶ Typically, the chief complaint is pain, usually associated with movement, whether from an overhead sport or attempting to lift heavy objects.
- ▶ Check for evidence of hyperextensibility or changes in the skin texture, such as velvety or loose skin, that could suggest hyperlaxity.
  - ▷ A careful history should be obtained to evaluate for different congenital and systemic disorders that could lead to capsular redundancy, such as Ehlers-Danlos, Marfan's, or benign joint hypermobility syndrome, which can be evaluated with the Beighton scoring system.[9]
  - ▷ Signs of generalized laxity include patellar instability, hyperextension of the elbow or knee, and the ability to touch the ground with one's palms while bending forward with the knees fully extended. These varied presentations underscore the need for the physician to define the underlying pathology and distinguish instability from laxity.
- ▶ History of multiple previous subluxating episodes or dislocation events caused by a traumatic or volitional event
  - ▷ Repetitive microtrauma to the labrum due to recurrent subluxation causes loss of chondrolabral restraint and further instability. These changes can lead to capsular stretching, which can present as symptomatic laxity.
- ▶ In addition to testing for multidirectional instability, one should evaluate for anterior and posterior instability as well as perform a thorough neurovascular exam.
- ▶ A sulcus sign is widely considered the gold standard test for evaluating multidirectional instability, although it has been shown to have a high specificity and a low sensitivity.[10]
  - ▷ The sign is observed by pulling axial traction of the patient's arm while the arm is resting on the patient's side.
  - ▷ A positive test will show dimpling, > 2 cm displacement from the acromion, and a palpable "sulcus" under the acromion as the arm is pulled inferiorly.[11] Matsen et al comment that a true positive sulcus test will reproduce the patient's symptoms.[2]

▷ When performing the sulcus test with the shoulder in external rotation, this can be a positive finding for a stretched rotator interval, commonly seen in patients with MDI.

► The load and shift test is performed with the patient supine on the exam table while the physician centers the humeral head by applying an axial force then translates the head.

▷ The exam is graded based on how much the humeral head shifts in relation to the glenoid. A classification of grade 1 occurs when the humeral head can be translated to the glenoid rim, grade 2 occurs when the humeral head can be dislocated and reduced spontaneously, and grade 3 occurs when the head can be dislocated but not reduced spontaneously.

▷ It is important to examine both shoulders for comparison.

► The Gagey hyperabduction test is most useful for evaluating inferior glenohumeral ligament translation. The test was originally described as being performed under anesthesia; however, currently it is most often tested in an upright awake patient while making comparative measurements to the asymptomatic shoulder.[12]

▷ A positive test occurs when the examiner is able to passively abduct the shoulder more than 105 degrees. It has been shown that an asymptomatic patient will typically abduct no more than 90 degrees.

PERTINENT IMAGING

► Although the diagnosis of MDI is typically a clinical determination, it is recommended to obtain standard radiographs at the office visit to evaluate the glenoid for dysplasia or hypoplasia.

► If bone loss is a concern, a computed tomography scan may be useful to help with surgical planning.

► Magnetic resonance imaging (MRI) will be the most useful tool in determining labral injury, the increased capsular volume, and glenohumeral ligament injury.

► Some surgeons prefer for this to be done with MR arthrography (MRA); however, the authors typically do not use MRA as it can be quite painful for the patient and often does not offer significant improvement in diagnosis from high-resolution MRI. Furthermore, in MDI, the pathology is often not capsulolabral detachment but capsular laxity.

EQUIPMENT

► Small glenoid anchors single- and double-loaded

► Cannulas, small 5.0 mm and large 7.5 mm

► Suture passing device

POSITIONING AND PORTALS

To proceed with this surgery, the authors prefer to place the patient in the lateral decubitus position, which can be accomplished with either a beanbag or a pegboard. After positioning the patient, the arm is hung using the arm holder. The surgery can also be performed in the beach chair position if preferred by the surgeon.

Figure 11-1. The double-loaded suture anchors in place at the most inferior point of attachment. The anchor is critical to ensure the IGHL is properly re-tensioned.

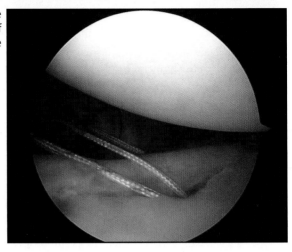

STEP-BY-STEP DESCRIPTION OF THE PROCEDURE

▶ The patient is examined in the supine position by performing the load and shift test while the patient is anesthetized to confirm the diagnosis. The authors recommend examining the contralateral shoulder to get an idea of the baseline to return the injured shoulder to.

▶ Patient is then placed in the lateral decubitus position using an axillary roll, ensuring all bony prominences are well padded and the peroneal nerve is free. Placing the patient in the lateral position will allow excellent access to the anterior, posterior, and inferior aspects of the glenohumeral joint, where the majority of the attention will be during the surgery.

▶ After the arm is prepped and draped and then hung with the preferred device by the surgeon, approximately 5 to 7 lbs of traction are used to suspend the arm. It is important to not overuse traction as this can cause neurologic complications.

▶ Create the posterior portal, which should be slightly more lateral than usual to allow for better angulation in the case that a posterior anchor will need to be placed.

▶ Complete a thorough inspection of the glenohumeral joint, with careful evaluation of the biceps anchor; the interval; and the anterior, inferior, and posterior capsule, documenting the appearance and laxity of the ligamentous structures.

▶ Placing the arthroscope in the anterior portal and viewing posteriorly is necessary for a complete evaluation and for the treatment of posterior pathology.

▶ Evaluate the anterior and posterior labrum and glenoid rim to assess bony loss and injury.

▶ Begin by repairing any displaced labral pathology by using an anchor to create a base to which the capsule can be plicated to. This is important to balance the joint and decrease the overall volume.

▶ Repair the labrum with double-loaded suture anchors at the most inferior point of attachment. This is the most critical spot to shift the displaced capsulolabral complex up to the glenoid and ensure that the IGHL is properly re-tensioned (Figure 11-1).

▶ Create an anteroinferior portal just above the subscapularis to assist in getting the proper angle for anchor placement (Figure 11-2).

▶ Simple or horizontal mattress suture configuration can be used and is helpful to keep the knots away from the glenohumeral joint to avoid symptoms of clicking and catching postoperatively.

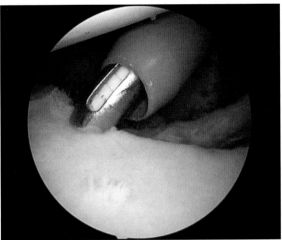

Figure 11-2. Portal placement above the subscapularis is essential for the correct angle of anchor placement.

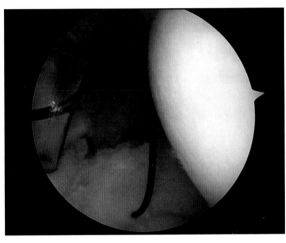

Figure 11-3. Placement of the PDS through the capsule and labrum to close the capsular-ligamentous complex.

▶ More superiorly, the authors typically use small single-loaded anchors as necessary. Once this is accomplished, the remaining capsular laxity is then addressed with pinch-tuck suture placement utilizing an absorbable PDS (polydioxanone) suture.

▶ To perform capsular plication, use the pinch-tuck technique to place sutures to decrease capsular volume

▶ If there is no labral pathology or after labral repair, start at the IGHL region approximately 1 cm off the edge of the intact labrum. Pierce the capsule using a suture-passing device.

▶ Come up through the capsule and then deliver the tip of the suture passer through the intact labrum, creating a fold of tissue, which will then be tied into the final position (Figure 11-3).

▶ If the labral complex appears intact but is of poor quality (eg, Kim lesion), the authors recommend augmenting the labrum-plication repair utilizing a 1.5-mm single-loaded all-suture anchor at the labral-cartilage interface.

▶ Once the anchor is placed, perform a routine pinch-tuck technique, delivering the suture-passing device through the labrum and then shuttling the suture from the anchor around (under) the labrum and capsular fold, then tie it into position (Figures 11-4 through 11-6).

▶ In this manner, the authors both plicate the capsule and repair any splits or weak points in the labrum.

Figure 11-4. After anchor placement, the stitch is passed through the capsule with a PDS suture, using the braided suture as a shuttle, to help perform the labral repair.

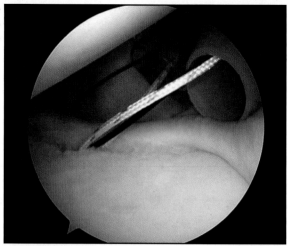

Figure 11-5. Use the knot pusher to help cinch the knot down creating the labral bumper.

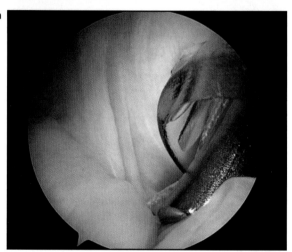

Figure 11-6. The final labral repair.

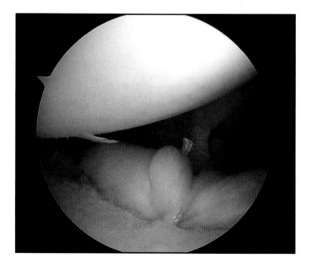

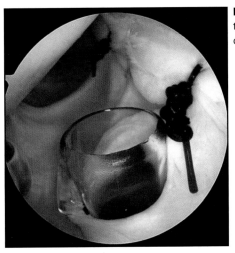

Figure 11-7. The use of PDS suture for the pinch-tuck technique to help assist in capsular tensioning, balancing of the joint, as well as to decrease the capsular volume.

▶ After completing the dominant instability pattern, attention should then be turned to balancing the capsule out by placing 2 or 3 pinch-tuck sutures on the other side of the joint, if necessary (Figure 11-7).

▶ In patients who have significant evidence of interval insufficiency and a positive sulcus sign that is not changed by external rotation, the authors will usually close the interval with 1 or 2 PDS sutures to augment the overall repair.

POSTOPERATIVE PROTOCOL

Protect the patient in an abduction pillow brace for 4 to 6 weeks, then instruct the patient to start performing active range of motion exercises on his or her own for 3 weeks. Physical therapy can be started at 8 weeks; at this time, formal physical therapy is begun where the patient works on active and active-assisted range of motion. However, the authors do not allow strict passive range of motion. In the third month, isometrics and scapular work begins. Full strengthening progresses in fourth month. It is typically 6 months before the patient is allowed to participate in contact sports.

POTENTIAL COMPLICATIONS

The posterior branch of the axillary nerve is at risk when placing the posteroinferior stitch and has shown to be injured in thermal shrinkage or capsular plication. This nerve divides into the superolateral brachial cutaneous branch and the nerve to the teres minor. Recent studies have shown that the posterior branch is 10 mm from the inferior aspect of the glenoid rim at the 6 o'clock position, while the nerve to teres minor was found to be located 12.4 to 18 mm from the inferior part of the glenoid rim in the 6 o'clock position with the patient in the standard lateral decubitus position. This study demonstrated that the nerve is on average 2.5 mm deep to the capsule.[13] A recent study described a rate of 0.2% to 3% complications that lead to neurological symptoms after arthroscopic shoulder surgery.[14] Thorough knowledge of the relationship of the axillary nerve to the glenohumeral joint is important in preventing injury during surgery.

TOP TECHNICAL PEARLS FOR THE PROCEDURE

1. The authors recommend that the surgeon not start at the most inferior portion of the capsule. Starting at the attachment of the IGHL complex creates a more inferior fold.

2. When the surgeon does go inferior to that first stitch, it is easier to work safely in that region because the created fold keeps him or her away from the branches of the axillary nerve, which could be at risk in this region.

3. Typically, the authors use 4 plication sutures for the capsular plication of dominant direction instability. Use 2 plication sutures for balancing the opposite capsular structures. Properly placed plication sutures have a significant effect on capsular volume. The use of 2 sutures in the front and 2 in the back in 5-mm bites has been shown to reduce capsular volume by 33% and allows for the surgeon to have direct control over the amount of capsular volume reduction.[15]

4. Utilize the 1.5-mm all-suture anchors to augment the labrum-capsular plication if there is any doubt about the quality of the labral tissue. A ball tip rasp is useful to roughen the capsular tissue prior to putting the plication sutures in order to stimulate healing.

5. In patients who have significant evidence of interval insufficiency and a positive sulcus sign that is not changed by external rotation, the authors will usually close the interval with 1 or 2 PDS sutures to augment the overall repair.

REFERENCES

1. Neer CS 2nd, Foster CR. Inferior capsular shift for involuntary inferior and multidirectional instability of the shoulder. A preliminary report. *J Bone Joint Surg Am*. 1980;62(6):897-908.
2. Matsen FA, Thomas SC, Rockwood CA. Anterior glenohumeral instability. In: Rockwood CA, Matsen FA, eds. *The Shoulder*. Philadelphia, PA: WB Saunders; 1994.
3. Pagnani MJ, Warren RF, Altchek DW, Wickiewicz TL, Anderson AF. Arthroscopic shoulder stabilization using transglenoid sutures. A four-year minimum followup. *Am J Sports Med*. 1996;24(4):459-467.
4. Savoie FH III, Miller CD, Field LD. Arthroscopic reconstruction of traumatic anterior instability of the shoulder: the Caspari technique. *Arthroscopy*. 1997;13(2):201-209.
5. Duncan R, Savoie FH III. Arthroscopic inferior capsular shift for multidirectional instability of the shoulder: a preliminary report. *Arthroscopy*. 1993;9(1):24-27.
6. Wichman MT, Snyder SJ. Arthroscopic capsular plication for multidirectional instability of the shoulder. *Oper Tech Sports Med*. 1997;5(4):238-243.
7. Ren H, Bicknell RT. From the unstable painful shoulder to multidirectional instability in the young athlete. *Clin Sports Med*. 2013;32(4):815-823.
8. Gerber C, Nyffeler RW. Classification of glenohumeral joint instability. *Clin Orthop Relat Res*. 2002;(400):65-76.
9. Beighton P, Horan F. Orthopaedic aspects of the Ehlers-Danlos syndrome. *J Bone Joint Surg Br*. 1969;51(3):444-453.
10. Walton JT, A J; Murrell, G AC. The Predictive Value of Clinical Tests for Shoulder Instability. Paper presented at: 47th Annual Meeting, Orthopaedic Research Society; February 25 - 28, 2001; San Francisco, California.
11. Warner JJ, Deng XH, Warren RF, Torzilli PA. Static capsuloligamentous restraints to superior-inferior translation of the glenohumeral joint. *Am J Sports Med*. 1992;20(6):675-685.
12. Gagey OJ, Gagey N. The hyperabduction test. *J Bone Joint Surg Br*. 2001;83(1):69-74.

13. Ball CM, Steger T, Galatz LM, Yamaguchi K. The posterior branch of the axillary nerve: an anatomic study. *J Bone Joint Surg Am.* 2003;85-A(8):1497-1501.

14. Carofino BC, Brogan DM, Kircher MF, et al. Iatrogenic nerve injuries during shoulder surgery. *J Bone Joint Surg Am.* 2013;95(18):1667-1674.

15. Flanigan DC, Forsythe T, Orwin J, Kaplan L. Volume analysis of arthroscopic capsular shift. *Arthroscopy.* 2006;22(5):528-533.

Please see videos on the accompanying website at

www.ArthroscopicTechniques.com

12

Arthroscopic Linked Double-Row Rotator Cuff Repair

Stephen S. Burkhart, MD and Patrick J. Denard, MD

INTRODUCTION

Rotator cuff repair has undergone dramatic advancements in recent years, progressing from an extensile open repair to an arthroscopic repair that can be performed in a minimally invasive fashion, maximizing restoration of anatomy. Initially, arthroscopic rotator cuff repair (ARCR) was performed with a single row of medial anchors. In an effort to improve footprint restoration and biomechanical strength, repairs transitioned from a nonlinked double-row repair to a suture-bridging double-row repair.

Biomechanically, the goal of a rotator cuff repair is to achieve high initial fixation strength, minimize gap formation, and maximize footprint contact area. In other words, while biology plays an important role in rotator cuff tendon healing, these biomechanical factors must be optimized by the surgeon at time 0 to provide the best chance for tendon healing.

The traditional double-row repair consisted of independent rows of medial and lateral anchors in which the medial sutures were placed in a mattress configuration and the lateral sutures were placed as simple sutures.[1] This repair improved footprint restoration[2] and fixation strength compared to single-row repairs.[3,4] The advancement of knotless suture anchors not only simplified the technical demand of ARCR but, more importantly, allowed the creation of suture-bridging constructs whereby the medial and lateral rows are linked. Suture-bridging repairs have improved footprint contact area and pressure as well as ultimate load to failure compared to traditional double-row repairs.[5,6] Moreover, because the medial and lateral rows of the suture-bridging double-row repair are linked, the construct exhibits self-reinforcing properties much like a Chinese finger trap (Figure 12-1).[7]

While there has been some debate in the literature regarding clinical outcomes after single-row repair versus double-row repair, several key factors should be considered and are briefly discussed here. (A more extensive review is available in the Burkhart and Cole article.[8]) The initial studies reported on the short-term functional outcome of single-row repairs compared to a traditional, nonlinked double-row repair.[9-11] With patient cohorts between 40 and 80 patients, these studies were underpowered and unable to detect differences between the 2 groups. A meta-analysis,

Ryu RKN, Angelo RL, Abrams JS, eds. *The Shoulder:*
AANA Advanced Arthroscopic Surgical Techniques (pp 133-145).
© 2016 AANA.

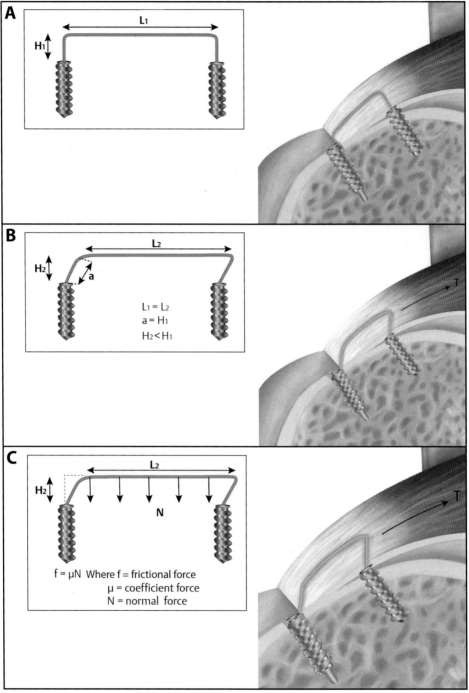

Figure 12-1. Schematic of self-reinforcing suture-bridge technique. (A) Linked double-row construct before loading. Inset: Free-body diagram of the construct. H_1, thickness of rotator cuff before loading; L_1, length of tendon beneath suture. (B) Loading of the linked double-row construct results in compression of the rotator cuff footprint. Inset: Free-body diagram of the construct. H_2, thickness of compressed rotator cuff under tensile load; L_2, length of tendon beneath suture; a, length of suture between tendon edge and lateral anchor; T, tensile loading force. (C) Up-close view of the linked double-row construct after loading. Inset: Free-body diagram showing normal force (N) distribution resulting from elastic deformation of tendon beneath the suture. The frictional force (f) increases as the normal force (N) increases under load. *(continued)*

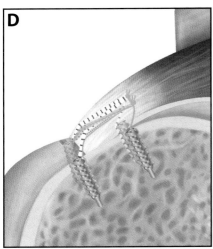

Figure 12-1 (continued). Schematic of self-reinforcing suture-bridge technique. (D) Linked double-row construct with 2 medial anchors linked to 2 lateral anchors provides maximal footprint compression under loading. Additionally, a medial double-mattress stitch in this case provides a seal to joint fluid. (Adapted from Burkhart SS, Lo IK, Brady PC, Denard PJ. *The Cowboy's Companion: A Trail Guide for the Arthroscopic Shoulder Surgeon.* Philadelphia, PA: Lippincott, Williams, & Wilkins, 2012.)

however, has revealed that healing rates are improved with double-row repairs. Duquin et al reviewed 23 articles with a total of 1252 rotator cuff repairs.[12] In their analysis of the pooled data, the recurrence rate for tears < 3 cm was 19% following single-row repair compared to only 7% following double-row repair. For tears larger than 3 cm, the re-tear rate increased to 45% following single-row repair vs 26% following double-row repair. These improved healing rates are important given that a healed rotator cuff repair is associated with a superior functional outcome at mid- and long-term follow-up.[13,14] Moreover, in addition to the short-term results (1 to 2 years) of the aforementioned studies, long-term follow-up has demonstrated that the functional outcome is also superior following a double-row compared to a single-row repair. Denard et al, for example, demonstrated that a traditional double-row repair of a massive tear was 4.9 times more likely to lead to a good or excellent functional outcome compared to a single-row repair at a mean of 99 months following repair.[15]

Excellent outcomes of suture-bridging double-row repairs have also recently been reported in several clinical studies. Frank et al reported an 88% rate of healing in 25 rotator cuff tears repaired with a suture-bridging construct.[16] Toussaint et al reported on 154 repairs and observed a 92% rate of healing in small tears as well as an impressive 84% rate of healing among massive tears.[17] Other studies have demonstrated similarly high rates of healing.[18-21] Based on these improved healing rates, the authors believe that a suture-bridging double-row repair is the current standard of care for rotator cuff repair.[22]

INDICATIONS

- ▶ Full-thickness rotator cuff tears
- ▶ Adequate tendon length
- ▶ Adequate tendon mobility (ie, the lateral tendon edge can reach to within 3 to 4 mm of the lateral edge of the greater tuberosity)

Controversial Indications

- ▶ Partial-thickness rotator cuff tears
- ▶ Small full-thickness rotator cuff tears (ie, 1-cm tears)

PERTINENT PHYSICAL FINDINGS

► Weakness in abduction

► Weakness in external rotation

► Positive impingement signs

PERTINENT IMAGING

► The authors routinely obtain 5 views of the shoulder: anteroposterior views in internal and external rotation, axillary view, outlet view, and 30-degree caudal-tilt view

► Magnetic resonance imaging (MRI) without contrast

► Computed tomography scan with intraarticular contrast in patients whom cannot have an MRI

EQUIPMENT

Much of the work can be performed with a standard 30-degree arthroscope. To improve visualization, particularly for concomitant subscapularis repair, biceps tenodesis, and placement of lateral row anchors, it is also very valuable to have a 70-degree arthroscope available. An arthroscopic pump beginning at 60 mm Hg is utilized to improve visualization. Dedicated outflow is avoided in order to decrease turbulence since this only hinders visualization. One or two 8.25-mm threaded clear cannulas are used for the working portals. The majority of suture passage is performed with a self-retrieving antegrade suture passer (Scorpion FastPass [Arthrex, Inc]), although a retrograde device (Penetrator [Arthrex]) is often useful for suture passage through the posterior aspect of the rotator cuff.

POSITIONING AND PORTALS

While the authors' preference is to perform all rotator cuff repairs in the lateral decubitus position, the beach chair orientation is a practical position for the patient as well. A towel is placed in the contralateral axilla and pillows are placed beneath the contralateral leg as well as between the legs. The operative shoulder is slightly reclined (20 degrees) toward the surgeon and the patient's position is secured with a beanbag and reinforced with tape. A warming blanket is draped over the torso. The arm is placed in 20 degrees of flexion and 20 to 30 degrees of abduction with 5 to 10 lbs of balanced suspension applied (Star Sleeve Traction System [Arthrex]). Alternatively, an articulated arm holder (SPIDER [Smith & Nephew]) is useful if a dedicated assistant to manipulate the arm is not available.

Portal placement is critical to provide an optimal angle of approach to the target tissues, and for that reason, with the exception of the initial posterior portal, an 18-gauge spinal needle is used to precisely establish all portals in an outside-in fashion. Posterior and lateral subacromial portals are used in all cases. An anterior portal can be used for portions of the diagnostic arthroscopy. An anterosuperolateral portal is also required for biceps tenodesis and can replace the anterior portal for diagnostic purposes. Accessory portals for anchor placement or suture passage should be employed if the standard portals (combined with manipulation of the arm) do not afford a proper angle of approach. For instance, the authors typically place anchors through small percutaneous incisions just lateral to the acromion to achieve the proper "deadman" angle for the suture anchors.

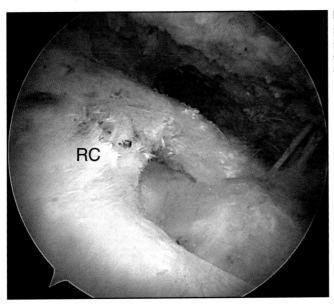

Figure 12-2. Right shoulder posterior subacromial viewing portal demonstrates a crescent-shaped rotator cuff tear amenable to a double-row rotator cuff repair. RC, rotator cuff.

The common portals are as follows:

▶ Posterior portal: The authors establish a posterior portal by palpating the soft spot of the glenohumeral joint and enter the joint at or just below the equator of the humeral head. The exact position varies from patient to patient but is approximately 4 cm inferior and 4 cm medial to the posterolateral corner of the acromion. This portal entry is used for the initial glenohumeral arthroscopy and working in the subacromial space.

▶ Anterior portal: This is established using an outside-in technique just superior to the lateral half of the subscapularis tendon for use during diagnostic glenohumeral arthroscopy.

▶ Lateral subacromial portal: Entry is approximately 4 cm lateral to the lateral aspect of the acromion, in line with the posterior border of the clavicle. Ensure that the portal is parallel to the undersurface of the acromion. This portal serves for viewing and working in the subacromial space.

▶ Anterosuperolateral portal: This portal is useful for a subscapularis repair or biceps tenodesis. It is established through the rotator interval just anterior to the supraspinatus tendon and directly above the long head of the biceps. The point of entry is approximately 1 to 2 cm lateral to the anterolateral corner of the acromion. Placement should be parallel to the subscapularis tendon and permit a 5- to 10-degree angle of approach to the lesser tuberosity.

STEP-BY-STEP DESCRIPTION OF THE PROCEDURE

When sufficient tendon mobility is present, the authors perform a suture-bridging repair of medium-sized crescent tears. When inadequate tendon mobility or length is present to permit a reasonably tension-free repair, the authors do not do a footprint reconstruction. When the quality of the tissue is good, the authors use a knotless SpeedBridge technique (Arthrex) with FiberTape (Arthrex) and 2 rows of BioComposite SwiveLock C suture anchors (Arthrex). For fair tissue, the authors utilize a SpeedBridge repair augmented with a medial double mattress suture (double-pulley technique[23]) since medial mattress sutures enhance the fixation of a knotless repair (Figure 12-2).[24] If the tissue quality is poor, additional suture passes through the tendon strengthen the construct (SutureBridge [Arthrex]). The authors describe their technique for a SpeedBridge repair

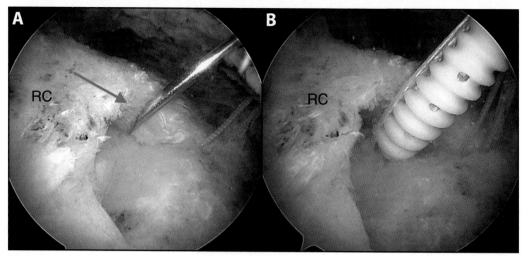

Figure 12-3. Right shoulder posterior subacromial viewing portal. (A) A spinal needle (blue arrow) is used as a guide to determine an adequate angle of approach for an anteromedial anchor. (B) Placement of an anteromedial anchor. A posteromedial anchor will subsequently be placed. RC, rotator cuff.

with a medial double-pulley. The steps for a SutureBridge repair are essentially the same, with the exception that more suture passes are performed medially and all sutures are tied before linking the sutures to the lateral row.

Prepare the Soft Tissues and Bone Bed

Following a diagnostic arthroscopy and completion of intra-articular and/or subscapularis work, the soft tissues and greater tuberosity bone bed are prepared. A bursectomy is completed and allows the surgeon to see the entire margin of the cuff tear. Any bursal leaders that attach to the internal deltoid fascia are debrided so that the tendon edge is clearly visible. The tear pattern is then assessed with a tissue grasper.

Soft tissue is removed from the greater tuberosity with an electrocautery device and a high-speed burr is used to lightly "dust off the charcoal." The greatest blood supply for rotator cuff healing enters from the bone.[25] Although a potential concern, it has been shown that the blood flow to the tendon is preserved with a suture-bridging repair.[26] Cannulated, side-vented suture anchors enhance the amount of blood and bone marrow products that reach the tendon-bone interface.

Medial Anchor Placement

A spinal needle identifies the proper approach from the lateral acromial boarder to the medial aspect of the footprint. A punch is then inserted via a percutaneous incision and used to create a bone socket for a SwiveLock C suture anchor. The bone socket is located just lateral to the articular margin and approximately 5 mm posterior to the bicipital groove (Figure 12-3). A SwiveLock anchor preloaded with FiberTape suture is placed through the same percutaneous portal used for punch insertion. Once the driver tip is fully inserted into the prepared bone hole, the screw is delivered. The insertion sheath is backed off to confirm that the top of the anchor is seated at or just below the bone surface. A posteromedial anchor is then inserted in the same fashion.

Suture Passage

It is important to restore the normal length-tension relationship of the tendon. The location of medial suture placement is critical and will determine the medial-to-lateral tension. Placing the

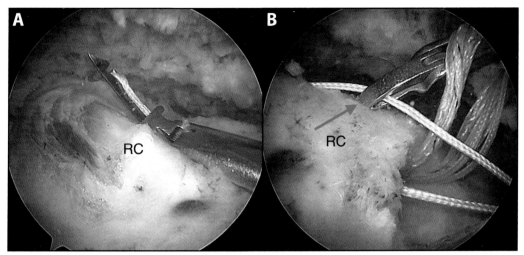

Figure 12-4. Right shoulder posterior subacromial viewing portal. (A) An antegrade suture passer is used to pass a FiberLink suture through the rotator cuff approximately 3 mm lateral to the musculotendinous junction. (B) The nonlooped end of the suture (blue arrow) is retrieved out of the same portal used for anchor placement. RC, rotator cuff. *(continued)*

sutures too far medially will result in overtensioning of the repair. The authors believe that such medial placement is in large part responsible for the reports of medial tendon failure following double-row repair. Conversely, if the medial sutures are placed too far laterally in the tendon, it will be undertensioned and the lateral tendon edge will not cover the footprint.

A grasper may be used to reduce the tendon so that the surgeon can identify the ideal location for placement of the medial sutures, usually 2 to 3 mm lateral to the musculotendinous junction. The ability to view this junction is afforded by the complete bursectomy. Once the medial-to-lateral location is determined, the anterior-to-posterior suture placement is evenly spaced relative to the anchor.

For the SpeedBridge repair, all sutures from a medial anchor are passed through the rotator cuff first. The FiberTape sutures can simply be passed through the rotator cuff with an antegrade suture passer (Scorpion) and retrieved. A FiberTape suture normally tapers to #2 FiberWire. In the SutureBridge kit, the 2 ends of the FiberWire are delivered together so that both FiberTape sutures limbs can be passed through the rotator cuff in a single pass. However, in most cases, the authors prefer to also pass the eyelet safety sutures through the same location so that a medial double-pulley repair can also be performed. This step is accomplished with a FiberLink suture, which is used to shuttle the FiberTape and the FiberWire eyelet sutures through the rotator cuff. FiberLink is a #2 FiberWire suture that has a closed loop on one end. The free nonlooped end of the FiberLink suture is loaded onto a Scorpion, inserted through a lateral working portal, and passed through the rotator cuff as previously described. The free end of the FiberLink is retrieved out of an anterior portal or the percutaneous portal used for anchor placement, while the looped end is held outside of the lateral portal. The FiberTape and FiberWire sutures from the antero-medial anchor are then retrieved out of the lateral portal and threaded through the looped end of the FiberLink. Finally, by pulling the free end the FiberLink, these sutures are shuttled through the rotator cuff at a single site. Alternating tension on the sutures limbs is used to confirm that slack is removed and that all of the suture has been shuttled through the rotator cuff. This step is repeated for the sutures from the posteromedial anchor (Figure 12-4).

Prior to obtaining lateral fixation, medial mattress stitches are tied with a double-pulley technique using the #2 FiberWire safety eyelet sutures from the SwiveLock anchors. This medial mattress stitch provides a medial seal between the glenohumeral joint and the rotator cuff and provides independent medial row fixation. A FiberWire suture limb is retrieved from both the anteromedial

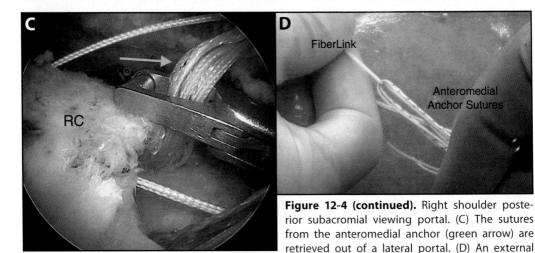

Figure 12-4 (continued). Right shoulder posterior subacromial viewing portal. (C) The sutures from the anteromedial anchor (green arrow) are retrieved out of a lateral portal. (D) An external view demonstrates how the sutures are passed through the loop end of the FiberLink and then turned back on themselves so that the sutures can be shuttled through the rotator cuff. The process is then repeated for the posteromedial sutures. RC, rotator cuff.

anchor and posteromedial anchor. Extracorporeally, a 6-throw surgeon's knot is tied over an instrument. The suture limbs beneath the knot are tensioned to ensure that the knot does not slide. The suture limbs above the knot are then cut. The knot is delivered into the subacromial space and seated onto the rotator cuff by pulling on the opposite ends of the sutures. Then, the opposite ends of the suture limbs are retrieved and the double mattress stitch is completed by tying a static knot in the subacromial space with a Surgeon's Sixth Finger Knot Pusher (Arthrex). The second knot must be tied as a static knot since sliding cannot occur through the anchor eyelet once the first knot has been tied. Knot security and loop security are optimized by tying a 6-throw surgeon's knot in which the fourth and sixth throws are flipped (optimizing knot security), and by tying the knot with a Surgeon's Sixth Finger Knot Pusher to optimize loop security (Figure 12-5).[27]

Reinforce the Rotator Cable

In 1993, the senior author (SSB) described the cable-crescent complex of the rotator cuff.[28] The posterior cable attachment corresponds to the attachment of the posterior infraspinatus. The anterior cable attachment bifurcates around the top of the bicipital groove with part of the anterior cable attachment corresponding to the anterior attachment of the supraspinatus and the other component corresponding to the upper attachment of the subscapularis. As long as the rotator cable attachments are intact, the cuff muscles can distribute the load along the cable that gets transferred to bone at the cable attachments. In this way, a torn rotator cuff can still function by load transmission through a construct that is analogous to a suspension bridge.

The authors strongly believe in reinforcing the rotator cable attachments during ARCR. Additionally, a standard suture-bridging repair (2 medial anchors and 2 lateral anchors) of a crescent tear will frequently leave "dog ears" at the anterior and posterior margins of the repair. The authors like to place cinch-loop sutures at or near the rotator cable attachments. In addition to reducing the dog ears, these cinch-loops reinforce the repair of the cable and thereby strengthen the most biomechanically important parts of the cuff.

Once the medial sutures have been placed, the anterior and posterior margins of the tear are assessed for the potential for dog ears following lateral row fixation. If this is anticipated, FiberLink sutures can be used to create cinch-loops at the apex of each dog ear. To place a cinch-loop, the free end of the suture is loaded onto a Scorpion and passed through the rotator cuff.

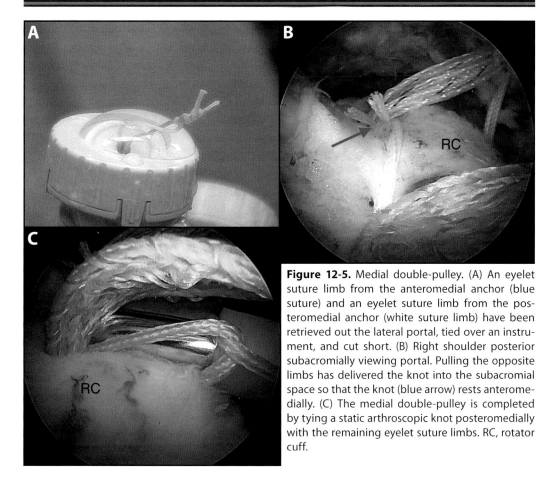

Figure 12-5. Medial double-pulley. (A) An eyelet suture limb from the anteromedial anchor (blue suture) and an eyelet suture limb from the posteromedial anchor (white suture limb) have been retrieved out the lateral portal, tied over an instrument, and cut short. (B) Right shoulder posterior subacromially viewing portal. Pulling the opposite limbs has delivered the knot into the subacromial space so that the knot (blue arrow) rests anteromedially. (C) The medial double-pulley is completed by tying a static arthroscopic knot posteromedially with the remaining eyelet suture limbs. RC, rotator cuff.

Then, the free end is retrieved and threaded through the looped end of the suture. Tensioning the free end delivers the loop down to the rotator cuff, creating a cinch-loop stitch (Figure 12-6). Note that for ease of placement, the authors typically pass these sutures prior to tying the medial double-pulley sutures.

Linked Lateral Fixation

To complete the repair, the FiberTape limbs are crisscrossed and secured laterally with 2 additional SwiveLock anchors. A FiberTape suture limb from the anteromedial anchor, a FiberTape suture limb from the posteromedial anchor, and the posterior dog ear reduction suture are retrieved out of a lateral portal. While maintaining tension on the suture limbs, the lateral cannula is used to determine the appropriate position for a posterolateral anchor. Abduction of the arm will facilitate visualization laterally and rotation of the arm is used to achieve the desired position of insertion that will restore the anatomy. It is sometimes necessary to clear the lateral gutter of soft tissue once again in order to optimize visualization prior to retrieving the sutures. Finally, a 70-degree arthroscope is frequently useful to see into the lateral gutter more clearly. A punch is inserted to create a bone socket. Extracorporeally, the FiberTape sutures are fed through the eyelet of the SwiveLock C anchor. The surgeon maintains visualization and holds the anchor while an assistant holds the cannula firmly in place and removes the punch. This ensures that the position of the bone socket is kept in view and allows the anchor to be directly inserted into the bone socket. As the anchor is held directly above the bone socket, the sutures are appropriately tensioned to remove slack from the construct and reduce the tendon to the tuberosity. The anchor

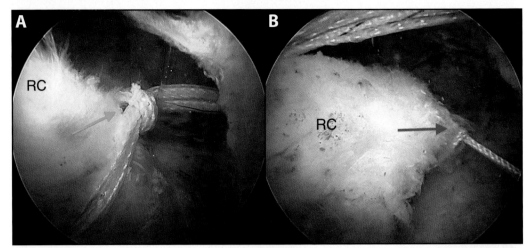

Figure 12-6. Right shoulder posterior subacromial viewing portal. FiberLink sutures are placed (A) posterior (green arrow) and (B) anterior (blue arrow) to the medial sutures for dog ear reduction and reinforcement of the rotator cable insertions. RC, rotator cuff.

Figure 12-7. Right shoulder posterior subacromial viewing portal demonstrates placement of a posterolateral anchor, which incorporates the posterior dog ear reduction suture and one suture tape limb each from the anteromedial and posteromedial anchors. RC, rotator cuff.

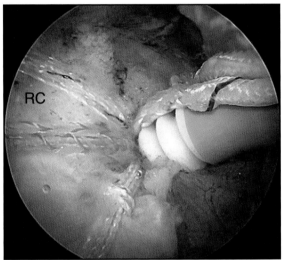

inserter is then advanced into the bone socket until the leading threads of the anchor begin to contact the bone. While holding the thumb pad on the SwiveLock driver, the anchor is inserted into the bone, the depth checked, and the suture limbs cut flush with the inserted anchor (Figure 12-7). The 2 remaining FiberTape suture limbs and the anterior dog ear reduction suture are then retrieved through the lateral portal and the steps are repeated with an anterolateral anchor. Both a subacromial and intra-articular view of the final repair is obtained. This repair creates both a low-profile transosseous equivalent repair and also provides a medial seal from the joint via the medial double mattress stitch (Figure 12-8).

POSTOPERATIVE PROTOCOL

Postoperatively, the involved arm is maintained in a sling for 6 weeks. During this time, the patient is allowed to do active wrist and elbow flexion and extension. Passive external rotation is

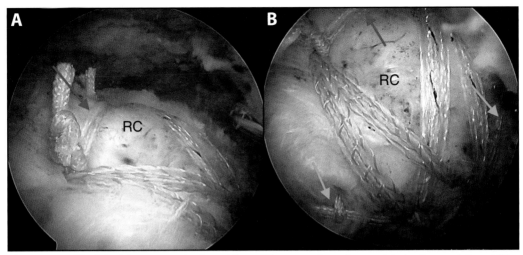

Figure 12-8. Final double-row repair viewed from (A) a posterior subacromial viewing portal, and (B) a lateral subacromial viewing portal. The medial double pulley (blue arrow) has created a double-mattress stitch, which provides a medial seal. The anterior and posterior cinch stitches (green arrows) provide dog ear reduction and reinforcement of the rotator cable insertions. RC, rotator cuff.

permitted if there is not an associated subscapularis tendon tear. Table slides are initiated immediately for single-tendon tears. At 6 weeks, the sling is removed and external rotation is initiated. Overhead passive forward flexion begins at this time with a rope and pulley. At 12 weeks, postoperative rotator cuff strengthening and internal rotation are allowed. Strengthening is delayed until 12 weeks following surgery as there is evidence that tendon healing takes approximately 12 weeks and the majority of re-tears occur within this early postoperative period.[14,29,30] Additionally, in the authors' opinion, there is no need to begin aggressive range of motion soon after the repair since the incidence of stiffness after an ARCR is exceeding low.[31] Full return to activity, including functions that accelerate the arm (tennis, golf, throwing), is allowed at 6 months following repair.

POTENTIAL COMPLICATIONS

Major complications following ARCR such as an infection or other need for readmission are extremely rare.[32] Overtensioning the repair may lead to medial row failure. This risk can be minimized by visualizing the musculotendinous junction. Neyton et al recently reported that when the musculotendinous junction was visualized and the medial sutures of a suture-bridging repair were placed lateral to the musculotendinous junction, the incidence of medial tendon failure was only 1 in 107 cases.[33] Additionally, recent biomechanical investigation has suggested that a medial mattress suture may reduce the potential for medial tendon failure. Overall, as described in the introduction, re-tear rates are dramatically decreased with a suture-bridge double-row repair. Patients with poor bone quality are at particular risk for greater tuberosity fracture due to improper placement of the lateral anchors. This problem is avoided by placing the anchors at least 5 mm distal to the lateral corner of the greater tuberosity and ensuring adequate space between the 2 lateral anchors (which is facilitated by clearly visualizing the lateral gutter). Postoperative cystic reaction was observed with first-generation absorbable anchors, but this has been substantially decreased with the newer calcium-composite materials.[34] Permanent postoperative stiffness, as noted previously, is low after ARCR.

Top Technical Pearls for the Procedure

1. Perform a complete bursectomy to clearly visualize the tear margins and musculotendinous junction.

2. Pass the medial sutures 2 to 3 mm lateral to the musculotendinous junction.

3. Reinforce the rotator cable and reduce dog ears with independent sutures anterior and posterior to the medial anchors.

4. Ensure adequate visualization of the lateral gutter prior to lateral anchor placement by performing an additional bursectomy and/or using a 70-degree arthroscope.

5. Cycle through the application of tension to the lateral sutures to ensure that all slack is removed from the construct prior to seating the lateral anchors.

References

1. Lo IK, Burkhart SS. Double-row arthroscopic rotator cuff repair: re-establishing the footprint of the rotator cuff. *Arthroscopy*. 2003;19:1035-1042.

2. Brady PC, Arrigoni P, Burkhart SS. Evaluation of residual rotator cuff defects after in vivo single- versus double-row rotator cuff repairs. *Arthroscopy*. 2006;22:1070-1075.

3. Ma CB, Comerford L, Wilson J, Puttlitz CM. Biomechanical evaluation of arthroscopic rotator cuff repairs: double-row compared with single-row fixation. *J Bone Joint Surg Am*. 2006;88:403-410.

4. Meier SW, Meier JD. The effect of double-row fixation on initial repair strength in rotator cuff repair: a biomechanical study. *Arthroscopy*. 2006;22:1168-1173.

5. Park MC, ElAttrache NS, Tibone JE, Ahmad CS, Jun BJ, Lee TQ. Part I: footprint contact characteristics for a transosseous-equivalent rotator cuff repair technique compared with a double-row repair technique. *J Shoulder Elbow Surg*. 2007;16:461-468.

6. Park MC, Tibone JE, ElAttrache NS, Ahmad CS, Jun BJ, Lee TQ. Part II: biomechanical assessment for a footprint-restoring transosseous-equivalent rotator cuff repair technique compared with a double-row repair technique. *J Shoulder Elbow Surg*. 2007;16:469-476.

7. Burkhart SS, Adams CR, Schoolfield JD. A biomechanical comparison of 2 techniques of footprint reconstruction for rotator cuff repair: the SwiveLock-FiberChain construct versus standard double-row repair. *Arthroscopy*. 2009;25:274-281.

8. Burkhart SS, Cole BJ. Bridging self-reinforcing double-row rotator cuff repair: we really are doing better. *Arthroscopy*. 2010;26:677-680.

9. Burks RT, Crim J, Brown N, Fink B, Greis PE. A prospective randomized clinical trial comparing arthroscopic single- and double-row rotator cuff repair: magnetic resonance imaging and early clinical evaluation. *Am J Sports Med*. 2009;37:674-682.

10. Grasso A, Milano G, Salvatore M, Falcone G, Deriu L, Fabbriciani C. Single-row versus double-row arthroscopic rotator cuff repair: a prospective randomized clinical study. *Arthroscopy*. 2009;25:4-12.

11. Franceschi F, Ruzzini L, Longo UG, et al. Equivalent clinical results of arthroscopic single-row and double-row suture anchor repair for rotator cuff tears: a randomized controlled trial. *Am J Sports Med*. 2007;35:1254-1260.

12. Duquin TR, Buyea C, Bisson LJ. Which method of rotator cuff repair leads to the highest rate of structural healing? A systematic review. *Am J Sports Med*. 2010;38:835-841.

13. Harryman DT 2nd, Mack LA, Wang KY, Jackins SE, Richardson ML, Matsen FA 3rd. Repairs of the rotator cuff. Correlation of functional results with integrity of the cuff. *J Bone Joint Surg Am*. 1991;73:982-989.

14. Kluger R, Bock P, Mittlbock M, Krampla W, Engel A. Long-term survivorship of rotator cuff repairs using ultrasound and magnetic resonance imaging analysis. *Am J Sports Med*. 2011;39:2071-2081.

15. Denard PJ, Jiwani AZ, Ladermann A, Burkhart SS. Long-term outcome of arthroscopic massive rotator cuff repair: the importance of double-row fixation. *Arthroscopy*. 2012;28:909-915.

16. Frank JB, ElAttrache NS, Dines JS, Blackburn A, Crues J, Tibone JE. Repair site integrity after arthroscopic transosseous-equivalent suture-bridge rotator cuff repair. *Am J Sports Med*. 2008;36:1496-1503.

17. Toussaint B, Schnaser E, Bosley J, Lefebvre Y, Gobezie R. Early structural and functional outcomes for arthroscopic double-row transosseous-equivalent rotator cuff repair. *Am J Sports Med*. 2011;39:1217-1225.

18. Kim KC, Shin HD, Lee WY. Repair integrity and functional outcomes after arthroscopic suture-bridge rotator cuff repair. *J Bone Joint Surg Am*. 2012;94:e48.

19. Mihata T, Watanabe C, Fukunishi K, et al. Functional and structural outcomes of single-row versus double-row versus combined double-row and suture-bridge repair for rotator cuff tears. *Am J Sports Med*. 2011;39:2091-2098.

20. Sethi PM, Noonan BC, Cunningham J, Shreck E, Miller S. Repair results of 2-tendon rotator cuff tears utilizing the transosseous equivalent technique. *J Shoulder Elbow Surg*. 2010;19:1210-1217.

21. Park JY, Siti HT, Keum JS, Moon SG, Oh KS. Does an arthroscopic suture bridge technique maintain repair integrity?: a serial evaluation by ultrasonography. *Clin Orthop Relat Res*. 2010;468:1578-1587.

22. Gartsman GM, Drake G, Edwards TB, et al. Ultrasound evaluation of arthroscopic full-thickness supraspinatus rotator cuff repair: single-row versus double-row suture bridge (transosseous equivalent) fixation. Results of a prospective, randomized study. *J Shoulder Elbow Surg*. 2013;22:1480-1487.

23. Arrigoni P, Brady PC, Burkhart SS. The double-pulley technique for double-row rotator cuff repair. *Arthroscopy*. 2007;23:675 e1-4.

24. Kaplan K, ElAttrache NS, Vazquez O, Chen YJ, Lee T. Knotless rotator cuff repair in an external rotation model: the importance of medial-row horizontal mattress sutures. *Arthroscopy*. 2011;27:471-478.

25. Gamradt SC, Gallo RA, Adler RS, et al. Vascularity of the supraspinatus tendon three months after repair: characterization using contrast-enhanced ultrasound. *J Shoulder Elbow Surg*. 2010;19:73-80.

26. Christoforetti JJ, Krupp RJ, Singleton SB, Kissenberth MJ, Cook C, Hawkins RJ. Arthroscopic suture bridge transosseus equivalent fixation of rotator cuff tendon preserves intratendinous blood flow at the time of initial fixation. *J Shoulder Elbow Surg*. 2012;21:523-530.

27. Lo IK, Burkhart SS, Chan KC, Athanasiou K. Arthroscopic knots: determining the optimal balance of loop security and knot security. *Arthroscopy*. 2004;20:489-502.

28. Burkhart SS, Esch JC, Jolson RS. The rotator crescent and rotator cable: an anatomic description of the shoulder's "suspension bridge". *Arthroscopy*. 1993;9:611-616.

29. Sonnabend DH, Howlett CR, Young AA. Histological evaluation of repair of the rotator cuff in a primate model. *J Bone Joint Surg Br*. 2010;92:586-594.

30. Miller BS, Downie BK, Kohen RB, et al. When do rotator cuff repairs fail? Serial ultrasound examination after arthroscopic repair of large and massive rotator cuff tears. *Am J Sports Med*. 2011;39:2064-2070.

31. Denard PJ, Ladermann A, Burkhart SS. Prevention and management of stiffness after arthroscopic rotator cuff repair: systematic review and implications for rotator cuff healing. *Arthroscopy*. 2011;27:842-848.

32. Martin CT, Gao Y, Pugely AJ, Wolf BR. 30-day morbidity and mortality after elective shoulder arthroscopy: a review of 9410 cases. *J Shoulder Elbow Surg*. 2013;22:1667-1675 e1.

33. Neyton L, Godeneche A, Nove-Josserand L, Carrillon Y, Clechet J, Hardy MB. Arthroscopic suture-bridge repair for small to medium size supraspinatus tear: healing rate and retear pattern. *Arthroscopy*. 2013;29:10-17.

34. Cobaleda Aristizabal AF, Sanders EJ, Barber FA. Adverse events associated with biodegradable lactide-containing suture anchors. *Arthroscopy*. 2014;30:555-560.

Please see videos on the accompanying website at

www.ArthroscopicTechniques.com

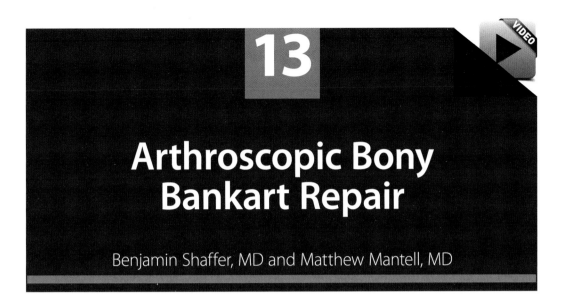

13

Arthroscopic Bony Bankart Repair

Benjamin Shaffer, MD and Matthew Mantell, MD

Introduction

Arthroscopic bony Bankart repair may be indicated in patients with anterior glenohumeral instability in which part of the bony glenoid has been fractured or avulsed along with the anteroinferior (AI) glenohumeral ligament/labrum complex. Seen in both the acute and chronic (recurrent) setting, bony Bankart lesions are relatively common with a reported incidence ranging from 4% to 70%.[1-4] Failure to restore normal structural integrity to the anterior glenoid has been convincingly shown to increase the risk of recurrent instability following conventional soft tissue arthroscopic repair alone.[5-9] Biomechanical studies have further reinforced the importance of preserving and/or re-establishing the normal architectural vault of the glenoid rim as critical to restoring normal shoulder stability.[10] Although the precise tolerance for glenoid bone loss (via fracture, erosion, or some combination) is not currently known, there seems to be an emerging consensus that anterior or AI bone defects approaching or exceeding 20% to 25% of the glenoid's normal diameter jeopardizes the effectiveness of an arthroscopic soft tissue repair alone.

The most commonly described and performed bony Bankart repair is the single-row technique, in which individually spaced anchors are placed along the rim or onto the face of the glenoid. Such an approach has been shown to be highly effective,[7,8,11-14] and is particularly appealing when dealing with fairly small fragments or when bone fragment quality is suboptimal (comminuted, crumbling, soft). (*Note:* Small here is defined as a fragment whose mediolateral dimensions are typically similar or less than the thickness of the labrum through which sutures will be passed [ie, 4 to 5 mm]. Bone fragments that are larger than this pose a greater challenge to encompass or pass through using various suture-passing devices, and may warrant consideration of a "bridge" or "2-row" technique.) The bone fragment(s) is/are incorporated into the repair itself using simple sutures to ensnare the bone within the capsuloligamentous complex.

Recent interest in achieving improved fixation has led to the evolution of a double-row procedure, first described by Zhang and Jiang[15] and further refined and popularized as a "bony Bankart bridge" technique by Millett et al.[16,17] Fixation is achieved by using suture anchors medial to the fragment on the glenoid neck, encircling the bone and adjacent capsulolabral tissue, and docking them into the anterior glenoid using knotless anchors. This ingenious approach offers the biologic advantage of eliminating sutures within the fragment/glenoid interface and, in the lab, has proven

Ryu RKN, Angelo RL, Abrams JS, eds. *The Shoulder:*
AANA Advanced Arthroscopic Surgical Techniques (pp 147-164).
© 2016 AANA.

biomechanically superior compared to the single-row technique, with improved compression and stability to mechanical loading.[18] This technique is particularly compelling in cases where the bony Bankart lesion constitutes a fairly large fragment or fragments, spanning a distance of more than 4 to 5 mm from the medial fracture plane to the glenoid rim. Large fragments can displace due to inadequate fixation using a single-point anchor fixation approach, whereas a double-row anchor construct can both achieve anatomic reduction and enhance fixation stability. However, double-row constructs are more technically challenging and can increase procedure time and anchor cost (2x as many anchors per bone fixation site). Passing sutures around or through a large fragment can be a tedious and difficult endeavor; therefore, due consideration ought to be given before undertaking the bone fragment repair.

Arthroscopic bone fixation using screws has been described and is conceptually appealing.[19] Several instrument sets are available for this purpose, one of which is the Percutaneous Pinning Set (Arthrex, Inc), which includes an array of devices used to target, drill, and fix bony fragments with cannulated variably sized screws. Offset guides, drill sleeves, and even flexible wires and drills have enhanced the authors' technical ability to achieve anatomic fixation using this approach. However, despite its compelling rationale, the reality is that the vast majority of bony Bankart lesions lack the size or sturdiness to permit percutaneous screw fixation. Even if they were large enough, rotational stability is not necessarily assured, requiring secure fixation at the superior and inferior aspect of the fragment, or a second screw above or below the first.

From a practical standpoint, most bony Bankart lesions will be fixed using either a single- or dual-row bridge suture anchor repair technique. How to proceed will be determined by a number of factors, including bone fragment size and the quality and ease with which the fragment can be manipulated and viewed for reduction and fixation. For smaller bone fragments, the authors will proceed with a single-row repair. Fragments greater than 4 to 5 mm from the medial glenoid neck to the rim are repaired with a double-row bone bridge technique. Currently, there are no clinical data that prove the superiority of dual-row bridge vs a single-row bony Bankart repair, but both single- and double-row techniques report a high rate of radiographic incorporation[20,21] and clinical success.[1,11-14,21] However, there are currently no studies comparing the clinical outcome of single- vs double-row bridge repairs.

The purpose of this chapter is to draw attention to this anterior instability variant, suggest indications for surgical treatment, and describe techniques by which this sometimes technically challenging problem can be successfully addressed using an arthroscopic approach.

INDICATIONS

► Patients with first-time or recurrent anterior instability associated with a glenoid rim fracture fragment that is less than 20% to 25% of the glenoid diameter

Controversial Indications

► Bony Bankart lesions exceeding 20% to 25% of glenoid involvement
► Presence of concomitant "significant" Hill-Sachs lesion or concomitant humeral avulsion of the glenohumeral ligament. (An "insignificant" Hill Sachs lesion is probably one that involves less than 10% depth of involvement of the humeral head and does not involve the underlying bone, but is more of a chondral lesion than an osteochondral impact zone. Humeral avulsion of the glenohumeral ligament lesions are uncommon but can accompany bony Bankart avulsions and technically may justify an open approach to satisfactorily address both sides of the capsuloligamentous pathology.)
► Bony Bankart lesion in a contact/collision athlete
► Failed prior arthroscopic stabilization in the face of poor quality anterior glenoid bone remnant

PERTINENT PHYSICAL FINDINGS

▶ Positive apprehension sign with the shoulder in the abducted externally rotated (ie, throwing) position

▶ Increased translation on anterior laxity testing via either load and shift test or anterior drawer test when compared to the opposite shoulder. Such testing may be accompanied by patients' subjective perception of instability or an objective palpable clunk during translation.

▶ Some patients with bony pathology of the glenoid may sense or exhibit instability only in the midrange of motion (rather than at the extremes), such as in 45 degrees of abduction/external rotation.

▶ Positive relocation sign

▶ Axillary nerve injury with sensory deficit to the overlying dermatome and/or deltoid weakness

▶ Although generalized ligamentous laxity and the sulcus sign are not specific or commonly present in patients with traumatic unidirectional instability, soft tissue laxity may be present even in this population and may require plication in addition to treating the bony lesion.

▶ Positive belly press test may reflect a subscapularis injury, which can (uncommonly) occur during a traumatic anterior instability event.

PERTINENT IMAGING

▶ High-quality radiographs are critical for preoperative planning purposes.

▶ Standard plain radiograph imaging (true anteroposterior in the plane of the glenoid [Grashey view], as well as an axillary and scapular Y view) are obtained in every patient.

▶ While it is much easier to see larger glenoid defects on plain films, one can assess for smaller lesions by loss of anterior cortical margin on the true anteroposterior or axillary view (Figure 13-1).

▶ Several radiographic studies have demonstrated improved detection of glenoid bony pathology using modified plain views such as the Bernageau[22] or West Point view.[23]

▶ However, 60% of bony lesions requiring operative treatment can be missed when radiographs are used alone preoperatively.[24]

▶ Because of the importance of detecting bony pathology, more sophisticated imaging, such as magnetic resonance imaging (MRI) or computed tomography (CT) scan, deserve consideration in patients with significant trauma or a history of multiple post-traumatic recurrences.

▶ MRI shows superior soft tissue detail and does not involve ionizing radiation, an advantage over CT imaging, particularly in the younger population with instability (Figure 13-2). However, no consistent scanner or sequencing currently demonstrates the ability to assess or measure bone involvement as accurately as CT scanning.

▶ CT scan enhances both detection and quantification of bony pathology, both on the glenoid and humeral side. A recent comparison study demonstrated that 3D CT was the most accurate imaging modality in predicting glenoid bone loss (Figure 13-3).[25] 3D CT scans, with or without contrast (depending upon acuteness of event), including views with and without digital subtraction of the humeral head, are the current imaging study of choice to assess bone involvement. CT scans permit bilateral glenoid morphology assessment during image acquisition, an advantage over MRI.

Figure 13-1. This axillary view demonstrates a slightly displaced bony Bankart lesion (arrows).

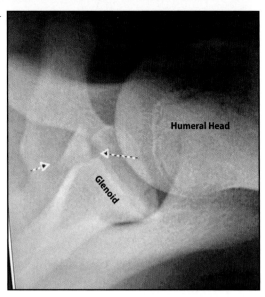

Figure 13-2. This axial MRI slice demonstrates the bony Bankart lesion (arrow head).

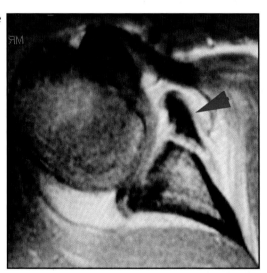

Figure 13-3. 3D CT imagine with humeral head digital subtraction allows precise determination of fragment size and location.

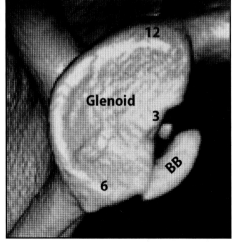

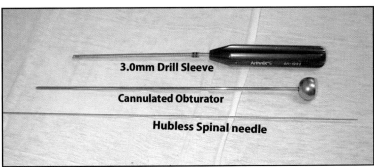

Figure 13-4. Percutaneous set for anchor insertion includes a long hubless spinal needle for targeting the glenoid, a cannulated obturator that dilates over the spinal needle, and a cannulated drill sleeve that passes over the obturator to establish a percutaneous portal.

EQUIPMENT

In addition to standard instruments used during shoulder arthroscopy, a number of specific instruments are critical in facilitating proper technique execution, including the following:

▶ A 70-degree arthroscopic lens, which when positioned in the posterior viewing portal, affords a nearly en-face view of the anterior glenoid.

▶ Multiple arthroscopic cannulae of various depths (7-cm length is usually sufficient, but must be considered in context of normal "working length" of hand instruments, such as rasps, shaver blades, drill sleeves, anchors, etc), widths (starting with a 5-mm outer diameter and changing to 8.25-mm outer diameter), and accommodation for instruments used during tissue manipulation, anchor insertion, suture passage, knot tying, and suture management.

▶ Percutaneous instrumentation specifically designed to permit accurate anatomic targeting around the "clock face" of the glenoid, typically at the 5, 6, or 7 o'clock positions. The authors have found that use of a system that utilizes a "hubless" spinal needle with accompanying nitinol wire and a series of small diameter metal dilation cannulae (Arthrex, Inc) are invaluable (Figure 13-4).

▶ Suture anchors of various sizes, with requisite drill/punch/tap instruments. The authors utilize 3-mm BioComposite SutureTak anchors (Arthrex), which are available single- and double-loaded with #2 Fiberwire (Arthrex). Occasionally, the authors will use smaller 2.4- or 2-mm implants (Arthrex). The authors prefer composite biocomposite (poly-L-lactic acid-based) or composite (polyetheretherketone) over metal anchors to minimize metallic debris, subsequent imaging distortion, loss of bone stock if/when requiring revision anchor placement, and risk of proud or loose metal anchor implants.

▶ Knotless anchors are also available, particularly helpful if using the bone bridge technique, relying on 2.9-mm BioComposite Pushlock Anchors (Arthrex), which employ metal cannula to permit implant passage.

▶ Multiple nondisposable and disposable suture-passing instruments, including those that shuttle suture through and around tissue (Figure 13-5). These most commonly include 0-, 45-, 60-, and 90-degree Spectrum hooks (Linvatec) or Suture Lassos (Arthrex). An additional helpful set of suture-passing devices is "Penetrators" (0-, 22.5-, and 45-degree upsweep tips [Arthrex], which can traverse soft tissue and bone and grasp and retrieve suture). Use of Jaw-designed suture passing instruments such as the Labral Scorpion (Arthrex) or Caspari Suture Punch (Linvatec) are particularly effective when passing suture through soft tissue. Use of a "Needle Punch" device (Arthrex), specifically modified with a 30-degree curve to facilitate passing sutures under the humeral head at the 6 o'clock position, can be extremely helpful in tough/thick ligament or labral tissue.

Figure 13-5. Two commonly used suture passing instruments, a Penetrator and a Caspari Suture Punch (Linvatec).

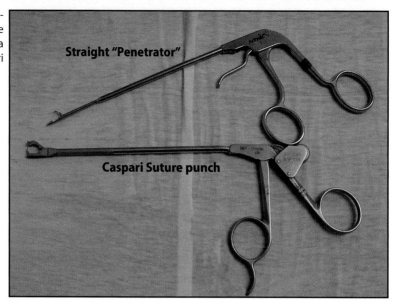

Straight "Penetrator"

Caspari Suture punch

▶ Instruments that permit suture passage through bone, such as the Bone Stitcher (Smith & Nephew)

▶ A set of cannulated percutaneous screw fixation instruments (Percutaneous Pinning Set, Arthrex) must be available in uncommon cases in which bony fragment fixation is achievable using screws.

▶ Open surgical tray should be available for use in cases where structural integrity cannot be restored arthroscopically and requires conversion to an open approach. This should include appropriate retractors as well as anchors that have suture needles to facilitate passage as possible alternatives to arthroscopic suture devices.

Positioning and Portals

Arthroscopic bony Bankart repair can be satisfactorily achieved in either the beach chair or lateral decubitus position. The latter is the authors' preferred approach as they have found that it affords superior visualization of the glenoid and labrum and does so without requiring much intraoperative shoulder manipulation or assistance. Care is taken to maintain the head and neck in neutral alignment and carefully pad the dependent extremity and protect bony prominences of the hip, fibular head, and lateral malleolus. The torso is maintained in this position using a vacuum-beanbag with support, with 5-lb sand bags positioned in the front and back in case of inadvertent beanbag insufflation during the case. Rolling the patient back approximately 15 to 20 degrees facilitates easier access to the front of the shoulder and gives the glenoid an orientation that is more parallel to the operating room floor. Failure to ensure the shoulder is rolled back can make anterior access more difficult. Although the authors do not routinely use an axillary roll, they are careful to ensure the axillary contents are well-protected. Once positioned, if any compression or concern exists, an axillary roll is placed. The arm is temporarily suspended by an IV pole for prepping and draping of the extremity from the shoulder girdle to the fingertips. During the procedure, the shoulder is suspended with a weight, which varies from as little as 7 to as much as 12 lbs based on patient size and tissue laxity. The authors use an ACUFEX Shoulder Positioner with the arm placed in approximately 30 degrees of abduction, 20 degrees of forward flexion, and neutral rotation.

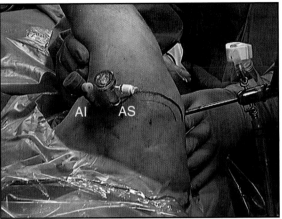

Figure 13-6. This view shows a right shoulder in the lateral decubitus position with the arthroscope in the posterior portal and the twin anterior portals. A clear 8.25-mm cannula is shown in the AS portal and a blue 5-mm cannula is in the AI portal.

Arthroscopic portals include the traditional posterior "soft spot" portal for initial shoulder arthroscopic viewing, placed approximately 2 to 3 cm inferior to and 2 cm medial to the posterolateral acromion. Rather than actually measuring placement, the authors try to identify the optimal placement for each patient by palpating the humeral head during anterior and posterior translation. By palpating directly over the anterior and posterior glenohumeral joints, one can discern a predictably accurate trajectory for posterior scope insertion. Anterior portals include "twin" anterosuperior (AS) and AI portals (Figure 13-6). The AS portal is established first, using an "outside-in" technique. A spinal needle is introduced just inferior and somewhat medial to the anterolateral margin of the acromion. This needle should enter the joint just under cover of the intra-articular long head biceps tendon and angle inferiorly toward the axillary pouch, roughly parallel to the anterior glenoid. Care should be taken to ensure proper cannula positioning just lateral to the glenoid rim. If the cannula is placed too laterally, instrument passage inferiorly may be challenging because of the sometimes obstructing humeral head. Upon a nick skin incision with a #11 blade, a straight clamp is used to spread soft tissue in a path parallel to the adjacent needle, followed by introduction of a blunt 5-mm cannula (Smith & Nephew Dyonics). The cannula's blue tip can be seen indenting the superior aspect of the rotator interval and, with gentle pressure, it usually "pops" into the joint. If the tissue is thick and difficult to penetrate, the blunt obturator can be replaced with a sharp one, which will easily puncture the joint capsule. The 5-mm cannula is next exchanged for an 8.25 mm x 7 cm fully threaded clear Fishbowl cannula (Arthrex), which will facilitate a variety of suture-passing instruments.

The AI portal is next established, again using an outside-in technique, and is placed immediately superior to the upper rolled tendon of the subscapularis tendon. Care should be taken to ensure that this portal is established a few centimeters from the AS portal to avoid instrument "sword fighting" when using both portals. Additionally, the AI portal must be directed from a lateral-to-medial angle to permit an accurate approach to the glenoid during glenoid drilling and anchor placement. Failure to ensure an accurate "angle of attack" may lead to articular cartilage damage due to subarticular tunneling of the drill and/or anchor, inadequate anchor purchase, or implant/device breakage due to unnecessary torque.

Under direct view, a second 5-mm cannula is introduced along the same trajectory as the spinal needle to establish the AI portal. The authors again replace the smaller cannula with a second 8.25 mm x 7 cm Fishbowl cannula. Both twin anterior portals have now been established.

Several other additional percutaneous portals are useful during arthroscopic bony Bankart repair. The most common is the accessory AI 5 o'clock portal.[26] Typically, this is placed from 1 to 3 cm inferior to the established AI portal, with a similar lateral-to-medial targeting angle determined with outside-in spine needle placement.

Occasionally, an accessory posteroinferior portal is helpful, particularly in cases of labral pathology that continues beyond the 6 o'clock position. This portal both facilitates anchor placement on the posteroinferior quadrant of the glenoid and provides an accessory portal for bony fragment manipulation and suture management. In cases of bony Bankart pathology, particularly when the fragment is large, this portal can make anchor placement and suture management easier.

STEP-BY-STEP DESCRIPTION OF THE PROCEDURE

Anesthesia and Exam

Following preoperative interscalene block anesthesia performed under ultrasound guidance in the holding area, the patient is brought to the operating room and undergoes general anesthesia. Exam under anesthesia is performed to assess the degree of translation in anterior, inferior, and posterior directions, and both shoulders are compared.

Positioning

The patient is then rolled into the lateral decubitus position as described previously, caring to ensure the patient is properly padded and rolled back such that the glenoid is parallel to the floor and the anterior shoulder readily accessible. The arm is prepped in a sterile manner from the chest wall to the fingertips and the shoulder is draped. Using a cord and a weight of 7 to 12 lbs (depending on arm size and joint distension), the arm is suspended using a forearm sleeve carefully wrapped with Coban (3M). The extremity is initially placed in 30 degrees of abduction and 20 degrees of flexion. Excessive force can actually decrease the ease of manipulation and visualization.

Portal Establishment and Diagnostic Arthroscopy

Diagnostic evaluation begins with placement of the 30-degree arthroscope in the posterior "soft spot" portal. A dual port cannula is used to facilitate irrigation and clearing of the joint using inflow through one port and suction through the other. Alternating inflow and suction permits optimal visualization, which is sometimes helpful following manipulation during the exam under anesthesia, which can stir up some bleeding and debris. Often, this initial viewing confirms expected pathology and is followed by establishment of the AS and AI portals as described previously. Occasionally, in cases of very small bony Bankart lesions, only a single anterior portal within the center of the rotator interval is necessary.

Diagnostic arthroscopy is performed systematically, viewing and palpating from both anterior and posterior portals. Concomitant pathology is identified and addressed at this time. The AS portal is often used as a viewing portal, permitting an en face view of the glenoid for anchor placement.

Assessment of Bony Bankart (and Other Associated Instability) Pathology

Although preoperative imaging should already have afforded preliminary evaluation of bone fragment size and position, careful intraoperative assessment is necessary. Visualization with a 70-degree lens from the posterior portal, while palpating and manipulating from the anterior portal(s), allows assessment of bone fragment dimensions, position, mobility, bone quality, and

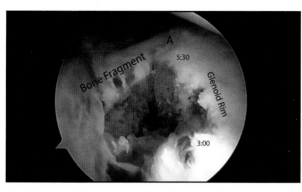

Figure 13-7. This arthroscopic view of a right shoulder, patient in the lateral decubitus position, 30-degree lens from the AS portal, demonstrates the bony Bankart fragment avulsed from the glenoid rim. The most inferior aspect of the labral detachment is seen just inferior to the 5:30 position, with the axilla of the lesion marked "A."

degree to which it has healed to the glenoid (and whether by fibrous or bony union). In addition, its relationship to the labrum/ligament complex (which often contains the avulsed fragment) and the degree, if any, of associated capsular patholaxity (Figure 13-7) is determined.

In addition to gauging the dimensions of the bony Bankart fragment, evaluation of the magnitude of glenoid deficiency is important at this step. It is most easily determined viewing with a 30-degree lens from the AS portal using a calibrated probe from the posterior portal to measure the amount of anterior glenoid bone loss relative to the "bare spot" technique as described by Burkhart et al.[27]

The posterolateral humeral head is inspected for evidence and extent of a Hill-Sachs lesion. The arm is often removed from traction and manipulated into an abducted and externally rotated "throwing" position, observing the degree to which the humeral head defect "engages" the glenoid. The ease of engagement may influence the decision to proceed with an arthroscopic bony Bankart repair and/or consider any adjunctive/alternative approaches, such as remplissage, humeral head bone grafting, open surgery, or a Bristow-Latarjet procedure.

Mobilize Fragment

Thorough soft tissue and bone fragment mobilization is critical for anatomic reduction of the bony Bankart, as well as allowing restoration of normal capsular tension. While viewing with a 70-degree lens from the posterior portal, a liberator rasp (Smith & Nephew) or other instrument (shaver or radiofrequency device) is brought in from the AS portal. This in-line approach permits mobilization of the bony Bankart lesion from the glenoid in the plane of the fracture. Further mobilization of the labrum from the glenoid rim can be exploited for the length of the soft tissue Bankart above and/or inferior to the bony Bankart lesion itself. The AI portal permits access to lesions extending inferiorly beyond the 5 o'clock position (right shoulder). Satisfactory mobilization is confirmed when the fragment and labral complex are easily translated superiorly and laterally, with visualization of the underlying subscapularis muscle.

Tissue Preparation

Thorough tissue preparation is essential to ensure biologic healing of the repaired lesion. With rare exception, most bony Bankart lesions are essentially nonunions and require debridement of interposed soft tissue and some method to try to generate a healing response. This is performed using a curved shaving blade, burr, and/or curette, addressing both the glenoid and bony fragment/labral faces of the fracture plane. Avoid overly aggressive bony Bankart debridement, which can inadvertently remove bone.

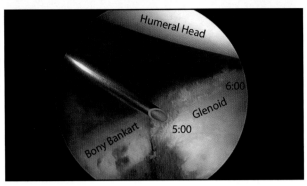

Figure 13-8. Arthroscopic viewing from AS portal with a 30-degree lens shows a spinal needle percutaneously directed at the axilla (A) of the labral detachment, just inferior to the 5 o'clock position. This is the most important anchor in securing anatomic reduction and fixation.

Plan Repair

At this point, one should have a reasonably clear perspective about how to best approach the observed pathology. The order of the repair includes the following:

1. Securing the inferior-most extent of the anterior bony Bankart lesion (usually at the 5 or 6 o'clock position for a right shoulder)

2. Fixing the bony Bankart lesion itself

3. Completing the construct with a final anchor at the superior-most extent of the Bankart lesion (usually at 2:30 or 3 o'clock position for a right shoulder)

Reduction of Bony Bankart Lesion

A traction suture is placed through the upper portion of the AI glenohumeral ligament just above the bony Bankart. This is best passed using the Labral Scorpion (Arthrex), NeedlePunch (Arthrex), or Caspari suture passing instrument via the AS portal. Tensioning the traction sutures through the AS portal facilitates superior translation of the inferiorly and medially displaced fragment, aiding in reduction and determining the optimal placement of sutures. Arthroscopic tissue graspers from the medial anchor (MA) portal further facilitate manipulation and reduction of the Bankart lesion. Occasionally, the authors have found a percutaneous spinal needle helpful as a "joystick" to manipulate the fragment.

First Anchor Placement

The first fixation point is the keystone of the repair. It serves to anchor the initial construct in an anatomically reduced position for the remainder of the case. It will also serve as perhaps the most important site of fixation through stress protection at the junction of normal and pathologic tissue (Figure 13-8). Although a knotless system can effectively achieve fixation at this point, the authors' preference is to use conventional suture anchors, which are more "forgiving" in terms of glenoid rim targeting.

Repair begins at the inferior-most extent of the detachment. The first anchor is placed at the inferior-most aspect of the tear, inferior to the bony Bankart fragment. The authors prefer a double-loaded 3-mm BioComposite SutureTak (Arthrex) anchor placed through the AI or 5 o'clock percutaneous portal, usually at the 5:30 to 6 o'clock position (right shoulder). Ideally, the anchor's double-loaded sutures emerge from the rim at the lesion's axilla. When drilling the anchor insertion site, make sure to have an appropriate "angle of attack" from lateral to medial to avoid undermining the articular cartilage (which occurs if one is too parallel to the joint). Also, be careful to avoid too vertical an approach, which can lead to inadvertent penetration of the inferior

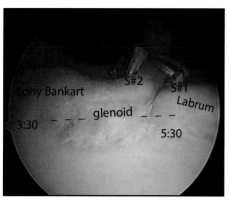

Figure 13-9. This arthroscopic view of a right shoulder, lateral decubitus position, shows the appearance following tying of the initial "keystone" anchor sutures at the axilla of the Bankart lesion, inferior to the bone fragment. A double-loaded suture anchor permitted simple suture capture of good capsulolabral tissue at 2 different sites at approximately the 5:30 position. This arthroscopic photo demonstrates fixation following suture passage for the bony Bankart repair. Tying these sutures before repairing the bony Bankart may compromise the ability to manipulate the bone fragment and cause undue stress on these important 2 first sutures, so they are clamped and final knot tying is delayed until the bony Bankart sutures have been passed.

glenoid rim and extraosseous anchor placement. A self-seating "fish mouth" type of drill sleeve (Arthrex) can be used to gently lever the humeral head out of the way while directly targeting the glenoid rim. Care is taken to avoid applying too much leverage to the drill sleeve. An assistant can help by laterally translating the humeral head for better visualization and access. The anchor should be open and ready for insertion so that drill sleeve position and in-line anchor insertion is maintained. The anchor must be firmly seated such that its eyelet is below the articular cartilage and tensioned to ensure it is secure within the bone.

First Anchor Suture Passage

Viewing from posteriorly, a limb of one of the inferior anchor sutures is then passed through either the AS or AI portal and through the ligament/labrum complex inferior to the bony Bankart fragment. This first suture is passed slightly inferior to the corresponding anchor point on the glenoid such that, when tied, it permits sufficient superior translation re-tension of the AI glenohumeral ligament complex, as is conventionally performed in a conventional soft tissue Bankart repair. A number of suture-passing instruments can be used for this first suture passage, though the authors find that the Labral Scorpion or NeedlePunch are particularly effective in achieving a robust capsular bite. Occasionally, this first suture can be passed from the posterior scope portal while viewing from the AS portal. The passed and unpassed first suture limb pair is retrieved through the AI cannula, and the first limb of the next suture pair is similarly passed. This next limb is placed 3 to 4 mm distant from the site of the first suture passage to ensure adequate tissue capture. The authors are now prepared to tie these 2 simple sutures. Sometimes, the construct will be modified, and one of the suture pairs will be passed twice to achieve a hybrid construct with one simple and one mattress configuration. Tying the second pair of sutures will establish and maintain fragment reduction for the remainder of the case (Figure 13-9). However, tying the sutures at this point can make subsequent anchor placement and suture passage challenging, especially if the bone fragment is large and/or the shoulder tight. Therefore, sutures are clamped and kept loose outside of the cannula at this time and tied only after the bone bridge construct anchors have been inserted and their sutures passed.

Bone Fragment Repair

The technique by which the bone fragment itself is fixed is determined by its size and quality. Fragments whose depth (medial-to-lateral dimension) is less than 3 to 4 mm can be fairly easily incorporated into a single-row repair as performed in a typical soft tissue Bankart procedure. Bone fragment(s) exceeding 4 to 5 mm in depth, however, may not be adequately secured with a single point of glenoid fixation and are better served with a double-row "bridge" construct.

Figure 13-10. This on-face view of the glenoid demonstrates a single-row fixation technique in which arthroscopic sutures or knotless anchors are used to secure the bony Bankart lesion by encircling it within the avulsed capsulolabral tissue. In this illustration, bony Bankart fixation has been achieved with 1 double-loaded suture anchor inferiorly and 3 single-loaded anchors proximally using simple configuration sutures.

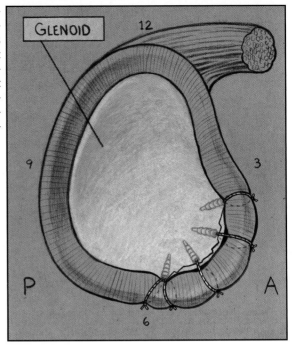

Single-Row Construct

Viewing from the posterior portal with a 70-degree lens, a single-loaded 2.4- or 3-mm BioSuturetac anchor (Arthrex) is seated at the glenoid rim 3 to 4 mm superior to the previously placed (sutures not tied) inferior-most anchor. A curved or 90-degree angle Spectrum hook through the AS portal is then used to shuttle a #1 polydioxanone (PDS) monofilament (Johnson & Johnson) underneath the bone fragment and labrum. This monofilament is retrieved and used as a suture shuttle to retrograde past one of the suture limbs of the anchor, with the other limb brought out on top of the labrum. The suture pair is retrieved and clamped outside of the AI portal and the remaining suture anchors are inserted at 4- to 5-mm intervals proximally along the length of the bony Bankart lesion, usually with 2 to 3 additional anchors. A single limb of each anchor is passed encircling the labrum with small bone fragment and with its paired limb brought out over the labrum/bone fragment. None of these sutures are tied until all bony Bankart/labral anchors and sutures have been seated and passed. All pairs are now tied in simple suture configurations, beginning inferiorly and proceeding up the glenoid. While suture tying, attention is placed on keeping the knot off of the articular face (Figure 13-10).

Double-Row "Bridge" Construct

Bony Bankart fragments exceeding 3 to 4 mm in height (measured from medial to lateral) are secured to the glenoid using a bone bridge double-row technique. Rather than single points of fixation along the glenoid rim, each attachment is secured with 2 points of fixation, one placed just medial to the bone fragment on the glenoid neck, and the other at the anterior glenoid rim (Figure 13-11).

Medial Anchor Placement

Viewing with a 30-degree lens from the AS portal, the first 3-mm single-loaded BioSuturetac Anchor is inserted through the AI portal or accessory AI (5 o'clock) portal into the medial glenoid. Anchor placement should be about 2 to 3 mm superior to the inferior aspect of the bone fragment

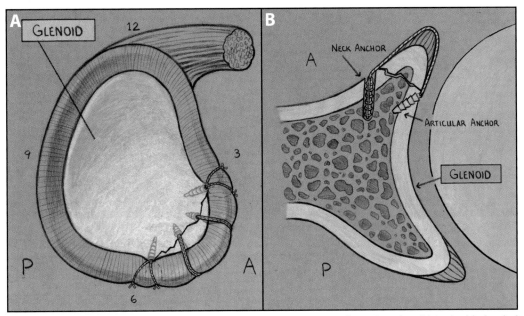

Figure 13-11. A double-row bony Bankart repair shows (A) an on-face view, in which double-loaded suture anchors capture the labral detachment superior and inferior to the bone fragment, and knotless anchors secure the bone fragment laterally. (B) An axial view demonstrates the double-row "bone bridge" construct.

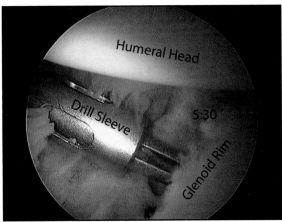

Figure 13-12. Viewing from the AS portal, a drill sleeve engages the medial glenoid neck just medial to the inferior aspect of the fracture fragment.

and should be just medial to the origin of the glenoid fracture fragment (Figure 13-12). Accurate medial anchor placement is critical to achieve anatomic bone fragment reduction. If the medial anchor is placed too medially, the buttress effect of this medial point is lost, permitting medial fragment displacement and malunion. If the medial anchor is placed too far laterally (toward the rim), the fragment will be translated laterally when securing the lateral row sutures. The anchor sleeve enters lateral to the fragment, essentially displacing the fragment medially while drilling and inserting the anchors.

Suture Passage

Each of the first medial anchors' 2 suture limbs are then passed around the bone fragment (Figure 13-13) and shuttled outside of the portal and clamped. Suture passage around the bone block is arguably the most demanding part of this procedure and can be achieved in a variety of

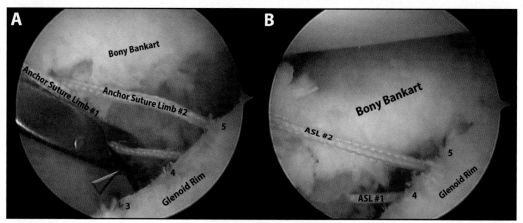

Figure 13-13. (A) In this arthroscopic view, a retriever grasps a limb of the blue monofilament suture passed around the bone fragment (arrowhead) and one of the anchor sutures limbs (anchor suture limb [ASL] #1). (B) After shuttling ASL #1 underneath and around the bone fragment, the other suture limb (ASL #2) is ready to be passed.

ways. The authors' preference is the use of a Spectrum crescent, straight, or curved hook delivered through the AI portal, which affords a direct shot deep to the bone block, emerging medially at the bony Bankart lesion/glenoid interface. A PDS suture is scrolled through the suture-passing instrument, grasped from the posterior (or accessory AI 5 o'clock) portal, and used to shuttle one limb from the medial anchor around the bone fragment. This step is repeated, penetrating the soft tissue/labrum medial to the bone block and 3 to 4 mm superior to the first suture pass (thereby achieving tissue capture between the suture passes and better construct fixation). Alternatively, one can use a Penetrator (0, 22.5, and 45 degrees) or Ideal Suture Grasper (DePuy Mitek) through the MA portal to grasp and retrieve the suture limbs. An alternative strategy to achieve suture passage is to drill and place the anchors through the soft tissue medial to the fragment, in situ, which prevents having to separately pass the suture limbs.

Before proceeding with lateral anchor placement to complete the "bridge," additional medial row anchors are first placed. This allows adjustment of anchor position placement to ensure an anatomic reduction of the fragment and also affords easier suture passage around the fragment. Usually, a total of 2 or 3 medial row anchors are required depending on the length (superoinferior dimension) of the fragment.

Lateral Anchor Placement and Suture Fixation

Next, the bone bridge is secured by inserting lateral anchors that correspond to each of the previously placed medial row anchors. Although conventional suture anchors can be used (tying their sutures to the corresponding medial row anchor sutures that have already been passed), the authors' preference is to use knotless anchors for the lateral row. This facilitates achieving a clean, low-profile, simple, yet strong, compressive fixation system, which can be fine-tuned during insertion.

When using a knotless system, accurate implant targeting is critical. The authors have found that the 5-mm metal cannula sleeve system used with the 2.9-mm Biocomposite Pushlock anchor to be ideally suited for this purpose. With the cannula positioned in the accessory inferior (5 o'clock) portal, a pilot drill hole is made at the anterior bony Bankart/glenoid interface for the most inferior bony Bankart knotless anchor. By pre-"painting" the drill bit with methylene blue, the hole margins are stained to ensure easy identification for subsequent anchor insertion. Next, the suture pair of the first (most inferiorly placed) medial anchor is retrieved and threaded through the 2.7-mm BioPushlock anchor. While reducing and maintaining reduction of the bony Bankart

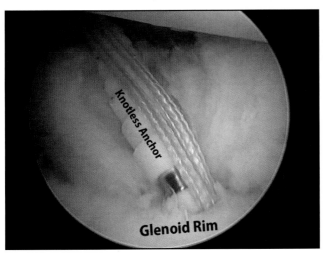

Figure 13-14. Following passage of the arthroscopic sutures around the captured bone block, they are threaded through a knotless anchor and seated directly at the interface between the bony Bankart fragment and the articular margin of the glenoid rim.

lesion either through previously placed traction suture, probe, or grasper from the AS portal and applying gentle superior translation with the traction stitch (previously placed in the AS portal), the first knotless anchor is seated onto the glenoid rim at a point directly lateral to the corresponding medially placed anchor pair (Figure 13-14). The first knotless anchor is gently seated and impacted into place.

These steps of drilling the next knotless anchor insertion site, retrieving the medial suture pair, threading the knotless anchor, and inserting the lateral anchor to tension the next step of the construct are repeated for each medial anchor.

Complete the Procedure

Upon completion of the bony Bankart repair, any labral detachment superior to the bony Bankart lesion is repaired using suture anchors. Because this repair is usually performed at the mid or superior aspect of the anterior glenoid, anchor placement and suture passage are usually achieved fairly easily using either the AS or MA portals. Labral repair anchors are placed at 3- to 5-mm intervals until the construct is complete (Figure 13-15).

Alternatives to the bone bridge construct are as follows:

► Suture passage through the bone block: There are several devices that permit transosseous suture passage across the fragment itself rather than around the fragment. This can prove challenging because of the difficulties sometimes encountered in penetrating a hard and sizable bone fragment, as well as the more common problem of iatrogenically comminuting the fragment into multiple "crumbs." If one does elect to drill across bone and pass a suture or use some bone-penetrating instrument, the hole in the fragment must be anatomically aligned with the placement of the anchor sutures. Failure to do so will cause fragment displacement and result in a nonanatomic repair. For these reasons, transosseous fixation is a less desirable manner of securing the bony Bankart lesion.

► Screw fixation through the bone block: Arthroscopic repair of a bony Bankart using screw fixation is conceptually appealing, and with today's instrumentation, technically achievable. However, the technique requires the ideal bone fragment that is robust enough to tolerate drilling without becoming fragmented, perfect anatomic reduction so that the bony Bankart will not be malreduced when fixed, and an ideal target angle for percutaneous screw placement across the fragment into good glenoid subchondral bone. In cases with large bony Bankarts, the authors have the instrumentation available (Bone Bankart Repair System [Arthrex]), but have not found the technique easy or satisfying.

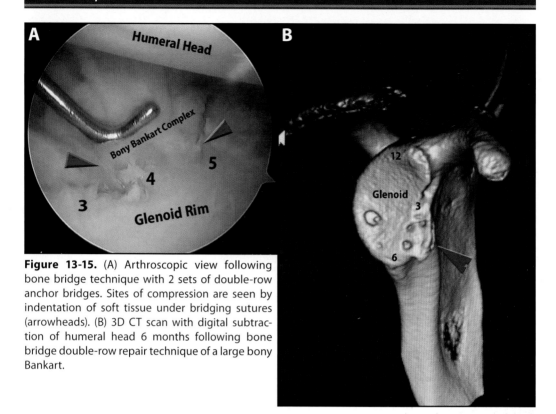

Figure 13-15. (A) Arthroscopic view following bone bridge technique with 2 sets of double-row anchor bridges. Sites of compression are seen by indentation of soft tissue under bridging sutures (arrowheads). (B) 3D CT scan with digital subtraction of humeral head 6 months following bone bridge double-row repair technique of a large bony Bankart.

POSTOPERATIVE PROTOCOL

Patients wear a shoulder sling with abduction pillow for 3 weeks. Skin sutures are removed in the office at 3 to 7 days postoperatively. Patients are allowed to come out of the sling twice daily for active elbow flexion/extension exercises and are instructed in scapular and rotator cuff strengthening exercises. Formal physical therapy starts at the 3-week mark, working to restore active and assistive range of motion with gentle strengthening of the cuff and scapular muscles advanced as tolerated. Combined abduction and external rotation is avoided until week 12. Patients are allowed to return to sport at 4 to 6 months.

POTENTIAL COMPLICATIONS

The most common complication of this procedure is failure to achieve anatomic reduction and secure fixation, with the potential for recurrent instability, and non- or malunion of the bony Bankart lesion. Other intraoperative risks include iatrogenic fragment comminution during suture passing or instrument penetration, inadequate fixation (single-row fixation with large fragment), and chondral damage during anchor drilling or insertion.

TOP TECHNICAL PEARLS FOR THE PROCEDURE

1. Evaluate for bony pathology in patients with anterior shoulder instability. Obtain appropriate radiographic imaging (MRI/CT) to detect and assess glenoid involvement.

2. Incorporation, rather than removal, of bony Bankart fragment(s) has been shown to increase the success rate in arthroscopic stabilization.

3. Attention to thorough tissue mobilization and debridement are requisite to achieving an anatomic reduction and biologic healing.

4. The key to repair begins at the inferior-most aspect of the bony Bankart lesion, where secure fixation at the axilla of the lesion ensures anatomic alignment during the remainder of the repair.

5. Single-row construct is adequate in many cases with small bone fragments, but double-row "bridge" technique affords enhanced compression and fixation in cases with fragments greater than 4 to 5 mm in mediolateral height.

REFERENCES

1. Porcellini G, Paladini P, Campi F, et al. Long-term outcome of acute versus chronic bony bankart lesions managed arthroscopically. *Am J Sports Med*. 2007;35(12):2067-2072.
2. Bigliani, LU, Newton, PM, Steinmann, SP, Connor, PM, McIlveen, SJ. Glenoid rim lesions associated with recurrent anterior dislocation of the shoulder. *Am J Sports Med*. 1998;26(1):41-45.
3. Griffith JF, Antonio GE, Yung PS, et al. Prevalence, pattern, and spectrum of glenoid bone loss in anterior shoulder dislocation: CT analysis of 218 patients. *AJR Am J Roentgenol*. 2008;190(5):1247-1254.
4. Edwards TB, Boulahia A, Walch G. Radiographic analysis of bone defects in chronic anterior shoulder instability. *Arthroscopy*. 2003;19(7):732-739.
5. Burkhart SS, DeBeer JF. Traumatic glenohumeral bone defects and their relationship to failure of arthroscopic Bankart repairs: significance of inverted pear glenoid and the humeral engaging Hill-Sachs lesion. *Arthroscopy*. 2000;16:677-694.
6. Boileau P, Villalba M, Héry JY, Balg F, Ahrens P, Newyton L. Risk factors for recurrence of shoulder instability after arthroscopic Bankart repair. *J Bone Joint Surg Am*. 2006;88(8):1755-1763.
7. Tauber M, Resch H, Forstner R, Raffl M, Schauer J. Reason for failure after surgical repair of anterior shoulder instability. *J Shoulder Elbow Surg*. 2004;13(3):279-285.
8. Sugaya H, Moriishi J, Dohi M, Kon Y, Tsuchiya A. Glenoid rim morphology in recurrent anterior glenohumeral instability. *J Bone Joint Surg Am*. 2003;85-A5;878-884.
9. Burkhart SS, Danaceau SM. Articular arc length mismatch as a cause of failed Bankart repair. *Arthroscopy*. 2000;16:740-744.
10. Itoi E, Lee SB, Berglund LJ, Berge LL, An KN. The effect of a glenoid defect on anterior-inferior stability of the shoulder after Bankart repair: a cadaveric study. *J Bone Joint Surg Am*. 2000;82(1):35-46.
11. Porcellini G, Campri F, Paladini P. Arthroscopic approach to acute bony Bankart lesion. *Arthroscopy*. 2002;18(7):764-769.
12. Sugaya H, Moriishi J, Kanisawa I, Tsuchiya A. Arthroscopic osseous Bankart repair for chronic recurrent traumatic anterior glenohumeral instability. *J Bone Joint Surg Am*. 2005;87:1752-1760.
13. Mologne TS, Provencher MT, Menzel KA, Vachon TA, Dewing CB. Arthroscopic stabilization in patients with an inverted pear glenoid. *Am J Sports Med*. 2007;35(8):1276-1283.

14. Kim YK, Cho SH, Son WS, Moon SH. Arthroscopic repair of small and medium sized bony Bankart lesions. *Am J Sports Med*. 2014;42:86.

15. Zhang J, Jiang C. A new "double pulley" dual row technique for arthroscopic fixation of bony Bankart lesion. *Knee Surg Sports Traumatol Arthrosc*. 2011;19(9):1558-1562.

16. Millett PJ, Braun S. The "bony Bankart bridge" procedure: a new arthroscopic technique for reduction and internal fixation of a bony Bankart lesion. *Arthroscopy*. 2009;25(1):102-105.

17. Millett PJ, Horan MP, Martstschlager F. The "bony Bankart bridge" technique for restoration of anterior shoulder instability. *Am J Sports Med*. 2013;41(3):608-614.

18. Giles JW, Puskas GJ, Welsh MF, Johnson JA, Athwal GS. Suture anchor fixation of bony Bankart fractures: comparison of single-point with double-point "suture bridge" technique. *Am J Sports Med*. 2013;41:2624.

19. Cameron SE. Arthroscopic reduction and internal fixation of anterior glenoid fracture. *Arthroscopy*. 1998;14:743-746.

20. Park JY, Lee SJ, Lee SH. Follow-up CT arthrographic evaluation of bony Bankart lesions after arthroscopic repair. *Arthroscopy*. 2012;28(4):465-473.

21. Jiang C-Y, Zhu YM, Liu X, Li FL, Lu Y, Wu G. Do reduction and healing of the bony fragment really matter in arthroscopic bony Bankart reconstruction? A prospective study with clinical and computed tomography evaluations. *Am J Sports Med*. 2013;41(11):2617-2623.

22. Pansard E, Klouche S, Billot N, et al. Reliability and validity assessment of a glenoid bone loss measurement using the Bernageau profile view in chronic anterior shoulder instability. *J Shoulder Elbow Surg*. 2013;22(9):1193-1198.

23. Pavlov H, Warren RF, Weiss CB Jr, Dines DM. The roentgenographic evaluation of anterior shoulder instability. *Clin Orthop Relat Res*. 1985;(194):153-158.

24. Bushnell CR, Herring MM. Bony instability of the shoulder. *Arthroscopy*. 2008;24(9):1061-1073.

25. Rerko MA, Pan X, Donaldson C, Jones GL, Bishop JY. Comparison of various imaging techniques to quantify glenoid bone loss in shoulder instability. *J Shoulder Elbow Surg*. 2013;22(4):528-534.

26. Davidson PA, Tibone JE. Anterior-inferior (5 o'clock) portal for shoulder arthroscopy. *Arthroscopy*. 1995;11(5):519-525.

27. Burkhart SS, Debeer JF, Tehrany AM, Parten PM. Quantifying glenoid bone loss arthroscopically in shoulder instability. *Arthroscopy*. 2002;18(5):488-491.

Please see videos on the accompanying website at

www.ArthroscopicTechniques.com

Benjamin Shaffer, MD is now deceased.

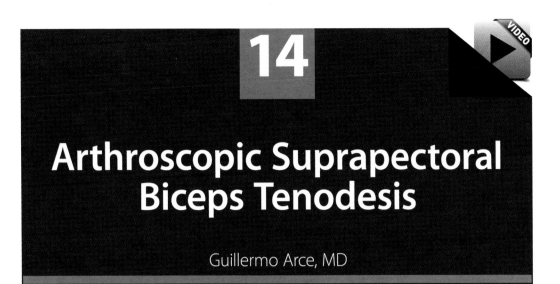

14

Arthroscopic Suprapectoral Biceps Tenodesis

Guillermo Arce, MD

INTRODUCTION

Lesions of the long head of the biceps tendon (LHBT) constitute a common cause of shoulder pain. For many years, surgical treatment of biceps disorders was limited to the removal of the LHBT intra-articular portion with either tenotomy or arthroscopic proximal tenodesis at the upper part of the bicipital groove. Tenotomy in young patients with high-demand activities has been largely unsatisfactory, leading to weakness, cramps, and cosmetic deformity.[1-4] During arthroscopic proximal tenodesis techniques, fixation occurs close to the articular cartilage, resulting in postoperative tenderness. The latter is mainly because a large segment of the degenerative tendon remains at the narrowest part of the groove after surgery.[5-8]

These limitations prompted surgeons to perform open subpectoral tenodesis.[9-11] Despite satisfactory results with this open procedure, neurological complications have occurred, whereas creating a wide socket at a narrow humeral shaft increases the risk of fracture. Furthermore, the use of an open approach is usually cumbersome in a muscular athletic shoulder.[12-14]

Even though a subpectoral fixation technique reduced postoperative pain, it did not eradicate the problem. Recent data suggest that free-nerve endings at the transverse ligament, tendon sheath, and bicipital groove left over after shoulder surgery can cause postoperative pain, especially in the setting of chronic inflammation. Surgical debridement and excision of those structures may mitigate pain by limiting the amount of residual free nerve-ending tissue, improving long-term surgical results.[15-20]

The arthroscopic suprapectoral biceps tenodesis (ASBT) technique emerged to accomplish the previously mentioned goals. This fully arthroscopic technique allows entire resection of the biceps proximal fragment along with the transverse ligament and the tendon sheath.

As expected, the procedure requires moderate-to-advanced arthroscopic skills. The surgeon should be able to recognize pertinent anatomical characteristics such as deeply vascularized areas (Figure 14-1). The area is well-vascularized by the ascending branch of the anterior circumflex artery. The surgeons need to be aware about the location of these structures and stay lateral to the LHBT in order to avoid intraoperative bleeding complications.

Ryu RKN, Angelo RL, Abrams JS, eds. *The Shoulder: AANA Advanced Arthroscopic Surgical Techniques* (pp 165-179). © 2016 AANA.

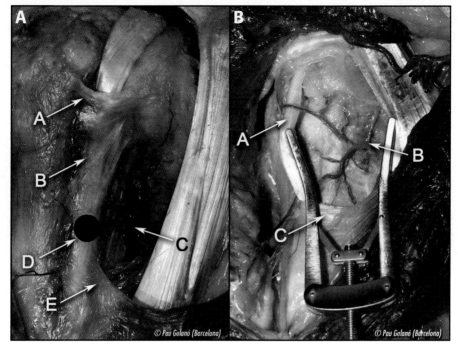

Figure 14-1. Dissected cadaveric right shoulder, anterior aspect. (A) [A] Transverse humeral ligament. [B] Bicipital sheath surrounding the LHBT. [C] Ascending branches of the circumflex artery and vein. [D] Suprapectoral fixation place. [E] Falciform ligament at the proximal edge of the pectoralis major tendon. (B) [A] LHBT. [B] Profuse vascularity medial to the LHBT. [C] Pectoralis major tendon. (Reprinted with permission of Pau Golano, MD, Barcelona, Spain.)

In the presence of moderate osteoporosis, the technique may be performed with suture anchors. However, fixing the tendon into a bone socket with an interference screw seems the best option to achieve faster healing and a shorter rehabilitation period.[21-26]

The objective of this chapter is to outline the technical details of this surgical procedure step-by-step and propose some pearls to guarantee a successful ASBT.

INDICATIONS

► Fraying and degenerative LHBT changes

► Biceps pulley lesions

► LHBT instability due to medial or lateral coracohumeral ligament bands tears

► LHBT dislocation/subluxation secondary to subscapularis tear

► Superior labral anteroposterior (SLAP) III or IV with LHBT involvement or SLAP II in patients over the age of 40 years[27]

► Significant LHBT tenosynovitis at the groove with positive physical and imaging findings

Contraindications

► Infection

► Severe osteoporosis

► Thin, fragile, and almost ruptured LHBT

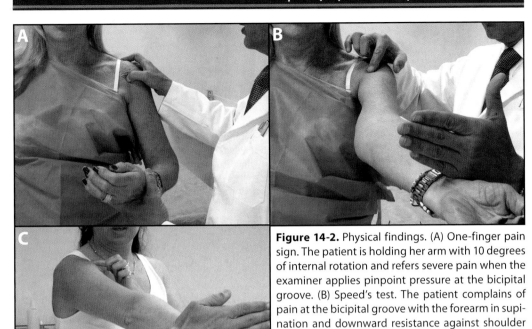

Figure 14-2. Physical findings. (A) One-finger pain sign. The patient is holding her arm with 10 degrees of internal rotation and refers severe pain when the examiner applies pinpoint pressure at the bicipital groove. (B) Speed's test. The patient complains of pain at the bicipital groove with the forearm in supination and downward resistance against shoulder flexion. (C) The O'Brien test. The patient complains of pain at the bicipital groove during resisted arm flexion with 30 degrees of arm adduction and the forearm in full pronation.

PERTINENT PHYSICAL FINDINGS

- ▶ Best LHBT tests:
  - ▷ "One-finger pain" at the bicipital groove, approximately 7 cm below the acromion with the arm in 10 degrees of internal rotation (Figure 14-2A)
  - ▷ Complete symptom relief after injection of local anesthetic at the bicipital groove
- ▶ Positive LHBT/SLAP tests:
  - ▷ Speed's test (Figure 14-2B)
  - ▷ O'Brien test (Figure 14-2C)

PERTINENT IMAGING

- ▶ X-rays: anteroposterior, axillary, and acromion outlet views
- ▶ Noncontrast magnetic resonance imaging (MRI) findings (Figure 14-3):
  - ▷ Fluid at the anterior bursa and bicipital groove
  - ▷ LHBT thickening and increased signal
  - ▷ Tendon subluxation out of the groove
- ▶ Ultrasound (Figure 14-4): Compare to the contralateral side; LHBT swelling and abnormal tendon signal within the groove.

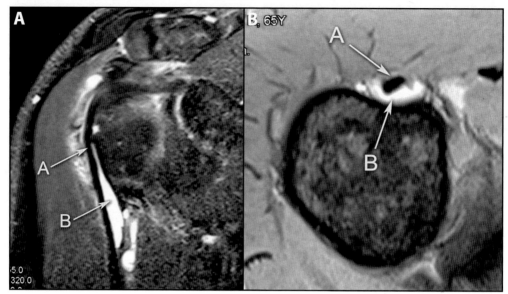

Figure 14-3. Preoperative imaging. Noncontrasted MRI. (A) Coronal view. Fluid at the anterior bursa and bicipital groove. (B) Axial view. LHBT thickening and increased signal.

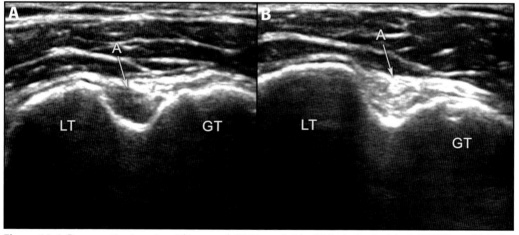

Figure 14-4. Preoperative imaging. Ultrasound. (A) Normal side. (B) Pathologic side. A, LHBT lies within the groove; GT, greater tuberosity; LT, lesser tuberosity.

EQUIPMENT

This procedure requires standard arthroscopic equipment with a 30-degree view arthroscope (Table 14-1). A radiofrequency device (VAPR VUE Radiofrequency System [Mitek Sports Medicine]) for coagulation and tissue vaporization is necessary to prevent bleeding and obtain clear visualization. In most cases, cannulas are not used. However, a specially designed cannula (PassPort Button Cannula [Arthrex]) can be useful for deltoid retraction, and an 8.25-mm cannula (Clear Cannula [Mitek Sports Medicine]) is recommended to stabilize the tendon and to avoid spinning during the interference screw insertion. There are many devices in the market to perform these techniques. Mainly 2 different systems are utilized to fix the biceps tenodesis at the suprapectoral area with interference screws. Both systems are suitable for LHBT fixation at the

Table 14-1. Required Equipment: Devices and Tools for the Long Head of the Biceps Tendon Tenodesis

SUPPLY	PRACTICE DETAILS
Ultrasound	Interscalene block and preoperative LHBT evaluation compared to the contralateral side
Brain oximetry	Safety management while the patient is in the beach chair position
Arthroscopic pump	Default pressure: 35 mm Hg. Flow: 80%. Increased up to 50 mm Hg during surgery based on blood pressure and visualization.
Standard shoulder instruments set	Suture and tissue management
Radiofrequency device	Coagulation and tissue vaporization
Cannula 8.25-mm wide	Prevent tendon spinning
Passport button cannula	Deltoid retraction to increase room and visualization

humerus and do not require whip stitched or externalization of the tendon. The Biceps SwiveLock (Arthrex) has a forked tip (built-in) that pushes the tendon into the socket, remaining inside the socket after delivering the screw, whereas in the MILAGRO BR Biceps Tenodesis System (Mitek Sports Medicine), a fork steers the tendon into the bone and then the system is withdrawn before screwing the final implant.

POSITIONING AND PORTALS

The beach chair position is preferred for any type of anterior shoulder extra-articular procedure because the patient can tolerate the procedure with only a plexus block, and the anatomic landmarks are easier recognized and 3D surgical orientation is less demanding. This position allows easier control of shoulder and elbow flexion and rotation during surgery. Furthermore, the fact that the scope is located at the lateral portal during the large part of the procedure further emphasizes the advantage of using the beach chair over the lateral decubitus position.

This outpatient procedure is performed under an interscalene block. During surgery, patients receive an intravenous infusion of propofol, titrated to achieve light sleep. For optimal surgical visualization, intraoperative systolic blood pressure is maintained at about 110 mm Hg. For safety reasons, the authors recommend measuring regional brain oxygen saturation with disposable scalp transducers.

STEP-BY-STEP DESCRIPTION OF THE PROCEDURE

Step 1: Portals and Tendon Evaluation

The entire scapula and arm are prepped and draped to allow unrestricted access to the anterior and posterior shoulder structures. After drawing the bony landmarks of the acromion lateral and anterior edge, acromion spine, and coracoid tip on the skin, 4 arthroscopic portals are established

Figure 14-5. Right shoulder. Arthroscopic portals. (1) Posterior portal. (2) Lateral portal. (3 and 4) Anterosuperior and anteroinferior portals.

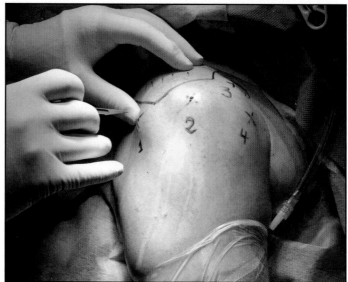

Figure 14-6. Right shoulder. Arthroscopic view of glenohumeral joint from the posterior portal. During the Ramp test, the LHBT looks frayed and degenerated. BT, biceps tendon; HH, humeral head.

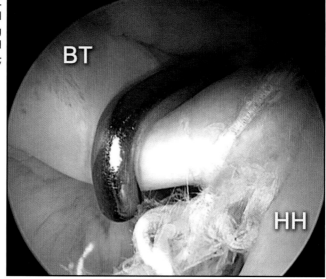

as follows. The posterior portal enables evaluation of the glenohumeral joint and LHBT. This portal is located 2 cm distal and 2 cm medial to the posterolateral corner of the acromion. The lateral portal is created between the middle and anterior third of the humeral head, 3 cm lateral from the acromion lateral edge. Two anterior portals are established with an outside-in technique at the proximal and distal points of the bicipital groove (Figure 14-5).

The shoulder is held in 30 degrees of flexion, approximately 10 degrees of internal rotation, and 30 degrees of abduction, allowing distension of the subacromial bursa and ensuring a clear view of the bicipital groove. The elbow is flexed 90 degrees to relax tension from the biceps tendon.

With the scope at the posterior portal and a probe through the anterosuperior portal, a thorough inspection of the glenohumeral joint is made. The Ramp test is performed for intra-articular LHBT examination (Figure 14-6). Furthermore, the LHBT is grabbed at the entrance of the bicipital groove with a suture manipulator clamp and the tendon is pulled into the glenohumeral joint, which improves access for tendon inspection (about 4 cm).

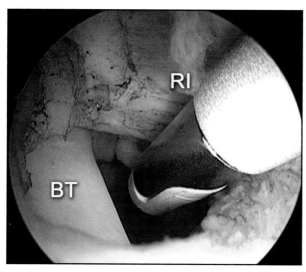

Figure 14-7. Right shoulder. Arthroscopic view of the subacromial space from the lateral portal. After opening the rotator interval, the LHBT is identified from above. BT, biceps tendon; RI, rotator interval.

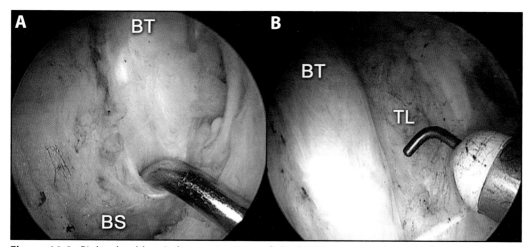

Figure 14-8. Right shoulder. Arthroscopic views of the bicipital groove from the lateral portal. The transverse ligament and the roof of the bicipital groove were detached with a radiofrequency device. BS, bicipital sheath; BT: biceps tendon; TL, transverse ligament.

When the rotator cuff is torn, the LHBT is readily recognized from the subacromial space. In the setting of an intact cuff, the surgeon scopes from the glenohumeral joint and a tiny opening of the rotator interval is made just anterior to the LHBT. Then, moving the scope to the lateral portal at the subacromial space, the tendon is identified from above (Figure 14-7).

Step 2: Tendon Release

With the scope at the lateral portal and using the anterosuperior portal for instrumentation, the roof of the bicipital groove, the transverse humeral ligament, as well as the tendon sheath are excised (Figure 14-8). Dissection requires special care due to the proximity of these structures with the underlying tendon. Typically, this maneuver is performed from proximal to distal up to the level of the falciform ligament at the upper part of pectoralis major tendon. An alternate way to dissect these structures is to go from distal to proximal. After an adequate anterior bursectomy, the surgeon can identify the pectoralis major tendon at its proximal edge and release the LHBT from this distal landmark to proximal (Figure 14-9).

Figure 14-9. Right shoulder. Arthroscopic view from the lateral portal. Proper debridement enables exposure of involved structures. BT, biceps tendon; PMT, pectoralis major tendon.

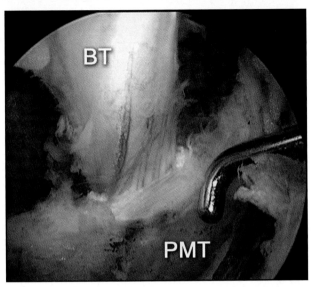

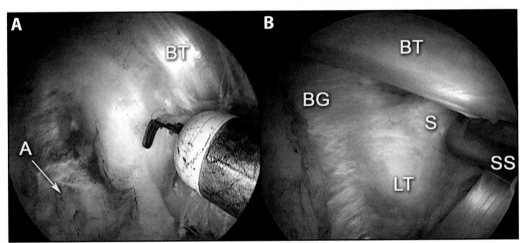

Figure 14-10. Right shoulder. Arthroscopic views of the bicipital groove from the lateral portal. Following LHBT displacement from the groove, the preferred location for LHBT tenodesis is determined and marked with radiofrequency. Working as a retractor, a switching stick through the subscapularis holds the LHBT out of the groove. BG, bicipital groove; BT, biceps tendon; LT, lesser tuberosity; S, subscapularis; SS, switching stick.

Step 3: Reaming the Bone Socket

After an adequate LHBT dissection, surgeon should be able to move the tendon freely. A switching stick is used through the subscapularis to retract the tendon medially out of the groove during the drilling process (Figure 14-10). With a bullet tip reamer, the surgeon drills a 20-mm deep bone socket approximately 10 mm above the pectoralis major tendon. A caliper determines tendon width. The drill bit diameter is oversized at 1 mm. Typically, a 9-mm diameter tunnel is drilled for female patients and a 10-mm diameter tunnel is drilled for male patients. Usually, screw diameters are 8 and 9 mm, respectively, for females and males. For both genders, screw length is approximately 20 mm (range 19.5 to 23 mm). Drilling at the bicipital groove should be precisely perpendicular to the bony surface because any angulation of the reamer may enlarge the tunnel outlet and jeopardize final fixation (Figure 14-11).

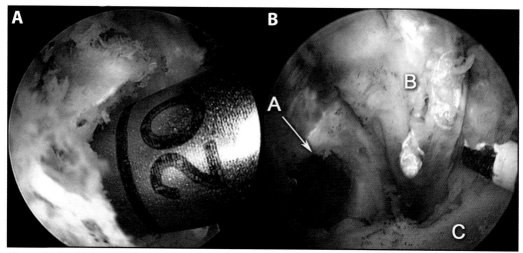

Figure 14-11. Right shoulder. Arthroscopic view from the lateral portal. (A) A 20-mm deep bone socket is drilled using a bullet tip reamer. (B) [A] Bone socket. [B] Biceps tendon. [C] Pectoralis major tendon.

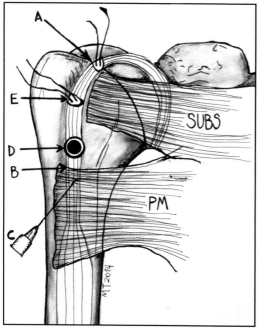

Figure 14-12. Right shoulder. Illustration indicating the relevant anatomy for an arthroscopic biceps tenodesis. (A) Tag stitch at the articular cartilage edge. (B) Superior border of the pectoralis major tendon. (C) Spinal needle fixes the LHBT distal segment to the pectoralis major tendon. (D) Bone socket. (E) Target level (TL), located either 2 to 2.5 cm above the socket level or halfway between the bone socket and the articular cartilage level.

Step 4: Restoring the Correct Length-Tension Relation

A main objective of the tenodesis procedure is to restore the normal length-tension relation of the tendon.[28-30] As the tunnel is 20-mm long and the tendon will run down and then up the socket, the LHBT segment that will be steered into the tunnel should be 40- to 45-mm long.

To obtain a normal length-tension relation, the buried segment must derive from the tendon proximal to the bone socket. Therefore, it is best to use a spinal needle to fix the biceps tendon to the pectoralis major immediately distal to the bone tunnel (Figure 14-12). By doing so, the authors prevent steering of the distal tendon segment into the socket. The latter frequently leads to overtensioning and, hence, technical failure.

Figure 14-13. Right shoulder. Intraoperative photograph of ASBT. (A) Arthroscope is located at the lateral portal. (B) A switching stick holds the LHBT out of the groove. (C) Anteroinferior portal. (D) A spinal needle stabilizes the LHBT distal segment. (E) Built-in forked tip implant.

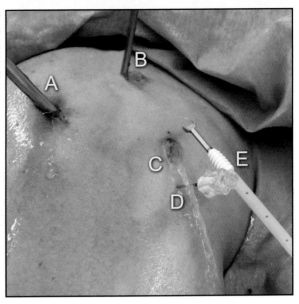

Despite the fact of patients' specific anatomy sizes and variations, based on Denard and colleagues' mean anatomic measurements,[30] the surgeon must take into account such distances to plan the correct tension. Average distances and strategic approach needed to ensure correct tension during tenodesis are detailed in Figure 14-12.

From LHBT origin at the labrum up to the articular cartilage edge, tendon length averages 25 mm. Before tenotomy, the authors perform a tag stitch through the tendon precisely at the level of the cartilage rim. This surgical gesture holds the tendon after tenotomy and acts as a useful landmark for additional measurements.

The mean tendon length from the level of the cartilage rim up to the superior border of the pectoralis major tendon is approximately 50 to 55 mm. Bone socket location should be 10 mm above the pectoralis major tendon. Therefore, the distance between the bone socket and the holding stitch is 40 to 45 mm. A sizer can be used to take the measurements; however, any instrument can work for this task as a caliper.

If the planned interference screw is 20-mm long, then the forked tip should grab the tendon 20 to 25 mm above the socket level or approximately halfway between the superior edge of the pectoralis major tendon and the articular cartilage rim. This place is defined as the *target level* (TL; see Figure 14-12).

Step 5: Tenotomy and Interference Screw Fixation

After retrieving the sutures of the superior tag stitch from the posterior portal, tenotomy is performed with radiofrequency right before interference screw fixation.

There are a number of systems for biceps tenodesis in the market; however, all of them share the same principles. Some implants have a polyetheretherketone forked tip as part of the insert to push the tendon inside the socket.[31] This tip stays inside the bone with the screw (Figures 14-13 and 14-14). In other devices, the fork is part of the instruments and it comes out before screw fixation.

In devices where the forked tip is cannulated and an integral part of the implant, additional tendon control can be obtained by delivering another tag suture through the tendon at the TL. By loading the sutures tails through the eyelets at the implant tip, the surgeon can easily steer the tendon inside the socket, obtaining an optimal length-tension relation.

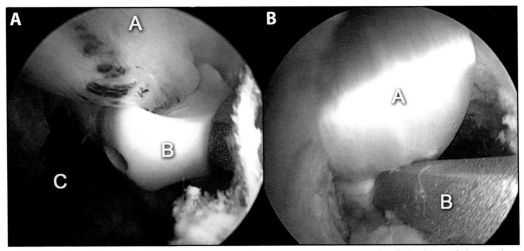

Figure 14-14. Right shoulder. Arthroscopic view from the lateral portal. The forked tip of the implant introduces the LHBT into the bone socket. (A) [A] LHBT. [B] Forked tip of the implant. [C] Bone socket. (B) [A] LHBT. [B] Implant shaft.

When the fork is part of the instruments, a pin can be used through the fork to pinch the tendon at the TL prior to steering the tendon into the bony socket. Use depth indicators on the distal end of the tendon fork to ensure the tendon is fully seated into the socket. A trocar tipped guide wire is placed through the fork to hold the tendon into the socket. After removing the fork, the implant is screwed in guided by the pin. An 8.25-mm wide cannula is used to press the tendon against the bone and prevent tendon spinning. The screw is left flush. Further depression of the screw into the socket can decrease fixation strength.[32,33]

If the authors have restored normal length-tension, the proximal tag suture would lay adjacent to the fixation site (Figure 14-15). The fixation is then probed with a hook and during elbow motion. The remaining tendon is trimmed and the arthroscopic portals are closed with figure-8 stitches (Figure 14-16).

POSTOPERATIVE PROTOCOL

The use of a shoulder brace is recommended for 4 weeks. Progressive range of motion exercises are allowed 3 weeks after surgery. Resisted elbow flexion and forearm supination are contraindicated for 2 months. Because symptom recovery is faster than the tissue-healing process, it is essential to emphasize patient compliance to postoperative protocol. Strengthening and gradual return to sports are expected between 3 and 5 months after surgery. Postoperative x-rays and MRI are required to determine adequate tendon healing before full return to high-demanding activities (Figure 14-17).

POTENTIAL COMPLICATIONS

There is a steep-to-moderate learning curve to achieve the adequate surgical skills to perform ASBT. Due to intraoperative bleeding and visualization problems, the procedure may require conversion to an open subpectoral tenodesis. During the last 3 years, the authors have performed 46 ASBT in 44 patients and no patient required conversion to open surgery. At medium-term clinical follow-up (mean 14 months, range 6 to 32 months), the authors observed fixation failure ("Popeye sign") in 4 cases (8.6%) and residual pain at the groove in 3 (6.5%) cases.

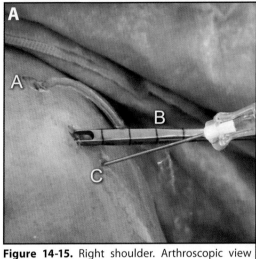

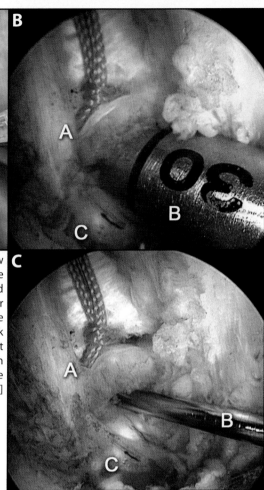

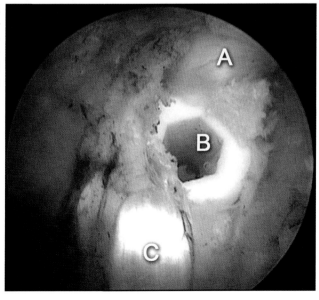

Figure 14-15. Right shoulder. Arthroscopic view from the lateral portal. (A) Different systems where the fork constitutes part of the instruments and comes out before final fixation. [A] Anterosuperior portal. [B] Forked instrument. [C] Spinal needle stabilizing the LHBT distal segment. (B) The fork steers the tendon into the socket. [A] Tag suture at the LHBT. [B] Forked instrument. [C] LHBT. (C) A pin holds the LHBT into the socket after retrieving the forked instrument. [A] Tag suture at the LHBT. [B] Pin. [C] LHBT.

Figure 14-16. Right shoulder. Arthroscopic view from the lateral portal. After trimming the redundant proximal segment, tendon stability is evaluated. (A) Biceps proximal segment. (B) Interference screw flushed to the bone surface at the socket outlet.

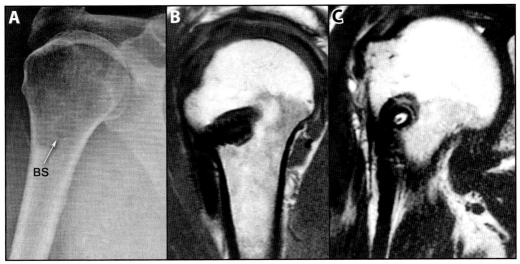

Figure 14-17. Postoperative imaging findings. (A) Anteroposterior x-ray showing the bone socket at the suprapectoral area. (B, C) MRI coronal slices demonstrating adequate tendon healing at the bone socket.

CONCLUSION

Even though the best place and technique to fix the LHBT at the proximal humerus is still controversial, ASBT constitutes a valuable surgical option for young patients or athletes. The procedure is safe and holds several advantages. Mainly, ASBT allows resection of the entire proximal segment of the LHBT and all of its associated structures that are often the source of residual pain. Furthermore, the open subpectoral tenodesis with distal fixation near a narrow diaphysis has a greater risk of humeral fracture.

Based on encouraging early results, the authors recommend the previously mentioned technique for the surgical management of the LHBT disorders of the patient with high-demanding activities.

TOP TECHNICAL PEARLS FOR THE PROCEDURE

1. To ensure a pleasant surgery, place the patient in the beach chair position, use the scope through the lateral portal, and create 2 anterior portals for introduction of surgical tools.

2. All of the dissections and tissue removal need to be done with a radiofrequency device. Surgeons should be aware of the vascular bundles medial to the LHBT in order to prevent bleeding complications.

3. Retract and hold the tendon out of the groove with a switching stick and use the reamer in a precisely perpendicular fashion to the bone. Perform oversize drilling (1 mm wider than the intended screw).

4. Only steer into the socket tendon segment that originated proximally to the socket. To do that, it is best to fix the distal biceps tendon to the pectoralis major with a spinal needle.

5. Defining a TL to pinch the tendon equidistant from the articular cartilage rim and the socket location is another important step to restore normal length-tension restoration.

REFERENCES

1. Slenker N, Lawson K, Ciccotti M, Dodson C, Cohen S. Systematic review. Biceps tenotomy versus tenodesis: clinical outcomes. *Arthroscopy.* 2012;28(4):576-582.

2. Wolf R, Zheng N, Weichel D. Long head biceps tenotomy versus tenodesis: a cadaveric biomechanical analysis. *Arthroscopy.* 2005;21(2):182-185.

3. Mariani EM, Cofield RH, Askew LJ, Li G, Chao E. Rupture of the tendon of the long head of the biceps brachii. Surgical vs non-surgical treatment. *Clin Orthop Relat Res.* 1998; 228:233-239.

4. Shank J, Singleton S, Braun S, et al. Comparison of forearm supination and elbow flexion strength in patients with long head of the biceps tenotomy or tenodesis. *Arthroscopy.* 2011;27(1):9-16.

5. Sanders B, Lavery K, Pennington S, Warner J. Biceps tendon tenodesis: success with proximal versus distal fixation. *Arthroscopy.* 2008;24(6):9.

6. Lemos D, Esquivel A, Duncan D. Outlet biceps tenodesis: a new technique for treatment of biceps long head tendon injury. *Arthrosc Tech.* 2013;2(2):e83-e88.

7. Jarrett CD, McClelland WB Jr, Xerogeanes JW. Minimally invasive proximal biceps tenodesis: an anatomical study for optimal placement and safe surgical technique. *J Shoulder Elbow Surg.* 2011;20(3):477-480.

8. Lutton D, Gruson K, Gladstone J, Flatow E. Where to tenodese the biceps: proximal or distal? *Clin Orthop Relat Res.* 2011;469(4):1050-1055.

9. Sethl P, Rajaram A, Beitzel K, Hackett T, Chowaniec D, Mazzocca A. Biomechanical performance of subpectoral biceps tenodesis: a comparison of interference screw fixation, cortical button fixation and interference screw diameter. *J Shoulder Elbow Surg.* 2013;22(4):451-457.

10. Richards D, Burkhart S. A biomechanical analysis of two biceps tenodesis fixation techniques. *Arthroscopy.* 2005;21(7):861-866.

11. Scully WF, Wilson DJ, Grassbaugh JA, Branstetter JG, Marchant BG, Arrington ED. A simple surgical technique for subpectoral biceps tenodesis using a double-loaded suture anchor. *Arthrosc Tech.* 2013;2(2):e191-e196.

12. Koch B, Burks R. Failure of biceps tenodesis with interference screw fixation. *Arthroscopy.* 2012;28(5):735-740.

13. Nho SJ, Reiff SN, Verma NN, Slabaugh MA, Mazzocca AD, Romeo AA. Complications associated with subpectoral biceps tenodesis: low rates of incidence following surgery. *J Shoulder Elbow Surg.* 2010;19(5):764-768.

14. Dickens J, Kilcoyne K, Tintle S, Giuliani J, Rue J. Subpectoral biceps tenodesis: an anatomic study and evaluation of at-risk structures. *Arthroscopy.* 2011;27(5):e40-e41.

15. Gothelf T, Bell D, Goldberg J, et al. Anatomic and biomechanical study of the biceps vinculum, a structure within the biceps sheath. *Arthroscopy.* 2009;25(5):515-521.

16. Mac Donald K, Bridger J, Cash C, Parkin I. Transverse humeral ligament: does it exist? *Clin Anat.* 2007;20(6):663-667.

17. Alpantaki K, McLaughlin D, Karagogeos D, Hadjipavlou A, Kontakis G. Sympathetic and sensory neural elements in the tendon of the long head of the biceps. *J Bone Joint Surg Am.* 2005;87(7):1580-1583.

18. Gleason PD, Beall DP, Sanders TG, et al. The transverse humeral ligament: a separates anatomic structure or a continuation of the osseous attachment of the rotator cuff? *Am J Sports Med.* 2006;34(1):72-77.

19. Soifer T, Levy H, Miller-Soifer F, Kleinbart F, Vigorita V, Bryk E. Neurohistology of the subacromial space. *Arthroscopy.* 1996;12(2):182-186.

20. Snow B, Narvy S, Omid R, Atkinson R, Vangsness T. Anatomy and histology of the transverse humeral ligament. *Orthopaedics.* 2013;36(10):1295-1298.

21. Arora A, Singh A, Koonce R. Biomechanical evaluation of a unicortical button versus interference screw for subpectoral biceps tenodesis. *Arthroscopy.* 2013;29(4):638-644.

22. Mazzocca A, Bicos J, Santangelo S, Romeo A, Arciero R. The biomechanical evaluation of four fixation techniques for proximal biceps tenodesis. *Arthroscopy.* 2005;21(11):1296-1306.

23. Golish R, Caldwell P, Miller M, et al. Interference screw versus suture anchor fixation for subpectoral tenodesis of the proximal biceps tendon: a cadaveric study. *Arthroscopy.* 2008;24(10):1003-1108.

24. Buchholz A, Martetschlager F, Siebenlist S, et al. Biomechanical comparison of intramedullary cortical button fixation and interference screw technique for subpectoral biceps tenodesis. *Arthroscopy.* 2013;29(5):845-853.

25. Kim SH, Yoo JC. Arthroscopic biceps tenodesis using interference screw: end-tunnel technique. *Arthroscopy*. 2005;21(11):1405.

26. Boileau P, Krishnan S, Coste JS, Walch G. Arthroscopic biceps tenodesis: a new technique using bioabsorbable interference screw fixation. *Arthroscopy*. 2002;18(9):1002-1012.

27. Werner B, Hakan P, Hart J, et al. Biceps tenodesis is a viable option for salvage of failed SLAP Repair. *J Shoulder Elbow Surg*. 2014;13(8):e179-e184.

28. David T, Schildhorn JC. Arthroscopic suprapectoral tenodesis of the long head biceps: reproducing an anatomic length-tension relationship. *Arthrosc Tech*. 2012;1(1):e127-e132.

29. Patzer T, Rundic J, Bobrowitsch E, Olender G, Hurschler C, Shofer M. Biomechanical comparison of arthroscopically performable techniques for suprapectoral biceps tenodesis. *Arthroscopy*. 2011;27(8):1036-1047.

30. Denard P, Dai X, Hanypsiak B, Burkhart S. Anatomy of the biceps tendon: implications for restoring physiological length-tension relation during biceps tenodesis with interference screw fixation. *Arthroscopy*. 2012;28(10):1352-1358.

31. Lorbach O, Trennheuser C, Kohn D, Anagnostakos K. The biomechanical performance of a new forked knotless biceps tenodesis compared to a standard knotless and suture anchor tenodesis. *Arthroscopy*. 2013;29(10):e91-e92.

32. Slabaugh M, Frank R, Van Thiel G, et al. Biceps tenodesis with interference screw fixation: a biomechanical comparison of screw length and diameter. *Arthroscopy*. 2011;27(2):161-166.

33. Slata M, Bailey J, Bell R, et al. Effect of interference screw depth on fixation strength in biceps tenodesis. *Arthroscopy*. 2014;30(1):11-15.

Please see videos on the accompanying website at

www.ArthroscopicTechniques.com

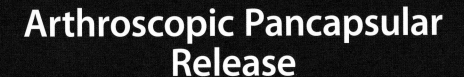

15

Arthroscopic Pancapsular Release

Katy Morris, MD and James Esche, MD

INTRODUCTION

In 1934, Codman inscribed that adhesive capsulitis was "difficult to define, difficult to treat, and difficult to explain from the point of view of pathology."[1] Today, idiopathic adhesive capsulitis remains a condition of unknown etiology where both passive and active range of motion are restricted, most notably in external rotation. Neviaser and Neviaser[2] described 4 stages of the condition. Romeo et al[3] later biopsied shoulders in each stage and reported their histological findings. Stage I is defined as the presence of night pain and loss of external rotation. Full range of motion returns after an intra-articular injection. No adhesions or capsular contractures are seen on arthroscopic evaluation. Capsular tissue is normal on biopsy, whereas the synovium is hypervascular and hypertrophic. In stage II, or the *freezing stage*, the pain remains and the degree of forward flexion, abduction, and internal and external rotation is reduced, even after an intra-articular injection. The biopsy of stage II shoulders has demonstrated the same degree of synovitis as stage I but with added perivascular and subsynovial capsular scarring. Stage III is referred to as the *frozen stage*. Patients complain mostly of stiffness and pain at the extremes of motion. On arthroscopic evaluation, there is a loss of the axillary fold. A hypercellular collagen-rich matrix with less synovitis is seen on biopsy. The *thawing stage*, or stage IV, is characterized by less pain and a gradual return of motion. Direct visualization of the capsule reveals mature adhesions. There have been no data on the histopathology of stage IV.

Treatment of idiopathic adhesive capsulitis ranges from skillful neglect to surgical intervention. Few studies have reported on nominal treatment. Grey[4] published successful results in 24/25 patients with use of simple analgesics at a minimum of 2 years. However, Hand et al[5] more recently published on 269 shoulders with adhesive capsulitis. They reported only 59% of patients having normal/near normal results using the Oxford Shoulder Score and 41% with ongoing symptoms, mostly mild in nature. These 2 studies most likely vary significantly because of the variable outcome measures used. Nonoperative treatments such as NSAIDs, oral steroids, intra-articular steroid injections, and physical therapy have been studied with varying results. Different NSAIDs and dosages have been compared to one another with no detectable dissimilarity in effect.[6,7]

Ryu RKN, Angelo RL, Abrams JS, eds. *The Shoulder:*
AANA Advanced Arthroscopic Surgical Techniques (pp 181-188).
© 2016 AANA.

The level I and II studies focusing on oral steroid efficacy suggest short-term pain relief when compared to control subjects, but this advantage was unsustainable long term.[8-10] Griesser et al[11] published a systematic review on the effectiveness of intra-articular steroid injections. The majority of the studies showed improved clinical outcome measures and passive shoulder motion at early follow-up. Similar to the oral steroid literature, these advantages over the comparison treatments were transient and equalized at latest follow-up.

Despite the limited literature showing its benefit, physical therapy is the most popular treatment modality for adhesive capsulitis. A Cochrane database review found no strong evidence to support the use of therapy alone as treatment.[12] Lower-level evidence does point to gentle stretching and painless active motion as a beneficial treatment option.[13-15]

Both manipulation under anesthesia (MUA) and arthroscopic capsular release are frequently utilized for patients who have failed nonoperative treatment. Based on a retrospective chart review, Levine et al[16] suggested patients were more likely to require operative intervention if their pain and range of motion were initially more severe, they were younger at time of onset, or they failed to respond to 4 months of therapy. Prior to the rise in arthroscopy, MUA was the standard of care for the management of adhesive capsulitis. Level IV studies by Dodenhoff et al[17] and Farrell et al[18] suggest that MUA provides sustainable symptomatic improvement in patients where other less invasive treatments had failed to provide relief. Conversely, the level I study published by Kivimaki et al[19] reported only slightly better forward flexion at 3 months when compared to the home exercise group.

Arthroscopic evaluation and capsular release has replaced MUA as the most utilized treatment of refractory adhesive capsulitis. It allows for complete inspection of the joint, confirmation of the diagnosis, and staging of the disease. The benefits of arthroscopic capsular release have been reported in many published studies. In a level III study, patients were twice as likely to have painless range of motion at 2-year follow-up when compared to MUA.[20] Both Ide and Takagi[21] and Le Lievre and Murrell[22] reported significant early improvements in pain and range of motion after capsular release with durable results at a mean of 7.5 and 7 years, respectively.

Currently, the degree of arthroscopic release is unresolved. Most are in agreement that release of the rotator interval, middle glenohumeral ligament, and anterior band of the inferior glenohumeral ligament is necessary. Resection of the posterior capsule arguably benefits patients with internal rotation deficits. However, Snow et al[23] challenge this benefit by reporting no difference in range of motion when a posterior release is incorporated. A 360-degree capsular release with or without a partial resection of the intra-articular portion of the subscapularis has gained popularity. Jerosch,[24] Le Lievre and Takagi,[22] and LaFosse et al[25] report satisfactory results utilizing slightly different circumferential capsular releases.

The goal for this chapter is to present the principal findings in the diagnostic evaluation of a patient with primary adhesive capsulitis as well as the step-by-step process the authors employ when performing a pancapsular release for refractory cases.

Indications

▶ Loss of passive and active range of motion refractory to at least 4 to 6 months of gentle progressive stretching (physical therapy or home therapy program)

Controversial Indications

▶ Single stage rotator cuff repair in a stiff shoulder
▶ Superior migration of humeral head with rotator cuff tear
▶ Capsular release coupled with debridement for glenohumeral osteoarthritis

PERTINENT PHYSICAL FINDINGS

- Loss of external rotation with arm at the side
- Pain at end ranges of shoulder motion and night pain (early findings)
- No specific areas of tenderness
- Referred pain to origin of deltoid
- Loss of both passive and active range of motion
- External rotation and abduction most notably affected
  - ▷ Mild: external rotation > 45 degrees
  - ▷ Moderate: external rotation < 45 degrees
  - ▷ Severe: external rotation < 10 degrees
- Extension and adduction rarely affected

PERTINENT IMAGING

- Radiographs: normal
- Magnetic resonance imaging: not necessary for diagnosis. May see thickening of coracohumeral ligament and capsule within rotator interval. Also, loss of axillary pouch volume can be seen on magnetic resonance arthrogram. This is reported more frequently by radiologist but with little clinical correlation.

EQUIPMENT

- 30- and 70-degree arthroscopes
- Arthroscopic shaver with oscillating feature
- Arthroscopic tissue biters/scissors
- Radiofrequency unit

POSITIONING AND PORTALS

- Positioning: Beach chair and lateral decubitus positions are acceptable for the arthroscopic capsular release. The authors prefer the lateral decubitus position with the arm placed in suspension at 50 to 60 degrees of abduction with 10 to 12 lbs of balanced suspension.
- Portals: posterior and anterior (established using outside-in method)

STEP-BY-STEP DESCRIPTION OF THE PROCEDURE

- Peripheral nerve block administered by anesthesia using ultrasound. Single injection vs continuous infusion via a catheter
- Examination under anesthesia: evaluate the passive range of motion of both the affected and unaffected shoulders. Document forward elevation, external rotation, and internal rotation in 0 degrees of abduction and 90 degrees of abduction and cross-body motion.

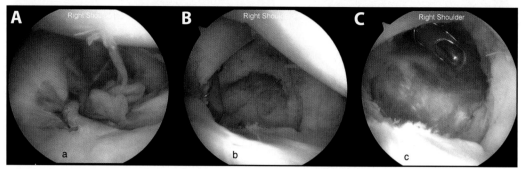

Figure 15-1. (A) Synovitis in rotator interval. (B, C) Removal of synovium.

▶ Place the patient in a lateral decubitus position with suspension/tension as outlined previously.

▶ Gentle MUA: Begin with flexion followed by rotation and then adduction. Usually, a patient's flexion, adduction, and external rotation improve. One does usually not obtain internal rotation with the arm at 90 degrees.

▶ Sterile preparation of the skin with sterile draping

▶ Establish posterior portal

▶ Anterior portal established using either the inside-out or outside-in technique

▶ Diagnostic intra-articular shoulder examination. Evaluate for findings of synovitis, thickened capsule, and loss of intra-articular volume.

▶ Complete the release of the rotator interval tissue, including the superior glenohumeral ligament. Identification of the coracoid process is key to avoiding debriding too far medially. Use of an arthroscopic shaver and/or radiofrequency device is acceptable. The coracohumeral ligament should also be released at this time (Figure 15-1).

▶ Complete the anterior release from the 1 to 6 o'clock position along the labrum. Care should be taken to stay in the capsule adjacent to the labrum to protect other structures. This will free the anterior capsule, subscapularis bursa, middle glenohumeral ligament, and anterior band of the inferior glenohumeral ligament. Underlying subscapularis tendon and muscle tissue is visible following adequate release. Use of a 70-degree arthroscope from the posterior portal can facilitate viewing the release as it proceeds to the inferior capsule (Figure 15-2).

▶ Complete the superior release from the 11 to 1 o'clock position. This includes the complete release of the superior glenohumeral ligament and superior capsule. Care is taken not to release the biceps or violate the rotator cuff/supraspinatus (Figure 15-3).

▶ Using switching sticks, place arthroscopic camera through anterior portal and shaver/radiofrequency device through the posterior portal.

▶ Complete the posterior release, resecting the capsule from the 11 to the 6 o'clock position. The release should be performed close to labrum. This will free the posterior capsule and posterior band of the glenohumeral ligament. The release should connect to the inferior extent of the anterior release. The axillary nerve can be visualized encased in adipose tissue in the interval between the infraspinatus and teres minor muscle tissue around the 6 o'clock position. Utilizing a 70-degree arthroscope from the anterior portal can facilitate visualization of the posterior-inferior capsular during the release (Figures 15-4 and 15-5).

▶ Subacromial evaluation: perform lysis of any adhesions if adhesions are present. Subacromial decompression is usually not necessary, and many patients with idiopathic frozen shoulder have a normal subacromial bursoscopy.

▶ Re-manipulate and document the range of motion achieved.

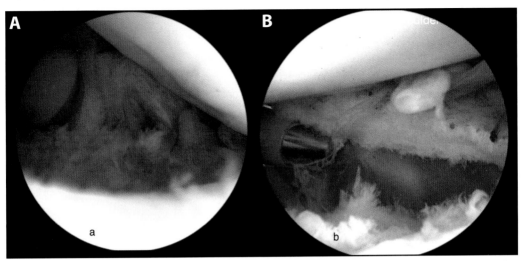

Figure 15-2. Anterior release. (A) Intact capsule and middle glenohumeral ligament. (B) Resected capsule/ middle glenohumeral ligament. Subscapularis muscle fibers are visible.

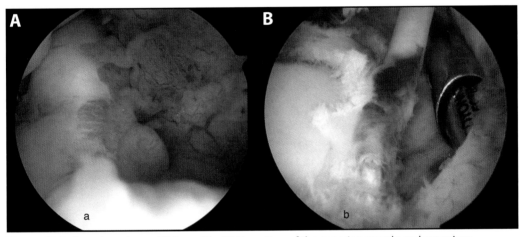

Figure 15-3. Superior release. (A) Synovitis. (B) Resection of the superior capsule and synovium.

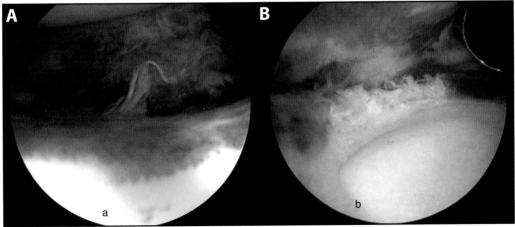

Figure 15-4. Posterior release. (A) Synovitis, capsular thickening. (B) Resection of posterior capsule and synovium.

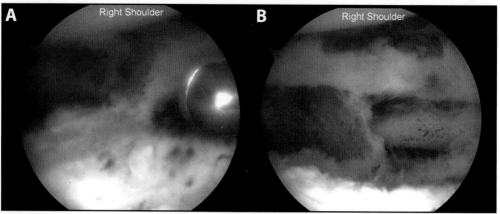

Figure 15-5. Inferior capsule. (A) Inferior capsule resection. (B) Axillary nerve encased in fat, visualized between the infraspinatus and teres minor muscle fibers.

POSTOPERATIVE PROTOCOL

Formal physical therapy program begins on postoperative day 0 or 1. This program includes a therapy session 5 days per week for 3 weeks. Therapy focuses on passive and active-assisted range of motion. Continuous passive motion devices are used between physical therapy sessions set for a comfortable range of motion. The most important element of the postoperative program is the avoidance of pain while going through the range of motion exercises. The exercises are performed 4 to 5 times per day for 5 to 6 minutes each. Strengthening is not initiated until a near full, painless range of motion is accomplished.

POTENTIAL COMPLICATIONS

► Recurrent stiffness

► Anterior dislocation

► Axillary nerve palsy

TOP TECHNICAL PEARLS FOR THE PROCEDURE

1. Arthroscopic pancapsular release should be performed only after failure of at least 4 to 6 months of gentle progressive stretching.

2. When releasing the capsule from the glenoid, remain within 1 to 2 cm of the labrum to avoid injury to significant structures (subscapularis, axillary nerve).

3. Utilizing the inside-out technique to establish the anterior portal is often helpful in an exceptional stiff shoulder when visualization of the subscapularis border is difficult due to the contractures and scarring.

4. Axillary nerve can be visualized surrounded in adipose tissue between the infraspinatus and teres minor at the 6 to 7 o'clock position.

5. Be aggressive in resecting the capsule. At the conclusion of a thorough release, muscle should be visible at all of the margins of the release.

REFERENCES

1. Codman EA. *The Shoulder: Rupture of the Supraspinatus Tendon and Other Lesions in or About the Subacromial Bursa.* Boston, MA: Thomas Todd Company; 1934:514.

2. Neviaser RJ, Neviaser TJ. The frozen shoulder: diagnosis and management. *Clin Orthop Relat Res.* 1987;223:59-64.

3. Rodeo SA, Hannafin JA, Tom J, Warren RF, Wickiewicz TL. Immunolocalization of cytokines and their receptors in adhesive capsulitis of the shoulder. *J Orthop Res.* 1997;15:427-436.

4. Grey RG. The natural history of "idiopathic" frozen shoulder. *J Bone Joint Surg Am.* 1978;60:564.

5. Hand C, Clipsham K, Rees JL, Carr AJ. Long-term outcome of frozen shoulder. *J Shoulder Elbow Surg.* 2008;17:231-236.

6. Rhind V, Downie WW, Bird HA, Wright V, Engler C. Naproxen and indomethacin in periarthritis of the shoulder. *Rheumatol Rehabil.* 1982;21:51-53.

7. Duke O, Zecler E, Grahame R. Anti-inflammatory drugs in periarthritis of the shoulder: a double-blind, between patient study of naproxen versus indomethacin. *Rheumatol Rehabil.* 1981;20:54-59.

8. Blockey NJ, Wright JK, Kellgren JH. Oral cortisone therapy in periarthritis of the shoulder: a controlled trial. *Br Med J.* 1954;1:1455-1457.

9. Buchbinder R, Hoving JL, Green S, Hall S, Forbes A, Nash P. Short course prednisolone for adhesive capsulitis (frozen shoulder or stiff painful shoulder): a randomized, double blind, placebo controlled trial. *Ann Rheum Dis.* 2004;63:1460-1469.

10. Binder A, Hazelman BL, Parr G, Roberts S. A controlled study of oral prednisolone in frozen shoulder. *Br J Rheumatol.* 1986;25:288-292.

11. Griesser MJ, Harris JD, Campbell JE, Jones GI. Adhesive capsulitis of the shoulder: a systematic review of the effectiveness of intra-articular corticosteroid injections. *J Bone Joint Surg Am.* 2011;93:1727-1733.

12. Green S, Buchbinder R, Hetrick S. Physiotherapy interventions for shoulder pain. *Cochrane Database Syst Rev.* 2003;CD004258.

13. Diercks RL, Stevens M. Gentle thawing of the frozen shoulder: a prospective study of supervised neglect versus intensive physical therapy in seventy-seven patients with frozen shoulder syndrome followed up for two years. *J Shoulder Elbow Surg.* 2004;13:499-502.

14. Vermeulen HM, Rozing PM, Oberman WR, le Cessie S, Vliet Vlieland TP. Comparison of high-grade and low-grade mobilization techniques in the management of adhesive capsulitis of the shoulder: a randomized controlled trial. *Phys Ther.* 2006;86:355-368.

15. Griggs SM, Ahn A, Green A. Idiopathic adhesive capsulitis: a prospective functional outcome study of nonoperative treatment. *J Bone Joint Surg Am.* 2000;82:1398-1407.

16. Levine WN, Kashyap CP, Bak SF, Ahmad CS, Blaine TA, Bigliani LU. Nonoperative management of idiopathic adhesive capsulitis. *J Shoulder Elbow Surg.* 2007;16:569-573.

17. Dodenhoff RM, Levy O, Wilson A, Copeland SA. Manipulation under anesthesia for primary frozen shoulder: effect on early recovery and return to activity. *J Shoulder Elbow Surg.* 2000;9:23-26.

18. Farrell CM, Sperling JW, Cofield RH. Manipulation for frozen shoulder: long-term results. *J Shoulder Elbow Surg.* 2005;14:480-84.

19. Kivimaki J, Pohjolainen T, Maimivaara A, et al. Manipulation under anesthesia with home exercises versus home exercises alone in the treatment of frozen shoulder: a randomized, controlled trial with 125 patients. *J Shoulder Elbow Surg.* 2007;16:722-726.

20. Ogilvie-Harris DJ, Biggs DJ, Fishtails DP, MacKay M. The resistant frozen shoulder: manipulation versus arthroscopic release. *Clin Orthop Relat Res.* 1995;(319):238-248.

21. Ide J, Takagi K. Early and long-term results of arthroscopic treatment for shoulder stiffness. *J Shoulder Elbow Surg.* 2004;13:174-179.

22. Le Lievre HM, Murrell GAC. Long-term outcomes after arthroscopic capsular release for idiopathic adhesive capsulitis. *J Bone Joint Surg Am.* 2012;94:1208-1216.

23. Snow M, Boutros I, Funk L. Posterior arthroscopic capsular release in frozen shoulder. *Arthroscopy.* 2009;25:19-23.

24. Jerosch J. 360 degrees arthroscopic capsular release in patients with adhesive capsulitis of the gle-nohumeral joint: indication, surgical technique, results. *Knee Surg Sports Traumatol Arthrosc.* 2001; 9:178-186.
25. LaFosse L, Boyle S, Kordasiewicz B, et al. Arthroscopic arthrolysis for recalcitrant frozen shoulder: a lateral approach. *Arthroscopy.* 2012;28:916-923.

Please see videos on the accompanying website at

www.ArthroscopicTechniques.com

16

Arthroscopic Anterior Glenoid Bone Block Stabilization

Hiroyuki Sugaya, MD

INTRODUCTION

Significant bone loss, often characterized by an inverted-pear glenoid or engaging Hill-Sachs lesion, is believed to be a main cause of failures after arthroscopic stabilization.[1-3] According to a 3-dimensionally reconstructed computed tomography (3DCT) study, the prevalence of glenoid bone defect has been reported as high as 90% in shoulders with chronic recurrent traumatic anterior instability, and an associated bony fragment is present in about half of shoulders with glenoid bone loss.[4] Further, bone loss in shoulders associated with a bony fragment is relatively significant compared to that in shoulders with attritional glenoid loss without a bony fragment.[4,5] According to the authors' previous study, although the fragment normally diminishes in size with time,[6] most of the shoulders with a significant glenoid defect retain a bony fragment when evaluated by 3DCT.[7,8] However, recently, many surgeons have tended to perform an open or arthroscopic Latarjet procedure regardless of the presence of a bony fragment. They believe they cannot rely on soft tissue repair alone or a bony Bankart repair using a relatively small fragment compared with the glenoid defect size.[9-13] This tendency occurs despite the fact that the Latarjet procedure is nonanatomic and has a potential risk of nerve injury.[14,15] The authors recently published a mid- to long-term follow-up of arthroscopic bony Bankart repairs for chronic shoulder instability in which more than 15% of glenoid bone loss was present. Follow-up revealed that glenoid morphology can normalize over time even when the retained glenoid fragment is relatively small.[16] Therefore, the majority of shoulders with significant bone loss and a retained fragment can be treated with an arthroscopic bony Bankart repair, which is a less invasive and more anatomic procedure.[5,16] However, although the prevalence is limited,[7,8] shoulders with little or no retained glenoid bone fragment do exist. The authors believe that these shoulders constitute the primary indication for bone grafting procedures, either with a free bone graft[8,17,18] or a coracoid transfer.[9-12] The stabilizing mechanisms in the coracoid transfer are a combination of restoring the glenoid arc and the sling effect of the conjoined tendon.[19,20] However, in the free bone grafting procedure, capsulolabral reconstruction is mandatory because stability is very dependent on the restoration of capsular integrity.[21,22] In this chapter, the arthroscopic bone block procedure combined with capsulolabral reconstruction using a "suicide" portal to insert screws parallel to the glenoid surface will be introduced in detail.

Ryu RKN, Angelo RL, Abrams JS, eds. *The Shoulder:*
AANA Advanced Arthroscopic Surgical Techniques (pp 189-197).

INDICATIONS

▶ Significant glenoid bone loss, which is more than approximately 20% to 25% loss of the inferior glenoid arc (diameter), with or without a very small bone fragment when associated with healthy capsule (robust with minimal evidence for attenuation or tearing)

Controversial Indications

▶ Significant glenoid bone loss with a relatively small bone fragment associated with a healthy capsule in a patient who is young and active (otherwise, arthroscopic bony Bankart repair is indicated)

▶ Significant glenoid bone loss with or without a very small fragment in association with an unhealthy capsule (in this instance, coracoid transfer is indicated since the normal capsular restraint to translation cannot be expected)

PERTINENT PHYSICAL FINDINGS

▶ Range of motion should be measured for both shoulders, especially external rotation with the arm at the side.

▶ Test for the presence of apprehension with the shoulder in abduction and external rotation.

▶ The most important and reliable physical examination for translational laxity can usually be obtained with the patient under anesthesia, comparing stability to the contralateral shoulder.

PERTINENT IMAGING

▶ A modified Bernageau view: a posteroanterior view with the patient lying on the affected axilla in his or her most relaxed position with the beam oriented 30 degrees caudally and directed toward the scapular spine. It is the most reliable and useful x-ray method.[8] In this method, clear x-ray images can be obtained more easily with a high probability of ascertaining bony pathology without using fluoroscopic imaging.[8,23]

▶ A 3DCT is the most accurate imaging study to assess glenoid morphology.[4,5,24] Determine whether the glenoid loss is attritional or due to a bony Bankart lesion. Quantify attritional bone loss or the size and shape of the bony glenoid fragment when present.[4,5,25]

▶ Although plain magnetic resonance imaging provides only limited information, magnetic resonance arthrography can be helpful when detecting soft tissue pathology such as a Bankart lesion, capsular damage, and/or a humeral avulsion of the glenohumeral ligament lesion. (However, the final diagnosis of soft tissue pathology can be made most accurately with a thorough diagnostic arthroscopy.)

EQUIPMENT

▶ Osteotomes for the iliac crest bone harvesting

▶ A 30-degree, 4-mm scope and standard shoulder arthroscopy tower

▶ Short 2- and 3.5-mm drill bits for graft preparation (Figure 16-1)

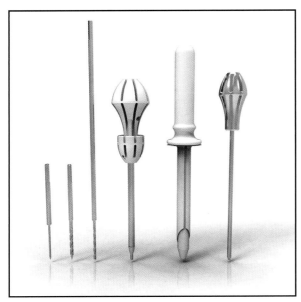

Figure 16-1. Free Bone Graft Kit (DePuy Synthes). From left to right, short 2- and 3.5-mm drill for graft preparation, cannula and cannulated obturator for screw insertion, slit graft introducer, and screwdriver.

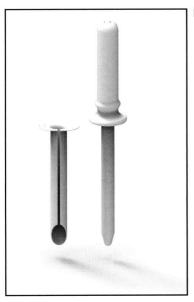

Figure 16-2. A slit graft introducer (left) and obturator (right).

- A long 2.7-mm drill bit (see Figure 16-1)
- Single-loaded suture anchor for a temporary bone graft fixation
- A slit graft introducer (see Figures 16-1 and 16-2)
- Cannula and cannulated obturator for screw insertion (see Figures 16-1 and 16-3)
- A long guide wire
- 3.5-mm screws
- A long screwdriver (see Figure 16-1)

Figure 16-3. Cannula and cannulated obturator for screw insertion. The tip of the obturator protrudes about 5 mm from the tip of the cannula so that the tip can be inserted to the hole in the graft providing for optimal control and positioning of the graft.

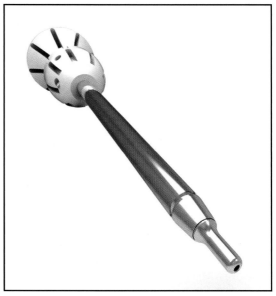

POSITIONING AND PORTALS

Patients are first placed on the beach chair positioner in the supine position under general anesthesia for harvesting a tricortical bone graft from the ipsilateral iliac crest. The patient is then raised to the beach chair position and joint laxity is assessed prior to insertion of the arthroscope into the glenohumeral joint. The entire arthroscopic procedure is carried out with the patients in the beach chair position.

STEP-BY-STEP DESCRIPTION OF THE PROCEDURE

Step 1: Harvesting the Iliac Bone Graft

An iliac tricortical bone graft 20 mm in length and 10 mm in depth is harvested from the iliac crest with the patient in the supine position prior to arthroscopy. The graft is then prepared for insertion in order to fit the configuration of the anteroinferior portion of the native glenoid as demonstrated on preoperative 3DCT. One drill hole is created using a short 3.5-mm drill to accommodate 3.5-mm cannulated screw insertion into the graft, and another 2 small holes are also created in the center of the graft using a short 2-mm drill for sutures from the suture anchor for temporary graft fixation (see Figures 16-1 and 16-4).

Step 2: Arthroscopic Evaluation and Mobilization of the Complex

A 4-mm arthroscope is introduced through a standard posterior portal and a diagnostic arthroscopy is performed. An anterior portal is then created through the rotator interval.[26] Inspection is performed from the anterior portal. The arthroscope is then returned to the posterior portal and, with working instruments inserted through the anterior portal, separation and mobilization of the labroligamentous complex from the glenoid neck is performed to around the 7:30 position (right

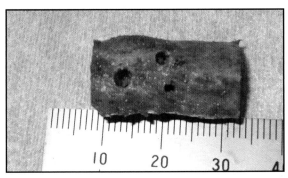

Figure 16-4. Iliac tricortical bone is harvested from the iliac crest. The graft is prepared for insertion in order to fit the configuration of the anteroinferior portion of the native glenoid. One large drill hole using the short 3.5-mm drill and 2 small holes using the short 2-mm drill are created prior to introduction of the graft into the joint.

shoulder) until the complex becomes completely free. The freed complex is retracted laterally with a retraction suture placed through the labrum percutaneously. Then, an anterosuperior portal is established at the anterosuperior margin of the rotator interval as the second working portal.[26]

Step 3: Introduction of the Bone Graft

First, the rotator interval capsule is partly resected in order to insert a slit graft introducer (see Figure 16-2), through the anterior portal to assist in graft delivery. A suture anchor loaded with #2 high strength suture, is inserted at the 3:30 position on the edge of the glenoid. Then the sutures are retrieved through the slit graft introducer. Both suture limbs are passed through the 2 previously prepared 2-mm holes in the center of the graft. The graft is then maneuvered into the glenohumeral joint through the slit graft introducer by pulling on these suture limbs while pushing on the graft itself. The graft is then fixed temporarily by knot tying of these sutures. The slit graft introducer is then removed.

Step 4: Making the Suicide Portal

The scope is introduced into the subacromial bursa from the posterior portal. Then, a postero-lateral portal (2 to 3 cm lateral to the posterolateral corner of the acromion) and anterolateral portal (2 to 3 cm lateral to the anterolateral corner of the acromion) are created exactly the same as for rotator cuff surgery. The scope is switched to the posterolateral portal and a shaver is introduced through the anterolateral portal. Bursal debridement continues until the coracoacromial ligament, base of the coracoid, and conjoined tendon become clearly visible. The scope is then introduced to the anterolateral portal and the glenoid and graft are clearly visible through the opening in the rotator interval (Figure 16-5A). Then, with the scope remaining in the anterolateral portal, the scope is redirected into the space between the conjoined tendon and the pectoralis major, and this space is debrided until the pectoralis minor tendon becomes visible using a shaver introduced from the anterior portal. Next, a switching rod is introduced from the posterior portal and the subscapularis is penetrated at the level of the center of the graft. The rod is then pushed through the subscapularis muscle and through the space between the conjoined tendon and the pectoralis minor (Figure 16-5B). Finally, the rod is pushed through the pectoralis major muscle and a small skin incision is made where the tip of the switching rod protrudes (Figures 16-5C and 16-6).

Step 5: Iliac Bone Graft Fixation

Next, a cannula for screw delivery is introduced over the switching rod and inserted into the glenohumeral joint through the subscapularis muscle by slowly withdrawing the rod while pushing on the cannula. A cannulated obturator is inserted into the cannula with the tip positioned at the screw hole of the graft (see Figure 16-3). A guide wire is then inserted through this cannulated

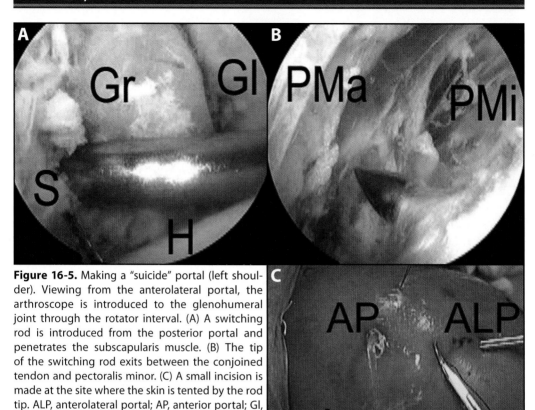

Figure 16-5. Making a "suicide" portal (left shoulder). Viewing from the anterolateral portal, the arthroscope is introduced to the glenohumeral joint through the rotator interval. (A) A switching rod is introduced from the posterior portal and penetrates the subscapularis muscle. (B) The tip of the switching rod exits between the conjoined tendon and pectoralis minor. (C) A small incision is made at the site where the skin is tented by the rod tip. ALP, anterolateral portal; AP, anterior portal; Gl, glenoid; Gr, bone graft; H, humeral head; PMa, pectoralis major; PMi, pectoralis minor; S, subscapularis. * indicates the exact location of the "suicide" portal.

Figure 16-6. The "suicide" portal in relation to other portals. The arthroscope is inserted in the anterolateral portal (ALP). The cannula for screw insertion is inserted at site of the "suicide" portal (SP). AP, anterior portal.

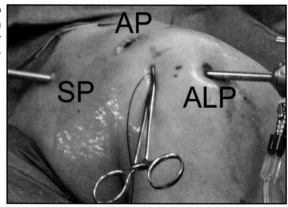

obturator, through the graft, across the glenoid neck, and out of the posterior skin where it is clamped. This prevents accidental removal of the guide wire after drilling. The cannulated obturator is then removed and a hole is drilled across the glenoid neck using the long cannulated 2.7-mm drill bit. After drilling, a 3.5-mm diameter cannulated cancellous screw of 30 mm in length (DePuy Synthes) is inserted through this cannula to the superior portion of the graft. The same procedure is then repeated in order to insert another screw into the inferior portion of the graft (Figure 16-7A).

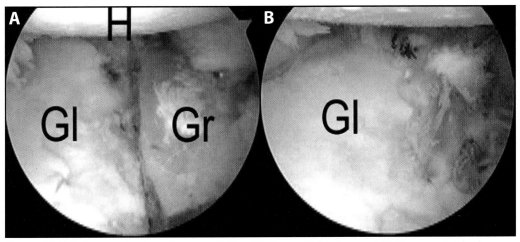

Figure 16-7. Arthroscopic view after completing (A) the graft fixation and (B) the capsulolabral reconstruction. Both images are views from the anterior portal. Gl, glenoid; Gr, graft; H, humeral head.

Step 6: *Anteroinferior Capsulolabral Repair*

The capsulolabral complex, which was previously mobilized, is then reattached to the native glenoid using another 3 to 4 biocomposite suture anchors loaded with #2 high strength suture in the same manner as a routine Bankart repair (Figure 16-7B).

POSTOPERATIVE PROTOCOL

The shoulder is immobilized for 3 weeks using a sling (Ultra Sling II [Donjoy]). At 3 weeks, passive and active-assisted exercises are initiated for forward flexion and external rotation while avoiding pain. After 6 weeks, the patient begins gentle strengthening exercises of the rotator cuff and scapular stabilizers. Three months after the operation, the patient is permitted to practice noncontact sports. Full return to throwing or contact sports is allowed after 6 months, according to the individual's functional recovery. The same postoperative protocol is used after a standard Bankart repair as well as that described previously for the iliac bone grafting of the glenoid.

POTENTIAL COMPLICATIONS

► Damage to neurovascular structures is a possible complication due to the proximity to these structures. Therefore, care should be taken when penetrating the subscapularis muscle and medial side of the conjoined tendon using a blunt switching rod.

► Other potential technical complications related to graft screw fixation such as graft fracture, inappropriate screw orientation, screw length discrepancy, and glenoid articular damage can be avoided by excellent visualization from the anterolateral portal

► Guide wire may cause posterior neurovascular injury when penetrating posterior skin if it is not inserted relatively parallel to the glenoid surface. However, since one of the great advantages in this anterior approach using the suicide portal is parallel fixation of the guide wires and screws, this risk can be minimized.

TOP TECHNICAL PEARLS FOR THE PROCEDURE

1. Recognize the configuration of the anteroinferior portion of the glenoid using preoperative 3DCT and trim the graft in order to fit the native glenoid.

2. Retract the released capsulolabral complex using a traction suture in order to keep enough working space during the graft fixation (see Figure 16-5).

3. Create the "suicide" portal safely and introduce the cannula and cannulated obturator as described.

4. Insert the first guide wire to the optimal position so that the graft becomes flush with the glenoid surface, then penetrate the posterior skin and clamp it. This prevents accidental removal of the guide wire after drilling.

5. Take care not to intersect and damage the screws used in the graft fixation while drilling for subsequent anchor insertion for the capsulolabral repair.

REFERENCES

1. Burkhart SS, De Beer JF. Traumatic glenohumeral bone defects and their relationship to failure of arthroscopic Bankart repairs: significance of the inverted-pear glenoid and the humeral engaging Hill-Sachs lesion. *Arthroscopy*. 2000;16:677-694.

2. Boileau P, Villalba M, Héry JY, Balg F, Ahrens P, Neyton L. Risk factors for recurrence of shoulder instability after arthroscopic Bankart repair. *J Bone Joint Surg Am*. 2006;88:1755-1763.

3. Lo, IY, Parten, PM, Burkhart, SS. The inverted pear glenoid: an indicator of significant glenoid bone loss. *Arthroscopy*. 2004;20:169-174.

4. Sugaya H, Moriishi J, Dohi M, Kon Y, Tsuchiya A. Glenoid rim morphology in recurrent anterior glenohumeral instability. *J Bone Joint Surg Am*. 2003;85:878-884.

5. Sugaya H, Moriishi J, Kanisawa I, Tsuchiya A. Arthroscopic osseous Bankart repair for chronic recurrent traumatic anterior glenohumeral instability. *J Bone Joint Surg Am*. 2005;87A:1752-1760.

6. Nakagawa S, Mizuno N, Hiramatsu K, Tachibana Y, Mae T. Absorption of the bone fragment in shoulders with bony Bankart lesions caused by recurrent anterior dislocations or subluxations: when does it occur? *Am J Sports Med*. 2013;41:1380-1386.

7. Maeda K, Sugaya H, Mochizuki T, Moriishi J. [The inverted-pear glenoid in recurrent anterior glenohumeral instability.] *Shoulder Joint (Katakansetsu)*. 2005;29:507-510.

8. Sugaya H. Instability with bone loss. In Angelo RL, Esch J, and Ryu RKN, eds. *AANA Advanced Arthroscopy: The Shoulder*. Philadelphia, PA: Elsevier; 2010:136-146.

9. Latarjet M. Techniques chirugicales dans le trairement de la luxation anteriointerne recidivante de l'epaule. *Lyon Chir*. 1965;61:313-318.

10. Lafosse L, Lejeune E, Bouchard A, Kakuda C, Gobezie R, Kochhar T. The arthroscopic Latarjet procedure for the treatment of anterior shoulder instability. *Arthroscopy*. 2007;23:1242.e1-5.

11. Dumont GD, Fogerty S, Rosso C, Lafosse L. The arthroscopic Latarjet procedure for anterior shoulder instability: 5-year minimum follow-up. *Am J Sports Med*. 2014;42:2560-2566.

12. Boileau P, Thélu CÉ, Mercier N, et al. Arthroscopic Bristow-Latarjet combined with Bankart repair restores shoulder stability in patients with glenoid bone loss. *Clin Orthop Relat Res*. 2014;472:2413-2424.

13. Bessière C, Trojani C, Carles M, Mehta SS, Boileau P. The open Latarjet procedure is more reliable in terms of shoulder stability than arthroscopic Bankart repair. *Clin Orthop Relat Res*. 2014;472:2345-2351.

14. Delaney RA, Freehill MT, Janfaza DR, et al. 2014 Neer Award Paper: neuromonitoring the Latarjet procedure. *J Shoulder Elbow Surg*. 2014;23:1473-1480.

15. Sastre S, Peidro L, Méndez A, Calvo E. Suprascapular nerve palsy after arthroscopic Latarjet procedure: a case report and review of literature. *Knee Surg Sports Traumatol Arthrosc*. 2014 May 18. [Epub ahead of print]

16. Kitayama S, Sugaya H, Takahashi N, et al. Clinical outcome and glenoid morphology after arthroscopic chronic bony Bankart repair: a 5 to 8 year follow-up. *J Bone Joint Surg Am*. 2015. In press.

17. Scheibel M, Kraus N, Diederichs G, Haas NP. Arthroscopic reconstruction of chronic anteroinferior glenoid defect using an autologous tricortical iliac crest bone grafting technique. *Arch Orthop Trauma Surg*. 2008;128:1295-1300.

18. Warner JJ, Gill TJ, O'hollerhan JD, Pathare N, Millett PJ. Anatomical glenoid reconstruction for recurrent anterior glenohumeral instability with glenoid deficiency using an autogenous tricortical iliac crest bone graft. *Am J Sports Med*. 2006;34:205-212.

19. Yamamoto N, Muraki T, An KN, et al. The stabilizing mechanism of the Latarjet procedure: a cadaveric study. *J Bone Joint Surg Am*. 2013;95:1390-1397.

20. Giles JW, Boons HW, Elkinson I, et al. Does the dynamic sling effect of the Latarjet procedure improve shoulder stability? A biomechanical evaluation. *J Shoulder Elbow Surg*. 2013;22:821-827.

21. Gelber PE, Reina F, Monllau JC, Yema P, Rodriguez A, Caceres E. Innervation patterns of the inferior glenohumeral ligament: anatomical and biomechanical relevance. *Clin Anat*. 2006;19:304-311.

22. Jerosch J, Castro WH, Halm H, Drescher H. Does the glenohumeral joint capsule have proprioceptive capability? *Knee Surg Sports Traumatol Arthrosc*. 1993;1:80-84.

23. Bernageau J. [Imaging of the shoulder in orthopedic pathology.] *Rev Prat*. 1990;40:983-992.

24. Chuang TY, Adams CR, Burkhart SS. Use of preoperative three-dimensional computed tomography to quantify glenoid bone loss in shoulder instability. *Arthroscopy*. 2008;24:376-382.

25. Mologne TS, Provencher MT, Menzel KA, Vachon TA, Dewing CB. Arthroscopic stabilization in patients with an inverted pear glenoid: results in patients with bone loss of the anterior glenoid. *Am J Sports Med*. 2007;35:1276-1283.

26. Sugaya H, Kon Y, Tsuchiya A. Arthroscopic Bankart repair in the beachchair position: a cannulaless method using an intra-articular suture relay technique. *Arthroscopy*. 2004;20(Suppl 2):116-120.

Please see videos on the accompanying website at

www.ArthroscopicTechniques.com

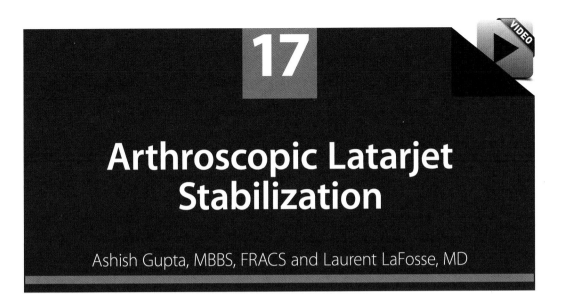

INTRODUCTION

Anteroinferior shoulder dislocation is a common shoulder injury that occurs in young patients. Numerous surgical advances have been made over the last 3 decades to manage this common and difficult condition. As shoulder arthroscopy has evolved, surgeons have started understanding the spectrum of different pathologies that may be included within the diagnosis of anterior shoulder instability. Arthroscopy and advanced radiological imaging has facilitated an understanding of glenoid and humeral bone loss, humeral avulsion of glenohumeral ligament lesions, anterior labral periosteal sleeve avulsion lesions, and glenoid erosions.

Bankart repair, the Bristow procedure, the Latarjet, and autogenous bone grafting of the glenoid have stood the test of time and remain viable options in treating this patient population. The challenge is choosing the most appropriate technique that is reproducible with the fewest complications, lowest revision rates, and early return to full function, combined with good long-term results.

A common belief exists that repair of the labrum and reinsertion of the capsule will stabilize the shoulder and restore normal function. However, the success of the Bankart repair depends on the strength of the often pathologic capsulolabral complex, commonly combined with a degree of glenoid bone loss, which is not addressed at the time of surgical repair.

Various authors have demonstrated that the arthroscopic Bankart procedure is prone to a high failure rate when performed in the wrong patient subset. Balg and Boileau reported a failure rate of 14.5% for Bankart repairs, which led them to propose the Instability Severity Index Score.[1]

Latarjet described a coracoid transfer procedure in 1954.[2] This procedure has since seen many modifications prior to the current stage. The subscapularis is no longer detached, 2 screws are utilized to fix the transferred coracoid to the glenoid rim, and the exact positioning of the graft has changed. Patte and Debeyre[3] explained the triple block effect of the Latarjet: the first is creating the labral capsular repair; the second is the coracoid increasing the surface area of the glenoid and thereby preventing a Hill-Sachs lesion from engaging; and third, but perhaps the most important, is the dynamic sling effect of the conjoined tendon and the subscapularis muscle preventing the

Ryu RKN, Angelo RL, Abrams JS, eds. *The Shoulder:*
AANA Advanced Arthroscopic Surgical Techniques (pp 199-217).
© 2016 AANA.

humeral head to dislocate in abduction and external rotation. These findings have been confirmed biomechanically.[4]

Why an Arthroscopic Latarjet?

The authors performed the first arthroscopic Latarjet in 2003. The technique has evolved significantly over the last 10 years with over 500 cases. It has become more streamlined, safer, and reproducible. Over this time frame, the arthroscopic Latarjet poses some distinct advantages over the open Latarjet, including the following:

► Arthroscopy allows the assessment of the quality of the ligamentous structures and assessment of chronic glenoid bone loss that is not apparent on imaging studies. Concomitant shoulder lesions such as superior labral anteroposterior (SLAP) tears, posterior labral tears, and loose bodies can be dealt with in the same setting.

► If the quality of the capsule labral structures is deemed poor or the bone defect is considered larger than anticipated preoperatively, the procedure can be easily converted to a Latarjet arthroscopically.

► The multiple views offered by the arthroscope enable the surgeon to quantify the glenoid and humeral bone loss better and thereby helps in proper placement of the coracoid bone graft.

► Complex bidirectional anterior and posterior instability can be dealt with in the same procedure.

► Arthroscopy offers the advantage of less postoperative scarring and pain, thereby enabling a quicker return to function.

INDICATIONS

► Glenoid bone loss: Most cases of recurrent anterior shoulder instability are associated with glenoid bone loss. This ranges from 70% to 90% in various studies.[5-7] Sugaya et al demonstrated that 90% of patients in their study group had a glenoid rim lesion.[8] The concept of "inverted pear glenoid" has been popularized by Lo et al.[9] In their study, Burkhart and Debeer demonstrated a large failure rate when a Bankart procedure was performed with > 25% bone loss.[10] This was further validated by Itoi et al.[6] Excessive bone loss (especially in active patients) has become a common indication to proceed with a Latarjet.

Bone loss can be quantified preoperatively by a Bernageau view (Figure 17-1).[11] This view has been validated to be an accurate measure of glenoid erosion/bone loss.[12,13] At the authors' institution, they routinely order bilateral Bernageau radiographs for both shoulders and compare the anteroposterior glenoid measurements (Figure 17-2).

In order to quantify the glenoid bone loss and assess the depth and size of the Hill-Sachs, a preoperative 3D computed tomography (CT) scan is routinely performed in all patients. An end "en face" view of the glenoid gives excellent visualization of the extent and location of the glenoid defect. Other authors have reported the same.[14]

Note: The authors believe that bone loss is common and an absolute number should not be used as the sole guide of an indication for a Latarjet. It should be considered in conjunction with the Hill-Sachs defect, quality of tissue, demands of the patient, and hyper laxity.

► Hill-Sachs defect: The size and location of humeral bone loss varies in each case. Saito et al demonstrated that the lesion usually exists between 0 to 24 mm from the top of the humeral head.[15] It is well-accepted that a large Hill-Sachs defect with or without glenoid bone loss is a significant contributor to recurrent instability. For small- to moderate-sized defects, both

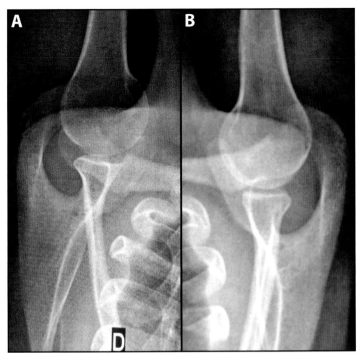

Figure 17-1. The Bernageau view demonstrates the chronic anterior glenoid bone loss in the left shoulder compared to the contralateral shoulder.

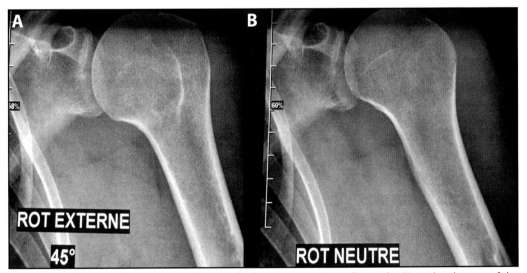

Figure 17-2. The same lesion is noted on standard anteroposterior radiographs. Note the absence of the anterior sclerotic rim of the glenoid inferiorly, demonstrating a chronic anterior rim erosion.

remplissage[16] and Latarjet have been proposed as treatment options.[17,18] For large-sized defects, osteochondral grafts and surface arthroplasty are surgical options.[19,20]

The Latarjet increases the joint surface area and the congruent arc, decreasing the joint surface contact pressure. There is no limitation to the range of external rotation, depending on how the anterior capsule is treated.

The remplissage procedure advances the capsule and infraspinatus into the defect, thus preventing anterior subluxation of the head. It does limit the degree of external rotation. The extent of this limitation depends on the technique utilized.[21] The clinical relevance of this reduced external rotation remains controversial.

Figure 17-3. Engaging Hill-Sachs noted along with glenoid bone loss during the initial examination.

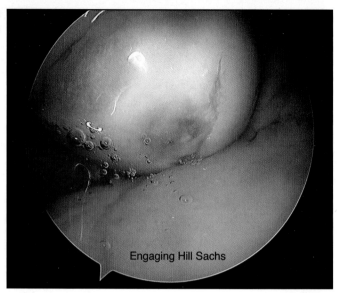

Engaging Hill Sachs

Figure 17-4. Glenoid bone loss noted, visualizing from the D portal.

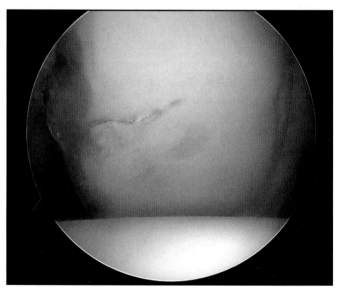

Note: The authors believe that a Latarjet increases the congruent arc and the dynamic sling effect provides significant stability without sacrificing external rotation.

▶ Engaging Hill-Sachs: A Hill-Sachs lesion occurring medial to the glenoid track is defined as an engaging Hill-Sachs as per Itoi et al (Figures 17-3 and 17-4).[6] As demonstrated by Burkhart and Debeer, an engaging Hill-Sachs, if left unaddressed, has an unacceptably high redislocation rate.

Note: The authors believe that identifying an engaging Hill-Sachs lesion intraoperatively is an indication for a Latarjet.

▶ Revision Bankart repair/revision surgery for instability: These patients can be separated into 2 subcategories:

1. Early failures: These are usually the result of undiagnosed bony defects, poor tissue quality, or excessive stresses posed on the repair (patients activity). A revision Bankart procedure has a higher failure rate than a Latarjet procedure in this setting.

2. Late failures: These occur because of repetitive stresses posed upon an already compromised capsule. Usually, the patients have a fairly sedentary lifestyle and redislocate upon commencing contact activity or sports. The primary pathology has been inadequately addressed in these patients and they develop progressive glenoid erosion over time.

▶ Contact athlete or high-risk occupation or sport: Contact athletes have a higher failure rate from a Bankart repair. The Latarjet offers more stability and return to sport. It has been validated that, for sportsmen in contact sports (eg, rugby, judo, wrestling), a Latarjet offers early return to sport, less stiffness, and a lower failure rate.[22,23]

Patients whose occupation puts them at risk, such as a high-rise building construction worker, where a sudden shoulder dislocation could be a life-threatening injury, a Latarjet is a good option.

▶ Quality of the capsulolabral structures: Patients who dislocate at a younger age (ie, age at onset) and who have numerous dislocations prior to the index operation have a significant bearing on the quality of the soft tissues. It is often noted that the capsule in these patients is never well-developed and often stretched due to the repetitive trauma. Trauma combined with generalized ligament laxity may benefit from the dynamic sling effect and increased arc of congruence offered by the Latarjet.

PERTINENT PHYSICAL FINDINGS

The patient undergoes a systematic shoulder exam. The following clinical signs are often seen:

▶ Forward elevation is almost normal. Only a mild reduction is noted. If the patient has significant bone loss or readily dislocates, he or she will not elevate the arm mainly due to apprehension than due to a fixed contracture.

▶ Lack of external rotation is commonly encountered.

▶ Internal rotation with the arm in abduction may be reduced.

▶ Apprehension tests are carried out.

▶ Both shoulders are assessed for asymmetric anterior and posterior drawer tests.

▶ Tests for generalized ligamentous laxity are carried out.

▶ The rotator cuff is tested. A traumatic shoulder dislocation can cause a concomitant cuff tear.

▶ Axillary nerve function is tested.

PERTINENT IMAGING

All patients undergo the following imaging:

▶ Bilateral shoulder anteroposterior radiographs in internal and external rotation

▶ Lateral scapular Y view

▶ Bernageau view (see Figure 17-1)

▶ CT Arthrogram or MRI

▶ 3D CT reconstruction of the "en face" view of the glenoid to evaluate for glenoid bone loss

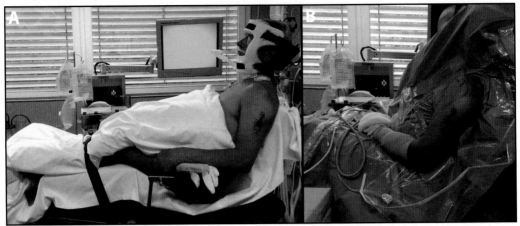

Figure 17-5. Setup in the beach chair position with the extremity free draped. No traction is used.

EQUIPMENT

▶ Standard shoulder arthroscopy equipment with a 30-degree viewing scope

▶ 2 #18 needles

▶ 2 rose-colored (18-gauge) spinal needles

▶ 2 switching sticks (Wissinger rods)

▶ Arthroscopic Latarjet instrumentation set designed by the senior author (DePuy Mitek)

▶ Electrocautery

▶ Shaver with fluid management system pump

POSITIONING AND PORTALS

Patient Setup

This procedure is carried out in the beach chair position under a general anesthetic with an ultrasound-guided interscalene block. A second-generation cephalosporin is used as antibiotic prophylaxis. All of the patients are monitored with a cerebral perfusion monitor to ensure adequate cerebral perfusion (in the beach chair position) throughout the procedure and a hypotensive anesthesia is administered (Figure 17-5).

The T-MAX Attachment (Smith & Nephew) is utilized. The torso is positioned to ensure that the medial edge of the scapula lies on the operating table and the scapula lateral to this edge is visible and accessible. The medial edge being supported enables protraction of the scapula, causing a seesaw effect.

The upper extremity is scrubbed with betadine or chlorhexidine and a sterile operating field is created with the hemithorax exposed and the upper limb freely draped. No traction is applied.

Portals

Multiple portals are created for various steps of this procedure (Figure 17-6). A standard 20-gauge spinal needle is used to guide correct portal placement. All portals are made using a #11 blade and only the skin is pierced. The soft tissue underneath the skin is perforated with the

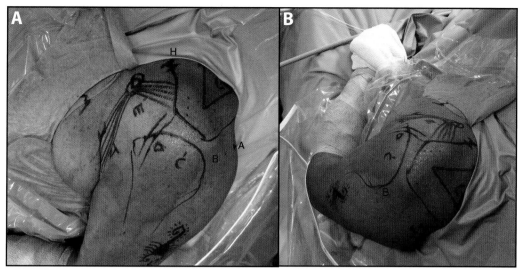

Figure 17-6. Various portals used.

help of the arthroscopic electrocautery, thereby enabling a clean passage for repetitive reinsertion of instruments; this prevents the portals from getting blocked by adjacent soft tissue swelling.

▶ A portal: Standard posterior portal through the soft spot of the shoulder. Used for intra-articular exam of the shoulder and passage of various instruments

▶ B portal: 2 cm lateral and inferior to the posterolateral edge of the acromion. Key portal for posterior labral repairs and SLAP repairs. Not usually used in an arthroscopic Latarjet unless a posterior labrum repair or a posterior bone block procedure is required to address persistent posterior or combined anteroposterior instability

▶ C portal: Standard Lateral portal made at the intersection of lines passing through the clavicle and the spine of the scapula. Must be lateral for ergonomic use of tools

▶ D portal: Made 2 cm inferolateral to the anterolateral edge of the acromion. This workhorse portal is made such that the instruments enter the shoulder directly over the biceps pulley. Portal is used for biceps tenodesis, cuff repairs, subscapularis repairs, and suprascapular nerve decompression. Used as a viewing portal throughout the arthroscopic Latarjet

▶ E portal: Standard anterior portal used for Bankart repairs. Utilized for all of the anterior capsular work

▶ I portal: Made 3 cm inferior to the coracoid just anterior to the anterior axillary fold. Invaluable portal used to obtain an end on view of the coracoid. Critical for coracoid harvesting and coracoid preparation

▶ J portal: Lateral to the I portal. Just lateral to the anterior axillary fold. Used for instrumentation

▶ H portal: Located superomedially to the coracoid and anterior to the clavicle. Is made under direct vision whilst viewing from the I portal. An electrocautery is used to establish the portal once the skin is incised because a tributary of the cephalic vein often needs to be coagulated. Portal is used in the preparation of the coracoid and for conducting the coracoid osteotomy

▶ M (medial) portal: A 2-cm–long portal made medially, lateral to the areola and the breast tissue in women; 5 cm inferior to the clavicle in line with the anteroposterior axis of the glenoid. The skin is incised and deeper dissection is carried out under direct vision to ensure that all of the deeper dissection is carried out lateral to the pectoralis minor, creating safe distance from the brachial plexus and axillary artery. One of the most utilized portals. Instrumental for coracoid preparation, harvesting, and graft placement and fixation

Figure 17-7. Engaging Hill-Sach on initial joint evaluation through the A portal.

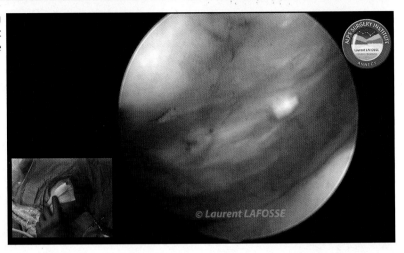

Step-by-Step Description of the Procedure

- ► First stage: Joint evaluation and evidence of engaging
- ► Second stage: Intra-articular joint preparation, capsulectomy, decortication, and marking 2 to 5 glenoid area
- ► Third stage: Coracoid preparation, pectoralis minor, coracoacromial ligament, and conjoined tendon release. MC nerve visualization, plexus visualization
- ► Fourth stage: Coracoid harvesting, Kirschner wires, drilling and top hats, stress riser, and final osteotomy
- ► Fifth stage: Anterior subscapularis preparation and split, axillary nerve visualization, switching stick from A
- ► Sixth stage: Glenoid exposure and final preparation
- ► Seventh stage: Coracoid retrieval with double cannula and final decortication
- ► Eighth stage: Coracoid placement
- ► Ninth stage: Coracoid fixation
- ► Tenth and final stage: Dynamic final joint evaluation

The following is a modification from the original technique previously published[24-26]:

- ► Initial joint visualization: The A portal is utilized and a standard shoulder arthroscopy is performed.
  - ▷ The size of the glenoid defect is established and the Hill-Sachs lesion is evaluated (Figures 17-7 and 17-8).
  - ▷ The shoulder is now abducted and externally rotated and the glenoid track is noted. The ease of the Hill-Sach lesion's engagement with the glenoid bone loss is evaluated; the persistence of dislocation is one of the most critical decision-making steps for deciding to proceed with a Latarjet procedure.
  - ▷ The quality of the anterior capsule is evaluated with a probe inserted through the E portal.
  - ▷ Associated SLAP tears or posterior Bankart lesions are probed.
  - ▷ Associated chondral injury and early arthritic changes are meticulously noted and documented. As the natural history of recurrent shoulder dislocation predisposes these patients to secondary degenerative arthritis.[27,28]
  - ▷ Once a decision is made to proceed with a Latarjet, a D portal is created.

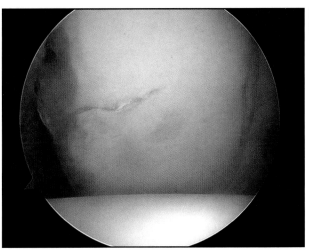

Figure 17-8. Glenoid bone loss noted (visualization through the D portal).

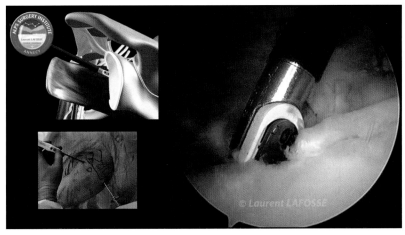

Figure 17-9. Location for the lower extent of the final graft is marked.

▶ Intra-articular joint preparation: With the camera in the A portal, the electrocautery is inserted in the D portal and the pathologic anteroinferior labrum is detached (2 to 6 o'clock; Figure 17-9). The rotator interval is opened and the superior border of the subscapularis is dissected. A transverse capsulotomy is performed in line with the fibers of the subscapularis. Only a small portion of the capsule is excised. This is different from the authors' earlier technique where the capsular excision was more extensive.

▶ Coracoid preparation: The switching stick is inserted in the D portal and is used to retract the deltoid superiorly. The assistant flexes the arm in neutral rotation throughout the coracoid preparation to increase visibility and create a working space.

Coracoid preparation involves a global visualization of the coracoid release and identification of the surrounding neurovascular structures. This is undertaken in 4 systemic steps:

1. Dissection lateral to the coracoid: The arthroscope is introduced into the D portal. A spinal needle is used to plan the I and J portals. Using the I portal, the coracohumeral and acromioclavicular ligaments are excised. Then, the subcoracoid bursa is excised using the electrocautery. This involves both ablation and a sweeping motion to dissect the tissue. Two small vessels, which pass into the muscle fibers of the subscapularis, are coagulated. Numerous small nerves can be seen entering the muscle belly of the subscapularis; vessels in the way of subscapularis split are cauterized. Care must always be taken to point the electrocautery toward the subscapularis and away from the brachial plexus.

Figure 17-10. Coracoid dissection. Visualizing through the J portal. The electrocautery (1 portal) is medial to the coracoid (on the inferior edge of the pectoralis minor).

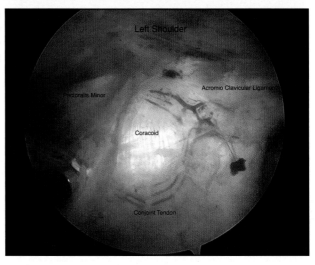

2. Dissection medial to the coracoid: The pectoralis minor tendon is identified and incised with the aid of an electrocautery, always keeping contact with bone. Distally, the junction between the pectoralis minor and the conjoined tendon is identified (Figure 17-10) and this plane is enlarged by blunt dissection. Laterally, the clavipectoral fascia is incised. The electrocautery is used as a blunt dissection probe and the soft tissue medial to the coracoid is teased away. The first structure to be identified is the musculocutaneous nerve. This nerve is always identified and protected. Followed by this, the posterior chord is visualized, which in turn guides the surgeon to the axillary artery. It must be noted that small punctate bleeding that occurs is coagulated using the electrocautery facing away from the plexus, thereby minimizing the risk of thermal injury to the nerves.

3. Dissection under the coracoid: Visualizing through the D portal and alternating between the I and J portals, the lump of fat under the coracoid is excised using cautery. The cautery is switched from the I to the M portal for complete visualization of the undersurface of the coracoid. Bleeders are encountered along the neck of the coracoid undersurface. These must be meticulously coagulated, as a good view of this region is crucial for completing a coracoid osteotomy.

4. Dissection on the superior surface of the coracoid: The superior surface of the coracoid consists of the remnant of the acromioclavicular ligament and bursal tissue. This is easily debrided without any hazard.

A global view of the coracoid must be attained while looking in from the I portal.

► Harvesting the coracoid: Using the spinal needle, the H portal is created. The first assistant controls the arthroscope and a second assistant flexes the arm in neutral rotation, allowing the surgeon to use both hands for completing the steps.

▷ Insertion of the top hats (Figure 17-11): The coracoid drill guide is inserted through the H portal. The ideal spot should be such that the tip of the guide is roughly 5 mm posterior to the tip of the coracoid. A superomedial-to-inferolateral direction is chosen. The guide wires are inserted through both cortices. First, the distal hole is drilled using the cannulated drill provided in the set. It must be inserted through the skin in oscillation mode to prevent injury to the cephalic vein. Once its end is visualized, the drill hole is made. The guide wire should be removed prior to advancing the cannulated drill to prevent injury to the plexus. The second hole is drilled (utilizing the guide) repeating the steps. The holes (9 mm apart) are then tapped using the tap provided and the top hats are inserted. Care must be taken not to overtighten the top hats and should be 2 fingers tight.

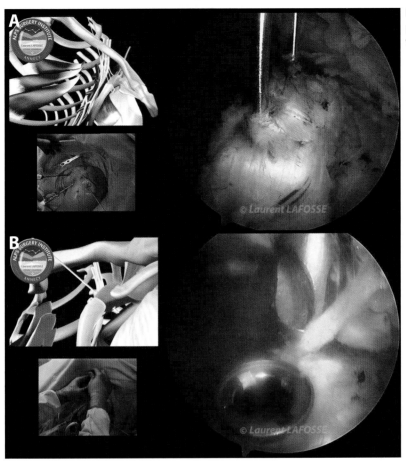

Figure 17-11. Coracoid preparation and harvesting.

Figure 17-12. Coracoid osteotomy.

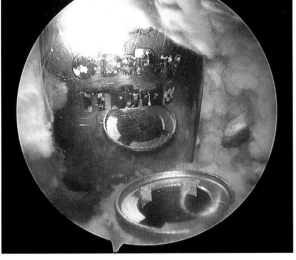

▷ Coracoid osteotomy: A 5-mm burr is introduced through the M portal while visualizing through the I portal, and the undersurface of the neck of the coracoid is burred to create a stress riser. The coracoid osteotome is used to perform a controlled osteotomy. Initially, the lateral cortex is osteotomized followed by the medial cortex (Figure 17-12) followed

Figure 17-13. Identification of the axillary nerve.

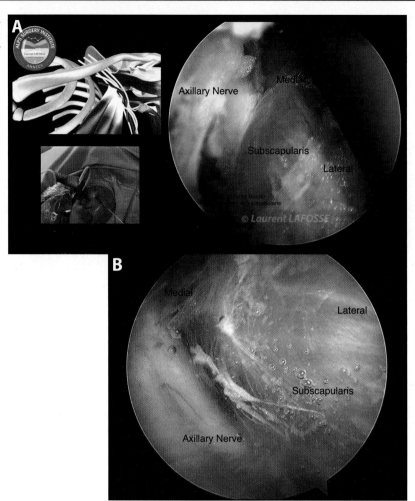

by inserting the osteotome superiorly and completing the controlled osteotomy. A fresh backflow of bleeding is attained and transient hyperpressure is attained using the pump. This is due to bone bleeding and will subside.

▶ Subscapularis split: The arm is adducted and held in neutral rotation without traction, visualizing through the J portal and working through the I portal.

▷ The shaver is used to excise the remainder of the subscapularis bursa.

▷ The electrocautery is used as a blunt probe and the medial surface of the subscapularis muscle is teased to clearly dissect the axillary nerve (Figure 17-13). This step is mandatory for protecting the axillary nerve and safely completing the subscapularis split.

▷ The superior border of the subscapularis is identified adjacent to the rotator interval, and its inferior margin is identified by the anterior circumflex artery and its 2 veins (3 sisters). The junction of the superior two-thirds and inferior one-third is marked.

▷ Creating internal and external rotation, the subscapularis split is made with the electrocautery always pointing away from the axillary nerve. The lateral extent of the dissection is to the edge of the bicipital groove, avoiding injury to the biceps tendon (Figure 17-14).

▷ A switching stick is inserted through the A portal traversing the joint and through the subscapularis split. Care must be taken to maintain a lateral direction such that the tip of the switching stick is always lateral to the plexus. This is then used as a retractor to retract

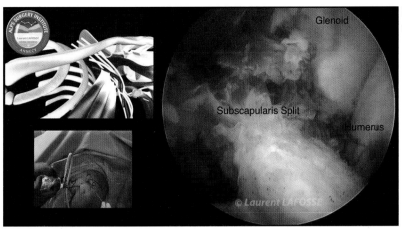

Figure 17-14. Sub-scapularis split.

the subscapularis fibers superiorly. The coracoid osteotome is now inserted through the M portal and positioned over the glenoid neck through the split and the second assistant now maximally externally rotates the arm to cause a blunt split of the medial fibers of the subscapularis. This step further safeguards against inadvertent injury to the axillary nerve.

► Glenoid exposure and drilling the screw holes: The arm is placed in internal rotation with no traction with the hand resting on the patient's lap to reduce the tension. Two switching sticks, one from the A portal and one from the J portal, are used to retract the superior and inferior fibers of the subscapularis. The I portal is used for visualization and the M portal is the working portal.

▷ The glenoid neck is contoured using the burr. Back bleeding is encountered from the bone and small perforators entering the bone through the subscapularis muscle belly are cauterized.

▷ The coracoid plastic cannulated guide is introduced through the M portal and the final position of the graft is ascertained. Ideally, this should be from 3 to 5 o'clock and the graft should never be positioned laterally. The guide is inserted and 2 guide wires are drilled into the glenoid neck with the tips of the wires exposed outside of the patient and held with artery forceps. These wires must be parallel to each other and the switching stick inserted through the A portal to ensure parallelism.

▷ The cannulated drill guide is used to assist drilling both cortices and the anticipated length of screws noted.

▷ The cannulated trocar from the Latarjet set is threaded over the inferior guide wire from the posterior skin puncture and is advanced anteriorly until it appears at the anterior glenoid neck.

▷ The guide wires are now removed from the posterior aspect of the patient, leaving behind the secured the cannulated trocar.

► Coracoid retrieval and final preparation: The arm is flexed and the double cannula is introduced (with the handle facing superiorly through the M portal). Visualizing from the I portal, the cannula and its 2 top hat screws are advanced in order to mobilize and transfer the coracoid.

▷ The coracoid is now oriented such that its undersurface faces the subscapularis.

▷ The surgeon eburnates the undersurface of the coracoid using a 5-mm burr through the J portal. Complete decortication of the undersurface of the coracoid is advisable to ensure union.

▷ It must be noted that the coracoid must be held still to prevent inadvertent slips causing damage to the critical neurovascular structures.

Figure 17-15. Introduction of the graft.

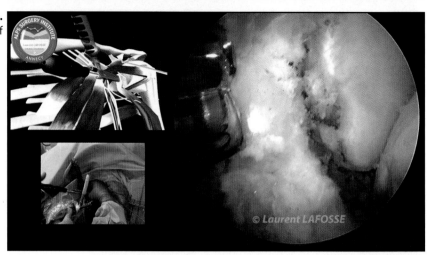

Figure 17-16. Graft is well fixed.

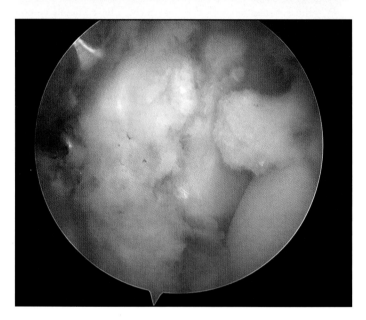

- ▶ Coracoid fixation: The arm is internally rotated and the coracoid is inserted through the subscapularis split. The inferior hole (adjacent to the origin of the conjoined tendon) in the coracoid is guided over the cannulated trocar.
  - ▷ The cannulated trocar is then advanced so that it passes through the top hat and the 2 guide wires reinserted anteroposteriorly trough the coracoid holes and the holes in the glenoid (Figure 17-15).
  - ▷ The visualization is changed between the J and the D portal to ensure that the graft is well in contact with the glenoid. Any failure of conformity can be addressed by burring the sharp edges through the E portal.
  - ▷ Once satisfied, 2 screws are inserted and the fixation of the graft attained.
  - ▷ Screws should be gently tightened as overtightening can lead to screw breakage and potential graft fracturing (Figure 17-16).
- ▶ Final inspection: The graft is viewed from the I , M, and A portals to ensure there is no graft prominence above the edger of the anterior glenoid. If prominent, the surface is visualized and

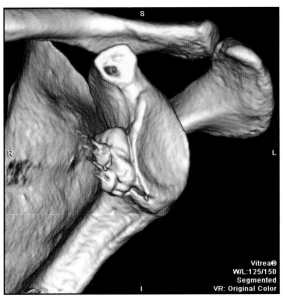

Figure 17-17. 3-month postoperative 3D CT demonstrating a well-positioned graft.

the elevated portion is burred down to ensure the graft is flush with the glenoid. The shoulder is taken through abduction and external rotation and evaluated for stability and graft fixation. The portals are all closed with subcuticular stitches and dressings applied. An abduction sling is utilized.

POSTOPERATIVE PROTOCOL

Most patients are discharged the next morning after their postoperative x-rays are checked. Patients are placed in an abduction sling for comfort. Follow-up is organized for a 2-week wound check and 6- and 12-week follow-up. No physiotherapy is recommended initially and patients are encouraged to actively elevate and move their arm. There is no limitation posed for internal or external rotation.

By 6 weeks, consolidation of the graft is noted radiographically and most athletes can return to contact sport at 3 months after the 3-month radiograph demonstrates union (Figure 17-17). A CT scan is obtained if there is

POTENTIAL COMPLICATIONS

The senior author has performed 500 arthroscopic Latarjet procedures. Complications encountered include the following:

▶ Hematoma postoperatively: Seen occasionally, patients usually complain of postoperative swelling of the hemithorax. This resolves after day 4 once the swelling subsides. This is a minor complication and is managed by reassurance, rest, analgesia, and cold packs.

▶ Infection: Superficial and deep infections have been encountered. Propionibacterium acnes has been the causative organism in most of the cases.

▶ Nerve injury: There are various reports of risks involved to the axillary and musculocutaneous nerve during the Latarjet procedure[29,30]; however, in the senior author's experience, due diligence and proper surgical technique helps minimize these risks. Despite best efforts, transient neuropraxias have been noted by the senior author.

▷ Transient suprascapular nerve palsy as a result of a long superior screw directed toward the spinoglenoid notch has occurred. This resolved with exchange of the screw to a shorter screw.

▷ Transient axillary nerve palsy: The author has experienced 1 case out of 500 patients who suffered from transient axillary nerve palsy, which recovered completely in 3 months.

▶ Graft positioning: This remains the "Achilles heel" of both open and arthroscopic Latarjet. The perfect position for positioning of the graft remains challenging. Various respected surgeons have proposed their ideologies; however, a consensus fails to exist. Nourissat et al demonstrated the 4 o'clock position to be the position of stability.[31] Yamamoto et al demonstrated that the 3 o'clock position is the site of maximal instability.[32] Saito et al have also found the most common position of the glenoid defect is from 2:30 to 4:30.[33] The following concerns do exist:

▷ Positioned too high: Risks the superior screw penetrating the spinoglenoid notch and damaging the suprascapular nerve

▷ Positioned too low: The inferior screw may miss the glenoid altogether

▷ Positioned too medial: May fail to have the biomechanical advantage of the bone block

▷ Positioned too lateral: Worst of the 4 scenarios, where the graft will cause chondral damage to the humeral head and pain. Usually, the patient complains of pain in the abducted external rotation position and an audible click may be heard

▶ Osteolysis: In the authors' retrospective review of cases, they have noted that the majority of grafts undergo osteolysis. The extent varies from patient to patient. The authors have noted in some patients with little preoperative glenoid bone loss to have more osteolysis. Some patients exhibit osteolysis as early as 6 months postoperatively. Osteolysis is universally noted to commence at the superior portion of the graft and progress inferiorly. DiGiacomo et al have found and reported a similar pattern in their patients.[34,35]

▶ Nonunion: Nonunion is uncommon and often present after significant trauma with broken screws. Due to the predominance of alpine sports in the authors' patient cohort, they often see these patients after a significant skiing or mountain climbing injury. Fracture of the graft is noted as well. These patients may need revision surgery with an iliac crest autograft.

▶ Stiffness postoperatively: The authors have noted stiffness to occur in acute shoulder dislocation cases, where the dislocation and surgery time frame was less than 10 days. These patients demonstrated a higher rate of postoperative stiffness compared to the patients who were operated on for their chronic pathology. Caution must be advised if surgery is contemplated in this early postoperative phase. A second subgroup of patients noted to have postoperative stiffness are the patients who have significant chondral loss of the humeral head. Early detection is important to avoid significant articular changes.

Results

The authors' 5-year results for a cohort of 100 patients who participated in the prospective study have recently been published.[36] Out of these, 64/89 shoulders were available for follow-up. There were no reported redislocations and one case of subluxation with a rate of recurrent instability of 1.59%. The mean aggregate Western Ontario Shoulder Instability (WOSI) index score was 90.6% +/− 9.4%. Mean WOSI domain scores were as follows: physical symptoms, 90.1% +/− 8.7%; sports/recreation/work, 90.3% +/− 12.9%; lifestyle, 93.7% +/− 9.8%; and emotions, 88.7% +/− 17.3% (Figure 17-18).

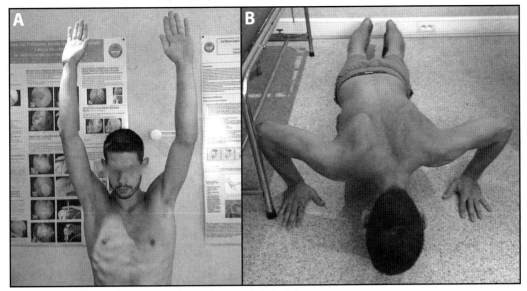

Figure 17-18. Six-week postoperative arthroscopic Latarjet.

The authors' earlier results were published in 2010.[24] These demonstrated early return to work and 91% excellent scores with 80% of the grafts positioned between 3 to 5 o'clock.

CONCLUSION

Arthroscopic Latarjet continues to evolve and remains a viable alternative in treating patients with shoulder instability. The arthroscopic nature of the procedure enables the surgeon to attend to simultaneous articular shoulder pathology. Good to excellent short- and long-term results have been noted. The graft positioning and osteolysis remain as topics for further research to improve the results of both the open and arthroscopic Latarjet.

TOP TECHNICAL PEARLS FOR THE PROCEDURE

1. Hypotensive anesthesia and an efficient fluid management pump system is mandatory.

2. Correct portal placement is critical.

3. Structures around the coracoid such as the clavipectoral fascia and the subscapularis bursa must be carefully dissected and excised.

4. Retraction of the scapula (utilizing a switching stick, through the D portal) will ensure correct placement of the graft.

5. The graft should be positioned parallel to the glenoid 3 to 5 mm medial to the anterior cartilage rim of the glenoid, thereby preventing the graft from being too proud.

REFERENCES

1. Balg F, Boileau P. The instability severity index score. A simple pre-operative score to select patients for arthroscopic or open shoulder stabilisation. *J Bone Joint Surg Br.* 2007;89(11):1470-1477.
2. Latarjet M. [Treatment of recurrent dislocation of the shoulder]. *Lyon Chirurgical.* 1954;49(8):994-997.
3. Patte D, Debeyre J. Luxations recidivantes de l'epaule. Encycl Med Chir. Paris-Technique chirurgicale. Orthopedie. 1980;44265:4.4-02.
4. Giles JW, Boons HW, Elkinson I, et al. Does the dynamic sling effect of the Latarjet procedure improve shoulder stability? A biomechanical evaluation. *J Shoulder Elbow Surg.* 2013;22(6):821-827.
5. Burkhart SS, Debeer JF, Tehrany AM, Parten PM. Quantifying glenoid bone loss arthroscopically in shoulder instability. *Arthroscopy.* 2002;18(5):488-491.
6. Itoi E, Yamamoto N, Kurokawa D, Sano H. Bone loss in anterior instability. *Curr Rev Musculoskelet Med.* 2013;6(1):88-94.
7. Moroder P, Tauber M, Hoffelner T, et al. The medial-ridge sign as an indicator of anterior glenoid bone loss. *J Shoulder Elbow Surg.* 2013;22(10):1332-1337.
8. Sugaya H, Moriishi J, Dohi M, Kon Y, Tsuchiya A. Glenoid rim morphology in recurrent anterior glenohumeral instability. *J Bone Joint Surg Am.* 2003;85-A(5):878-884.
9. Lo IK, Parten PM, Burkhart SS. The inverted pear glenoid: an indicator of significant glenoid bone loss. *Arthroscopy.* 2004;20(2):169-174.
10. Burkhart SS, Debeer JF. Traumatic glenohumeral bone defects and their relationship to failure of arthroscopic Bankart repairs: significance of the inverted-pear glenoid and the humeral engaging Hill-Sachs lesion. *Arthroscopy.* 2000;16(7):677-694.
11. Bernageau J, Patte D. [The radiographic diagnosis of posterior dislocation of the shoulder (author's transl)]. *Revue de Chirurgie Orthopedique et Reparatrice de L'appareil Moteur.* 1979;65(2):101-107.
12. Pansard E, Klouche S, Billot N, et al. Reliability and validity assessment of a glenoid bone loss measurement using the Bernageau profile view in chronic anterior shoulder instability. *J Shoulder Elbow Surg.* 2013;22(9):1193-1198.
13. Murachovsky J, Bueno RS, Nascimento LG, et al. Calculating anterior glenoid bone loss using the Bernageau profile view. *Skeletal Radiol.* 2012;41(10):1231-1237.
14. Sugaya H. Techniques to evaluate glenoid bone loss. *Curr Rev Musculoskelet Med.* 2014;7(1):1-5.
15. Saito H, Itoi E, Minagawa H, Yamamoto N, Tuoheti Y, Seki N. Location of the Hill-Sachs lesion in shoulders with recurrent anterior dislocation. *Arch Orthop Trauma Surg.* 2009;129(10):1327-1334.
16. Purchase RJ, Wolf EM, Hobgood ER, Pollock ME, Smalley CC. Hill-Sachs "remplissage": an arthroscopic solution for the engaging Hill-Sachs lesion. *Arthroscopy.* 2008;24(6):723-726.
17. Degen RM, Giles JW, Johnson JA, Athwal GS. Remplissage versus Latarjet for engaging Hill-Sachs defects without substantial glenoid bone loss: a biomechanical comparison. *Clin Orthop Rel Res.* 2014;472(8):2363-2371.
18. Di Giacomo G, De Vita A, Costantini A, de Gasperis N, Scarso P. Management of humeral head deficiencies and glenoid track. *Curr Rev Musculoskelet Med.* 2014;7(1):6-11.
19. Giles JW, Elkinson I, Ferreira LM, et al. Moderate to large engaging Hill-Sachs defects: an in vitro biomechanical comparison of the remplissage procedure, allograft humeral head reconstruction, and partial resurfacing arthroplasty. *J Shoulder Elbow Surg.* 2012;21(9):1142-1151.
20. Armitage MS, Faber KJ, Drosdowech DS, Litchfield RB, Athwal GS. Humeral head bone defects: remplissage, allograft, and arthroplasty. *Orthop Clin North Am.* 2010;41(3):417-425.
21. Elkinson I, Giles JW, Boons HW, et al. The shoulder remplissage procedure for Hill-Sachs defects: does technique matter? *J Shoulder Elbow Surg.* 2013;22(6):835-841.
22. Cerciello S, Edwards TB, Walch G. Chronic anterior glenohumeral instability in soccer players: results for a series of 28 shoulders treated with the Latarjet procedure. *J Orthop Traumatol.* 2012;13(4):197-202.
23. Neyton L, Young A, Dawidziak B, et al. Surgical treatment of anterior instability in rugby union players: clinical and radiographic results of the Latarjet-Patte procedure with minimum 5-year follow-up. *J Shoulder Elbow Surg.* 2012;21(12):1721-1727.
24. Lafosse L, Boyle S. Arthroscopic Latarjet procedure. *J Shoulder Elbow Surg.* 2010;19(2 Suppl):2-12.
25. Lafosse L, Lejeune E, Bouchard A, Kakuda C, Gobezie R, Kochhar T. The arthroscopic Latarjet procedure for the treatment of anterior shoulder instability. *Arthroscopy.* 2007;23(11):1242 e1241-1245.

26. Rosso C, Bongiorno V, Samitier G, Dumont GD, Szollosy G, Lafosse L. Technical guide and tips on the all-arthroscopic Latarjet procedure. *Knee Surg Sports Traumatol Arthrosc.* 2014 May 10. [Epub ahead of print].

27. Hovelius L, Saeboe M. Neer Award 2008: Arthropathy after primary anterior shoulder dislocation—223 shoulders prospectively followed up for twenty-five years. *J Shoulder Elbow Surg.* 2009;18(3):339-347.

28. Hovelius L, Olofsson A, Sandstrom B, et al. Nonoperative treatment of primary anterior shoulder dislocation in patients forty years of age and younger. A prospective twenty-five-year follow-up. *J Bone Joint Surg Am.* 2008;90(5):945-952.

29. Shah AA, Butler RB, Romanowski J, Goel D, Karadagli D, Warner JJ. Short-term complications of the Latarjet procedure. *J Bone Joint Surg Am.* 2012;94(6):495-501.

30. Delaney RA, Freehill MT, Janfaza DR, Vlassakov KV, Higgins LD, Warner JJ. 2014 Neer Award Paper: neuromonitoring the Latarjet procedure. *J Shoulder Elbow Surg.* 2014;23(10):1473-1480

31. Nourissat G, Radier C, Aim F, Lacoste S. Arthroscopic classification of posterior labrum glenoid insertion. *Orthop Traumatol Surg Res.* 2014;100(2):167-170.

32. Yamamoto N, Itoi E, Abe H, et al. Effect of an anterior glenoid defect on anterior shoulder stability: a cadaveric study. *Am J Sports Med.* 2009;37(5):949-954.

33. Saito H, Itoi E, Sugaya H, Minagawa H, Yamamoto N, Tuoheti Y. Location of the glenoid defect in shoulders with recurrent anterior dislocation. *Am J Sports Med.* 2005;33(6):889-893.

34. Di Giacomo G, de Gasperis N, Costantini A, De Vita A, Beccaglia MA, Pouliart N. Does the presence of glenoid bone loss influence coracoid bone graft osteolysis after the Latarjet procedure? A computed tomography scan study in 2 groups of patients with and without glenoid bone loss. *J Shoulder Elbow Surg.* 2014;23(4):514-518.

35. Di Giacomo G, Costantini A, de Gasperis N, et al. Coracoid bone graft osteolysis after Latarjet procedure: a comparison study between two screws standard technique vs mini-plate fixation. *Int J Shoulder Surg.* 2013;7(1):1-6.

36. Dumont GD, Fogerty S, Rosso C, Lafosse L. The arthroscopic Latarjet procedure for anterior shoulder instability: 5-year minimum follow-up. *Am J Sports Med.* 2014;42(11):2560-2566.

Please see videos on the accompanying website at

www.ArthroscopicTechniques.com

18

Arthroscopic Suprascapular Nerve Release
The Transverse Scapular Ligament and Spinoglenoid Notch

Kevin D. Plancher, MD, MS and Stephanie C. Petterson, MPT, PhD

INTRODUCTION

The etiology of posterior shoulder pain can be elusive for the treating physician. Compression of the suprascapular nerve at either the transverse scapular ligament or the spinoglenoid ligament leads to resultant posterior shoulder pain, muscle weakness, and permanent muscle atrophy if left untreated.[1,2] Suprascapular nerve compression is often localized to a discrete portion of the length of the nerve which, because of its anatomical position, makes it susceptible to entrapment. Early literature noted the nerve, when compressed at the transverse scapular ligament, was affected by trauma such as a fracture through the scapular notch or even a proximal humerus fracture caused by a direct blow to the shoulder. It has been reported that the suprascapular nerve is the second most common isolated nerve injury seen in shoulder dislocations, second to the axillary nerve.[3] Tumors, whether benign or malignant, are other potential causes with encroachment of the suprascapular notch by intrinsic or extrinsic masses. The most common benign lesion is a ganglion, either continuous or separate from the articular labrum.

Arthroscopic release of the suprascapular nerve can result in a dramatic, immediate reversal of the patient's pain profile as well as improvements in shoulder strength; however, in long-standing cases in patients with chronic symptoms, reversal of muscle atrophy has not been well-documented. The arthroscopic technique increases the ability to visualize anatomy, allows for a faster return to sports or activities of daily living, and is the preferred approach when surgery is indicated. The morbidity and postoperative recovery following arthroscopic releases is also less traumatic for the patient.

INDICATIONS

► Visible atrophy to the supraspinatus, infraspinatus, or both proven in a patient with suprascapular nerve entrapment on physical examination often with a chronic ache or pain in the posterior periscapular region (Figure 18-1)

Ryu RKN, Angelo RL, Abrams JS, eds. *The Shoulder: AANA Advanced Arthroscopic Surgical Techniques* (pp 219-231). © 2016 AANA.

Figure 18-1. (A) Clinical photo of bilateral shoulders, right affected more than left, with supraspinatus and infraspinatus atrophy implying compression at the transverse scapular ligament. (B) Clinical photo of a weightlifter with pain, weakness, and EMG-proven compression of the suprascapular nerve at the transverse scapular ligament in the left shoulder. (Reprinted with permission from KD Plancher.)

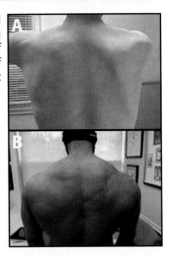

▶ Patients with a space-occupying lesion, with a negative magnetic resonance imaging (MRI) for atrophy, and a negative electromyography (EMG) often with chronic ache or pain located 4 cm medial from the glenohumeral joint and inferior to the scapular spine

Controversial Indications

▶ Patients with a large or massive, irreparable rotator cuff tear with or without EMG findings of suprascapular neuropathy
▶ Patients with labral tear and/or associated paralabral cyst around the suprascapular nerve at the spinoglenoid notch

PERTINENT PHYSICAL FINDINGS

▶ Compression at the transverse scapular ligament demonstrates atrophy of both the supraspinatus and infraspinatus fossa in chronic conditions when compared to the unaffected, opposite side (see Figure 18-1). Beware that atrophy may be masked by the overlying trapezius and muscle bulk of the deltoid muscles in well-developed individuals such as bodybuilders who participate in a weight-training program (see Figure 18-1B).
▶ Compression at the spinoglenoid ligament results in chronic conditions of atrophy of only the infraspinatus.
▶ Painless weakness in shoulder external rotation and abduction will be detected in patients with spinoglenoid ligament compression. In patients with long-standing disease, the teres minor and serratus anterior muscle can compensate for weakness of the infraspinatus to obtain near-normal strength.
▶ Tenderness will be present in the suprascapular notch between the clavicle and scapular spine, 3 cm medial and anterior to Neviaser's portal with compression of transverse scapular ligament.
▶ The suprascapular nerve sends a branch to the acromioclavicular (AC) joint. Therefore, the cross arm adduction test may also be used to help make the diagnosis of suprascapular neuropathy at the spinoglenoid ligament. The examiner moves the elbow to the nonaffected side in order to cross the body of the patient, who has placed his or her hand on the opposite

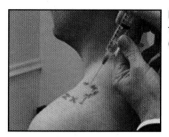

Figure 18-2. Clinical photo of a lidocaine injection to be placed at the transverse scapular ligament, 3 cm medial to Neviaser's portal. (Reprinted with permission from KD Plancher.)

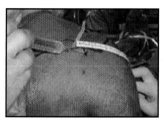

Figure 18-3. Clinical photo of a lidocaine injection to be placed at the spinoglenoid ligament, 4 cm medial to the posterolateral corner of the acromion. (Reprinted with permission from KD Plancher.)

shoulder. When suprascapular nerve compression is present, this maneuver will provoke pain in the AC joint, even in the absence of AC joint degeneration on x-ray or profound tenderness on palpation. The pain must be felt in the posterior aspect of the shoulder to distinguish it from pain associated with the AC joint.[4]

▸ Selective injections: A 1% lidocaine anesthetic injection (5 to 10 cc) can be injected into the spinoglenoid notch or the transverse scapular ligament notch to help accurately diagnose suprascapular nerve compression. Aspiration is performed to avoid the suprascapular artery (Figures 18-2 and 18-3). The cross arm adduction test can once again be performed following the injection. If previously positive, the test must now be a nonprovocative maneuver. If pain is still present at the AC joint after this injection, then the physician should consider an alternative diagnosis and not one of suprascapular nerve compression.

PERTINENT IMAGING

▸ Electrodiagnostic testing with myography and nerve conduction studies, while the best objective measure for a suspected diagnosis, are often negative as this is a dynamic and not a static diagnosis.

▸ Plain radiographs should include a true (Grashey) anteroposterior, axillary lateral, Y or supraspinatus outlet, Stryker notch, and a Zanca view to observe the AC joint.[5] *Note*: The anteroposterior scapular view with the beam aimed 15 to 30 degrees cephalad obliquely at the transverse scapular ligament can aid in detecting any calcifications, exostosis, or previous trauma in the form of callous formation at the notch or osseous notch variants.[5,6]

▸ MRI is the best imaging modality to detect suprascapular nerve pathology with a T2-weighted sagittal oblique image. Presence or absence of supraspinatus and infraspinatus muscle atrophy and fatty infiltration may be noted. Chronic denervation, seen best on T1 spin echo with increased signal intensity within the muscle mass, will demonstrate muscle atrophy with fatty infiltration. Detection of muscle edema, which has been suggested to be one of the earliest signs of suprascapular nerve entrapment, may also be noted with MRI.[7] Some patients will demonstrate increased signal intensity on T2 fast spin echo fat saturation sequence with a normal muscle mass, implying subacute denervation of the nerve caused by neurogenic edema.

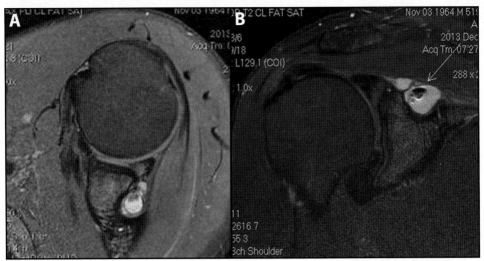

Figure 18-4. Two MRI slices demonstrating a classical finding of a ganglion cyst compressing the suprascapular nerve. (Reprinted with permission from KD Plancher.)

Table 18-1. Rengachary Classification System of Anatomic Suprascapular Notch Variants

NOTCH TYPE	DESCRIPTION
Type I	Wide depression of the entire superior border of the scapula
Type II	Blunted V-shaped notch occupying the middle one-third of the superior border of the scapula
Type III	U-shaped notch in the superior border of the scapula with symmetrical, parallel lateral borders
Type IV	A small, V-shaped narrow groove in the superior border of the scapula
Type V	U-shaped notch in the superior border of the scapula with partial ossification of the medial aspect of the transverse scapular ligament. The diameter of the notch along the superior border is narrow as a result
Type VI	Complete ossification of the transverse scapular ligament creating a foramen

Adapted from Rengachary SS, Burr D, Lucas S, Hassanein KM, Mohn MP, Matzke H. Suprascapular entrapment neuropathy: a clinical, anatomical and comprehensive study. Part 2: anatomical study. *Neurosurgery.* 1979;5(4):447-451.

► The MRI can identify a ganglion with a homogenous signal, low T1 intensity, high T2 intensity, and rim enhancement if contrast is placed (Figure 18-4).[8] Computed tomography detects notch variants previously been described by Rengachary (Table 18-1).[9] Evidence of an ossified transverse ligament can also be identified with computed tomography.

► Ultrasound may be helpful to identify ganglion cysts.

EQUIPMENT

- ► 30-degree video arthroscope
- ► 18-gauge spinal needle
- ► 3.5-mm mechanical full radius shaver
- ► Radiofrequency coagulation wand
- ► 1/8" and 1/4" Lambotte osteotome
- ► #15 blade
- ► Inflow pump
- ► Beach chair or lateral decubitus positioner
- ► Arthroscopic scissors
- ► Mallet
- ► 3.5-mm arthroscopic burr
- ► Arthroscopy probe
- ► Arthroscopic switching stick

POSITIONING AND PORTALS: ARTHROSCOPIC RELEASE OF THE TRANSVERSE SCAPULAR LIGAMENT

While the lateral decubitus position may be used, the authors have found the beach chair position easier when performing a suprascapular nerve decompression.[10] The patient is placed in a beach chair position with arm placed at its side for arthroscopic release of the transverse scapular ligament. The patient should be prepped and draped from the midsternum to the midposterior spine with the neck and scapular areas included. The anesthesiologist should maintain a systolic blood pressure slightly below 100 mm Hg. To avoid unnecessary swelling and to increase visibility, the pump pressure is kept low at 45 mm Hg maximum. This procedure should precede any additional procedures performed on the same shoulder that day.

STEP-BY-STEP DESCRIPTION: ARTHROSCOPIC RELEASE OF THE TRANSVERSE SCAPULAR LIGAMENT

Step 1

The standard subacromial portals, including posterior, anterolateral, and lateral subacromial portals, are used for decompression at the transverse scapular ligament. An additional portal for successful completion of the decompression is a portal made from outside-in, first with an 18-gauge spinal needle, 3 cm medial and slightly anterior to Neviaser's portal. This portal is created and altered with visualization located anterior to the leading edge of the supraspinatus. The portal is approximately 6 to 8 cm medial to the anterolateral border of the acromion in between the clavicle and scapular spine (Figure 18-5).

The arthroscope is introduced into the subacromial space and a subacromial decompression is completed, if needed, and encouraged for the surgeon attempting this procedure for the first few

Figure 18-5. Intraoperative photo of a left shoulder prepped and draped in preparation for a transverse scapular ligament and spinoglenoid ligament release. The portals are labeled as follows: (A) working portal for spinoglenoid ligament release; (B) viewing portal with 30-degree arthroscope for spinoglenoid ligament release; (C) standard posterior portal for intra-articular glenohumeral arthroscopy; (D) Neviaser's portal; and (E) portal for release of the transverse scapular ligament. The round circle anteriorly is the coracoid. Anterior to portal D is the AC joint. The arthroscopic shaver or thermal device will be placed at the anterolateral edge of the acromion with the viewing portal shown as the solid purple line laterally off of the acromion to allow the surgeon to release the transverse scapular ligament. (Reprinted with permission from KD Plancher.)

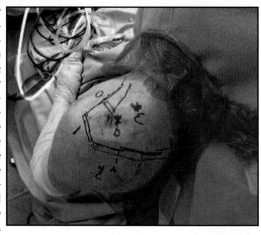

Figure 18-6. Arthroscopic inside view of a left shoulder showing the supraspinatus, its leading edge anterior to the left, with the trochar inside pointing to the coracoacromial ligament. (Reprinted with permission from KD Plancher.)

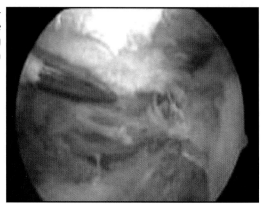

times, to allow for adequate visualization. Release of the coracoacromial ligament is performed and is helpful for enhanced visualization. The arthroscope is moved midway to two-thirds of the way posterior along the lateral edge of the acromion. The authors avoid placing it at the posterolateral corner (Figure 18-6). The shaver is introduced in the portal created at the anterolateral edge of the acromion. This entry point will allow for adequate clearance of all soft tissue necessary to complete this operation. The shaver is introduced into the anterolateral portal at the edge of the acromion, far enough anterior to avoid crowding with the arthroscope.

Step 2: Moving From the Coracoacromial Ligament to the Coracoclavicular Ligament

A spinal needle is placed in the center of the AC joint and a second spinal needle is placed in Neviaser's portal to help guide the procedure (Figure 18-7). Identify and follow the coracoacromial ligament to its medial side of the coracoid. Soft tissue is either ablated with a radiofrequency device or removed with a mechanical shaver while ensuring hemostasis and unrestricted visualization occurs throughout the procedure (Figure 18-8A). The anterior edge of the supraspinatus must always be maintained in view while proceeding medially in the subacromial space when attempting to release the transverse scapular ligament. Upon identification of the coracoid, the coracoclavicular ligaments are identified first, the trapezoid laterally, and subsequently the more medial conoid ligament (Figure 18-8B). The conoid is always more posterior in position and there

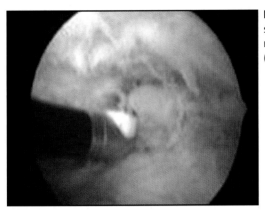

Figure 18-7. Radiofrequency device clearing the soft tissue as it heads medially to identify the spinal needle coming from outside-in of Neviaser's portal. (Reprinted with permission from KD Plancher.)

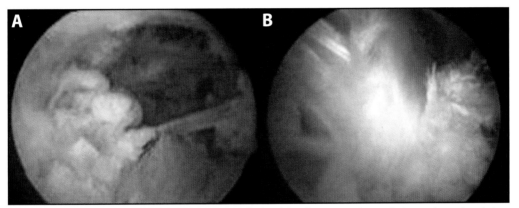

Figure 18-8. (A) Arthroscopic view of the same left shoulder demonstrating soft tissue cleared and visualization often with small tributaries of the suprascapular artery left unharmed. (B) The conoid ligament, recognized as the most lateral attachment of the transverse scapular ligament, now with the transverse scapular ligament in sight but covered by soft tissue and the artery and nerve not protected. (Reprinted with permission from KD Plancher.)

is usually an area of fat surrounding this ligament. It is recommended to clear this space with the use of a radiofrequency wand. The spinal needle placed in the AC joint will remind the surgeon of the location of conoid ligament, and the needle in Neviaser's portal will keep visualization in the correct orientation as the arthroscope is placed more medially and remains anterior to the supraspinatus. The most medial border of the conoid ligament is the most lateral attachment of the transverse scapular ligament. The arthroscope needs to be turned 180 degrees when the conoid ligament is found and the transverse scapular ligament will come into view. When dealing with any soft tissue mass that exists in the supraspinatus fossa, the mass must be evacuated as one continues the release and moves medially to the transverse scapular ligament. The stalk of the soft tissue mass will almost assuredly be located alongside the transverse scapular ligament (Figure 18-9). The original 18-gauge spinal needle that was placed 3 cm medial to Neviaser's portal should be in view and is moved to be placed directly on the transverse scapular ligament.

Step 3: Release of the Transverse Scapular Ligament
Final Steps

An additional portal is created with the 18-gauge spinal needle that was placed approximately 3 cm medial to Neviaser's portal (Figure 18-10). The skin incision is made large enough to introduce the blunt obturator from the arthroscope that will aid in gently pushing away tissue

Figure 18-9. Decompressed ganglion cyst at the spinoglenoid notch prior to complete excision of its root. (Reprinted with permission from Jonathan Ticker, MD.)

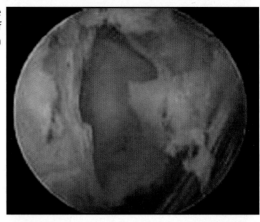

Figure 18-10. Arthroscopic view of the same needle heading toward the transverse scapular ligament to aid in visualization of an accurate landmark. (Reprinted with permission from KD Plancher.)

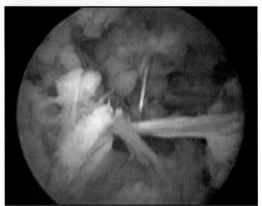

Figure 18-11. A blunt obturator/trochar retracting the artery out of harm's way, revealing the suprascapular nerve adhered to the calcified and thickened transverse scapular ligament. (Reprinted with permission from KD Plancher.)

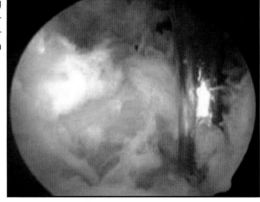

to visualize the transverse scapular ligament and keep the suprascapular nerve out of harm's way. A 180-degree rotation of the arthroscope to look inferiorly from the conoid ligament will also identify the artery and/or vein normally overlying the transverse scapular ligament. The blunt obturator is used to retract any supraspinatus muscle and fat posteriorly, allowing for an excellent view of the transverse scapular ligament as well as the suprascapular artery (Figure 18-11). The obturator is positioned to retract the nerve more medially so that the transverse scapular ligament is isolated. Another small incision is made next to the already made, newly created medial portal. An arthroscopic scissor is used to divide the transverse scapular ligament close to the lateral extent

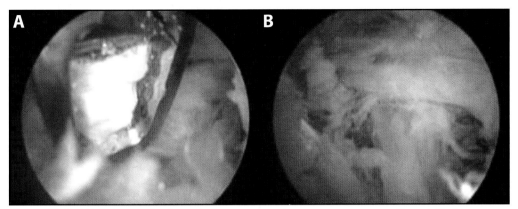

Figure 18-12. (A) Arthroscopic view of scissors attempting to cut and remove the calcified transverse scapular ligament. In this case, a Lambotte osteotome was introduced to help remove the calcified transverse scapular ligament. (B) Arthroscopic view of the successful release of the transverse scapular ligament, revealing the suprascapular nerve to the right and the remnant of the calcified transverse scapular ligament to the left. Note the suprascapular artery superiorly and running diagonally to the right. (Reprinted with permission from KD Plancher.)

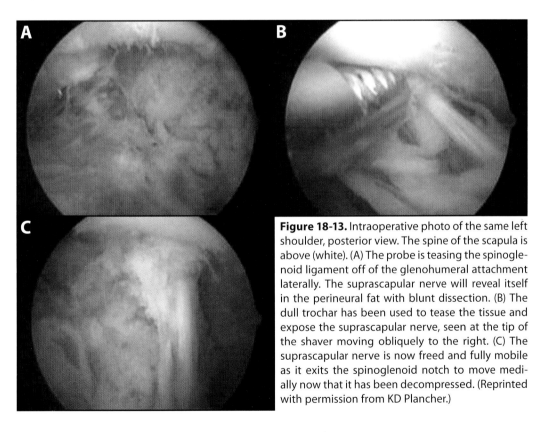

Figure 18-13. Intraoperative photo of the same left shoulder, posterior view. The spine of the scapula is above (white). (A) The probe is teasing the spinoglenoid ligament off of the glenohumeral attachment laterally. The suprascapular nerve will reveal itself in the perineural fat with blunt dissection. (B) The dull trochar has been used to tease the tissue and expose the suprascapular nerve, seen at the tip of the shaver moving obliquely to the right. (C) The suprascapular nerve is now freed and fully mobile as it exits the spinoglenoid notch to move medially now that it has been decompressed. (Reprinted with permission from KD Plancher.)

of the suprascapular notch (Figure 18-12). If the ligament is calcified, a 1/8" Lambotte osteotome is used through this second small incision. A 3.5-mm burr or small 3.5-mm full radius shaver may be used to safely smooth any protuberance of bone that may be encountered as long as the nerve and artery are carefully protected. The blunt tip trocar is then utilized to assess the mobility and adequacy of the release of the suprascapular nerve (Figure 18-13). All portals are routinely closed by surgeon preference.

POSITIONING AND PORTALS: ARTHROSCOPIC RELEASE OF THE SPINOGLENOID LIGAMENT

While the lateral decubitus position may be used, the authors have found the beach chair position easier when performing a suprascapular nerve decompression at the spinoglenoid ligament.[11,12] The patient is placed in a beach chair position with arm placed at its side for arthroscopic release of the spinoglenoid ligament. The patient should be prepped and draped from the midsternum to the midposterior spine with the neck and scapular areas included. The anesthesiologist should maintain a systolic blood pressure slightly below 100 mm Hg. To avoid unnecessary swelling and to increase visibility, the pump pressure is kept low at 45 mm Hg maximum.

STEP-BY-STEP DESCRIPTION: ARTHROSCOPIC RELEASE OF THE SPINOGLENOID LIGAMENT

Arthroscopic release of the suprascapular nerve at the spinoglenoid notch should be approached from the posterior shoulder. The authors utilize a posteromedial and posterolateral portal in the infraspinatus fossa. A subacromial approach can also be used as previously described by others, but the authors have found the following described technique quite simple.[13]

Step 1

The portals selected include 2 portals: 1) the viewing portal, which is placed 8 cm medial to the posterolateral corner of the acromion, just inferior to the scapula spine, and 2) the working portal, which is placed 4 cm medial to the posterolateral corner of the acromion, just inferior to the scapula spine. Measurements are adjusted by 1 mm for the size of the patient, large or small.

The blunt trocar is introduced into the viewing portal and is directed toward the infraspinatus fossa inferior to the spine and gently moved anatomically posterior until it makes contact with the infraspinatus fossa and bone. The infraspinatus fibers must be swept away, and the trocar is directed medially, passing over the suprascapular nerve and falling into the spinoglenoid notch. Riding the fossa always keeping bone in sight is an easy way to land in the spinoglenoid notch. The key step that allows for visualization is to ensure that the trocar sweeps tissue under the roof of the infraspinatus spine, feeling the curvature of the infraspinatus fossa.

The arthroscope replaces the trocar and the spinoglenoid ligament is visualized.

Step 2: Triangulation for Working Portal

An 18-gauge spinal needle is placed to triangulate with the arthroscope. The trocar is now introduced into the working portal and the soft tissue is teased away laterally, as the course of the nerve can always be located at the medial aspect of the spinoglenoid notch. A radiofrequency wand or a small radius, nonaggressive shaver with the suction turned off can be utilized at this point to clear the tissue superior and, more specifically, the spinoglenoid ligament (Figure 18-14). This ligament resembles ligamentum mucosa seen in the knee. Resection is similar to resection in the knee as a ligamentum mucosa may be excised leaving the anterior cruciate ligament alone. The spinoglenoid ligament laterally resected will leave the nerve seen heading medially untouched. The ligament can be followed to the glenohumeral joint at its insertion to understand and visualize safely the complete resection of the ligament. By staying on the spine of the scapula during resection, bleeding will be minimized.

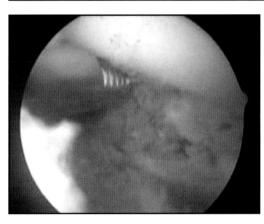

Figure 18-14. Intraoperative photo of the same left shoulder, posterior view. The spine of the scapula is above. The shaver is taking the spinoglenoid ligament directly off the spine of the scapula. All work is being completed lateral to the suprascapular nerve. This is no different than resecting the ligamentum mucosa/infrapatellar plica in a knee; all work is done on the bone or the notch (the knee), thereby safely avoiding injury to the nerve anteriorly and medially. (Reprinted with permission from KD Plancher.)

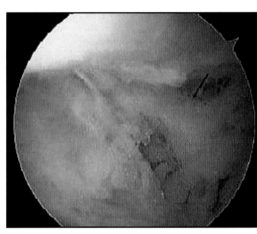

Figure 18-15. Arthroscopic view of the left shoulder, posterior view, with the arrow pointing to the suprascapular nerve heading medially. Note the bulging tissue to the left, representing a ganglion cyst not yet decompressed. The spine of the scapula (white) is above. (Reprinted with permission from KD Plancher.)

Step 3

The spinoglenoid notch should now be evaluated for any variations in anatomy such as the presence of a ganglion cyst or a bifid nerve that may be compressing the suprascapular nerve (Figure 18-15). The portals are closed by surgeon preference.

POSTOPERATIVE PROTOCOL

Rehabilitation is affected by any additional procedures performed in conjunction with the suprascapular nerve release. Patients are discharged from the hospital on the same day as surgery. Patients are instructed in the use of a sling for comfort for the first postoperative week routinely. If a concomitant superior labral anteroposterior repair is performed, then the patient must remain in a sling for 3 to 4 weeks, and then the surgeon's superior labral anteroposterior protocol is followed. For isolated suprascapular nerve releases, patients are seen in the office postoperative day 1, and pendulum exercises and progressive range of motion exercises are initiated. Patients are then permitted to increase their activity as tolerated with return to full overhead activities within 6 weeks. Patients are routinely seen for follow-up evaluation at 6, 12, 24, and 52 weeks. Repeat EMG and nerve conduction studies are conducted at 6 months to assess suprascapular nerve function per surgeon request. A full therapy strengthening program can begin at 6 weeks if a suprascapular nerve decompression is the only procedure performed on the shoulder.

POTENTIAL COMPLICATIONS

With a thorough understanding of the pertinent anatomy surrounding the suprascapular nerve, few complications have been reported. The ability to restore muscle strength and reverse the muscle atrophy is very difficult if not impossible. Patients should be clearly informed of the limitation to not be able to restore normal strength prior to surgery. When releasing the transverse scapular ligament, identification of the artery is always performed to avoid laceration. When releasing the spinoglenoid ligament, there is no need to locate any artery or vein unless aberrant anatomy occurs. The joint space is never violated in both procedures and, therefore, the risk of arthrofibrosis has been minimized. No series to date has reported any infection postoperatively from either of these procedures. Restoration of muscle atrophy on the other hand, as discussed previously, is quite difficult; however, as reported by Fabre et al, they had a resolution of muscle atrophy in 52% of their patients with isolated suprascapular muscle atrophy, which has been the authors' finding as well.[14]

CONCLUSION

The authors' experience with this technique has been exceptionally successful when a patient has failed conservative treatment for no more than 6 to 12 weeks and has EMG-proven compression and visible atrophy in the supraspinatus or infraspinatus fossa or both. The patient's pain profile the next day after release is reliably extinguished. While the authors have not been successful in restoring the muscle bulk in those patients whose disease has not been present for more than 2 years, some measurable external rotation strength has been restored. This technique is safe and effective as a minimally invasive solution for suprascapular nerve entrapment.

TOP TECHNICAL PEARLS FOR THE PROCEDURE

1. Accurately identify the surface landmarks and draw out with a ruler the exact location of all portals.

2. Keep the systolic blood pressure below 100 mm Hg to allow for optimal visualization and the pump pressure at a low setting (eg, ≤45 mm Hg) to avoid unnecessary swelling.

3. Perform the release of the suprascapular nerve at the transverse scapular ligament and spinoglenoid ligament first, prior to any other additional procedure, to ensure swelling in the shoulder is kept to a minimum.

4. When releasing the transverse scapular ligament, protect the nerve with a blunt trocar through a portal 3 cm medial to Neviaser's portal.

5. Manage the expectation and goals for the patient if atrophy is visibly present.

REFERENCES

1. Plancher KD, Johnston JC, Peterson RK, et al. The dimensions of the rotator interval. *J Shoulder Elbow Surg.* 2005;14(6):620-625.
2. Plancher KD, Luke TA, Peterson RK, et al. Posterior shoulder pain: a dynamic study of the spinoglenoid ligament and treatment with arthroscopic release of the scapular tunnel. *Arthroscopy.* 2007;23(9):991-998.
3. Visser CP, Coene LN, Brand R, et al. The incidence of nerve injury in anterior dislocation of the shoulder and its influence on functional recovery. A prospective clinical and EMG study. *J Bone Joint Surg Br.* 1999;8 (4):679-685.
4. Fehrman DA, Orwin JF, Jennings RM. Suprascapular nerve entrapment by ganglion cysts: a report of six cases with arthroscopic findings and review of the literature. *Arthroscopy.* 1995;11(6):727-734.
5. Post M, Mayer J. Suprascapular nerve entrapment. Diagnosis and treatment. *Clin Orthop Relat Res.* 1987;(223):126-136.
6. Yoon TN, Grabois M, Guillen M. Suprascapular nerve injury following trauma to the shoulder. *J Trauma.* 1981;21(8):652-655.
7. Ludig T, Walter F, Chapuis D, et al. MR imaging evaluation of suprascapular nerve entrapment. *Eur Radiol.* 2001;11(11):2161-2169.
8. Fritz RC, Helms CA, Steinbach LS, Genant HK. Suprascapular nerve entrapment: evaluation with MR imaging. *Radiology.* 1992;182(2):437-444.
9. Rengachary SS, Neff JP, Singer PA, Brackett CE. Suprascapular entrapment neuropathy: a clinical, anatomical, and comparative study. Part 1: clinical study. *Neurosurgery.* 1979;5(4):441-446.
10. Plancher KD, Petterson SC. Posterior shoulder pain and arthroscopic decompression of the suprascapular nerve at the transverse scapular ligament. *Op Tech Sports Med.* 2014;22(1):58-72.
11. Plancher KD, Peterson RK, Johnston JC, et al. The spinoglenoid ligament. Anatomy, morphology, and histological findings. *J Bone Joint Surg Am.* 2005;87(2):361-365.
12. Ghodadra N, Nho SJ, Verma NN, et al. Arthroscopic decompression of the suprascapular nerve at the spinoglenoid notch and suprascapular notch through the subacromial space. *Arthroscopy.* 2009;25(4):439-445.
13. Plancher KD, Petterson SC. Posterior shoulder pain and arthroscopic decompression of the suprascapular nerve at the spinoglenoid notch. *Op Tech Sports Med.* 2014;22(1):73-87.
14. Fabre T, Piton C, Leclouerec G, Gervais-Delion F, Durandeau A. Entrapment of the suprascapular nerve. *J Bone Joint Surg Br.* 1999;81(3):414-419.

Please see videos on the accompanying website at

www.ArthroscopicTechniques.com

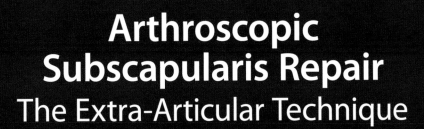

19

Arthroscopic Subscapularis Repair
The Extra-Articular Technique

Richard K. N. Ryu, MD and Matthew T. Provencher MD

INTRODUCTION

Isolated subscapularis tears are uncommon and are usually associated with a traumatic event in younger patients. Most subscapularis tears are discovered in older patients in combination with the anterosuperior tear pattern in which the anterolateral supraspinatus tendon, biceps, and rotator interval are also involved.[1] It is noteworthy that, because of the complex anatomy of the rotator interval, subscapularis tears can often be underappreciated and therefore underdiagnosed. For the practicing clinician who encounters biceps and anterior cable injuries of the supraspinatus, a careful examination of the subscapularis tendon is mandated.

Most subscapularis tears result from age-related degeneration with loss of cellularity, vascularity, and tissue thinning. A less common etiology can arise from subcoracoid impingement and the "roller-wringer" effect, in which the coracohumeral distance is narrowed (less than 7 mm), predisposing to a mechanical injury from the tip of the coracoid.[2] Pain and weakness, especially in internal rotation, are the common complaints as the subscapularis tear is often only one component of a broader rotator cuff disease pattern.

The subscapularis accounts for 50% of rotator cuff strength, and because it possesses the largest footprint (averaging 26 mm x 18 mm in dimension), a double-row transosseous equivalent repair, if adequate tissue is present, provides for a reliable repair construct.[3] Numerous clinical reports have verified the excellent healing potential of the subscapularis, although residual weakness has been a common postoperative finding.[4-9] In one study, fatty infiltration and muscle atrophy were improved following magnetic resonance imaging (MRI)-documented healing of the repaired isolated subscapularis tear.

When tasked with a subscapularis repair, isolated or in tandem with other cuff pathology, a step-wise approach to the repair should be rehearsed, focusing on the individual steps in sequence that allow for the successful implementation of a robust construct. The steps are as follows:

▶ Preoperative determination and recognition of the tear pattern based on physical examination and corroborated with diagnostic imaging (MRI as modality of choice)

Ryu RKN, Angelo RL, Abrams JS, eds. *The Shoulder:*
AANA Advanced Arthroscopic Surgical Techniques (pp 233-244).
© 2016 AANA.

- Determine if the tear is compatible with repair; assess fatty infiltration, retraction, tendon size, revision status, and condition of the axillary nerve
- Appropriate, strategic portal placement
- Assess and treat the biceps if indicated (inferior suprapectoral tenodesis or tenotomy in selected cases); some degree of biceps injury or instability is commonplace (medial subluxation or dislocation)
- Subscapularis mobilization
- Subcoracoid decompression, if warranted
- Footprint preparation
- Anchor insertion; one triple-loaded anchor per centimeter of tear
- Retrograde suture passage with suture hook or retriever
- Medial row vertical mattress knot-tying followed by completion of lateral double-row knotless anchor insertion
- Complete supraspinatus and infraspinatus tendon repair as needed
- Subacromial smoothing if pathologic subacromial changes are observed

INDICATIONS

While there may be some controversy regarding treatment when partial tears of the subscapularis are encountered,[10] there is little doubt regarding the following:

- Full thickness subscapularis tear should be repaired in order to restore the balanced force couples provided by the functional subscapularis and infraspinatus tendons. Classification of subscapularis tear patterns generally reflect the condition of the bulky superior portion of the tendon that, when detached, renders the tendon much less effective.
- In clinical situations in which a massive, irreparable tear is encountered, partial repairs that include the subscapularis and some or all of the infraspinatus may provide adequate functional results with regard to improved motion and some enhancement of strength and pain relief.[11,12]

Controversial Indications

- Significant Goutallier changes of muscle atrophy and fatty infiltration are associated with a higher failure rate with attempted rotator cuff repair,[13] including the subscapularis. Some investigators contend that, despite significant atrophy and fatty infiltration, repair of a compromised subscapularis still provides a beneficial tenodesis effect, arguing that the degree of fatty infiltration should not preclude an attempted repair.[14]
- Fraying of the superior intra-articular border of the subscapularis is a phenomenon of unknown significance. While fraying can be associated with a missed, clinically significant intrasubstance lesion and associated biceps instability, the possibility of asymptomatic fraying should be considered before embarking on a repair.

PERTINENT PHYSICAL FINDINGS

The principal physical findings on examination are weakness on stress testing of the subscapularis.

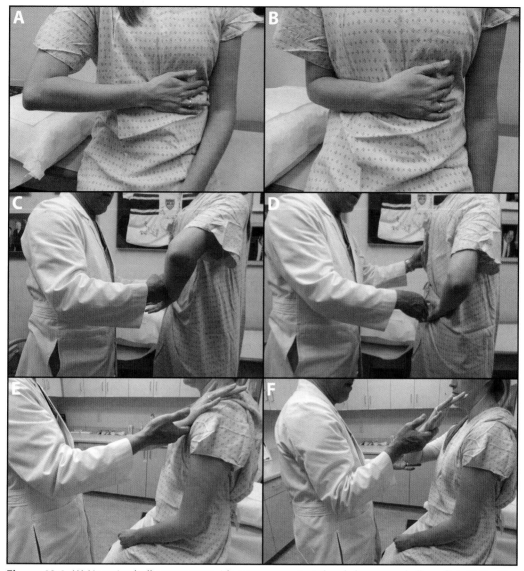

Figure 19-1. (A) Negative belly press test with pressure against the abdomen and elbow flat. (B) Positive belly press test with the wrist flexed and the elbow at the side. (C) Negative lift off test with the arm lifting the examiner's hand away from the low back. (D) Positive lift off test with the patient unable to lift the arm away from the body. (E) Negative bear hug test with the upper arm resisting force from its position on the opposite shoulder. (F) Positive bear hug examination with the arm lifted away from its position on the opposite shoulder.

▶ The belly press, lift off, and bear hug tests remain the tests of choice with each potentially providing more specific data (Figure 19-1).[15,16] The belly press test offers a potential means of quantifying the degree of tearing while focusing on the upper one-half of the subscapularis while the lift off exam theoretically evaluates the lower half of the tendon. The bear hug can also verify the integrity of the upper one-half of the subscapularis. Although there remains controversy regarding the segment of the subscapularis tested in these 3 positions, pain and weakness are consistent with a subscapularis tear.

▶ Hyper-external rotation when compared to the contralateral side can also signal a massive, retracted subscapularis tear.

Figure 19-2. Axial MRI of a left shoulder retracted subscapularis tear (large arrow). White arrow points to the empty bicipital groove. Biceps is intra-articular and medial to the subscapularis tendon edge (curved arrow).

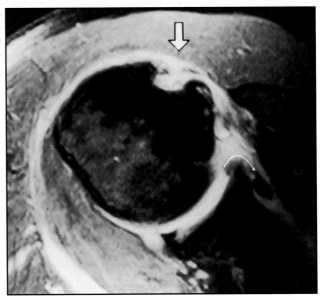

Pertinent Imaging

▶ Plain x-rays may reveal anterior subluxation of the humeral head or a possibly compromised coracohumeral distance, implying subcoracoid stenosis; these films are of limited value in establishing the diagnosis.

▶ While ultrasound in experienced hands has been described as a valuable tool in visualizing subscapularis pathology, MRI remains the modality of choice when assessing the presence of a subscapularis tear with the added value of establishing associated biceps and rotator cuff tendon involvement as well as the degree of retraction and condition of the muscle tendon unit (Figure 19-2).[17-19] Unless the axial views are carefully evaluated, the subscapularis tear can be easily missed by the reviewing surgeon.

Equipment

As with most operations, there are many different tools available to accomplish the task at hand. With the authors' technique, they prefer retrograde suturing. Additionally, whenever feasible, a double-row transosseous repair is the authors' preferred construct. The robust nature of the upper one-half of the subscapularis and the large footprint lend themselves to this repair method, assuming that residual tendon length is adequate.[20]

▶ 70- and 30-degree arthroscopes

▶ Ring curette (prepare lesser tuberosity)

▶ Radiofrequency unit for soft tissue debridement

▶ Switching stick(s): narrow diameter

▶ Motorized shaver and burr

▶ Cannulae: 8.25, 7.5, and 5.5 mm in diameter

▶ Suture hooks: Crescent, angled (45 degrees left and right) hooks; #1 polydioxanone (PDS) suture for retrograde shuttling

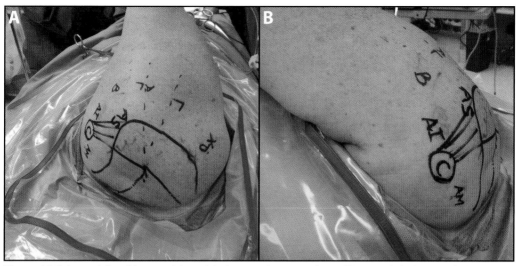

Figure 19-3. Lateral decubitus position with the portals mapped out. AI, anteroinferior portal; AL, antero-lateral portal (viewing); AM, anteromedial portal (medial to the coracoid); AS, anterosuperior portal; B, biceps portal; C, coracoid landmark; L, lateral portal; P, standard posterior portal.

▶ Suture anchors: Triple-loaded with #2 braided, high strength suture; appropriately sized bone punch or tap for anchor insertion. Knotless suture anchors for lateral row fixation in double-row construct

▶ Grasper: Circle tip and locking jaw types

▶ Knot pusher

STEP-BY-STEP DESCRIPTION OF THE PROCEDURE

The authors' preferred position is the lateral decubitus with 2 posterior kidney rests and one anteriorly. The patient is tilted posteriorly 10 to 15 degrees to align the glenoid with the floor. During the case, the table is tilted back another 15 to 20 degrees to make the anterior shoulder more accessible from a posterior position. The arm is positioned in 20 to 30 degrees of abduction, slight internal rotation, and 10 to 15 degrees of forward flexion with 10 lbs of balanced suspension.

Step 1

The landmarks and portals are drawn first with a skin scribe followed by local anesthetic injections into the portal sites (Figure 19-3). Several portals must be established: the standard posterior viewing portal (PP); an anterolateral viewing and working portal (ALP); a biceps portal (BP) for direct instrumentation of the biceps and lesser tuberosity; an anteroinferior portal (AIP) for access to the glenohumeral joint as well as the subscapularis and biceps; an anterosuperior portal (ASP; anterolateral corner of the acromion), which can be used to grasp and manipulate the subscapularis and biceps as well as serve as a portal for a switching stick functioning as a retractor; and an anteromedial portal (AMP), through which a suture hook is utilized to retrograde sutures through the torn edge of the subscapularis. It is noteworthy that the suture hook is used in the subdeltoid plane and travels medial to lateral underneath the coracoid arch.

A standard PP (2 to 3 cm inferior and 1 cm medial to the posterolateral corner of the acromion) is used to evaluate the glenohumeral articulation and the subacromial space. Intra-articular structures are assessed for their integrity. The subscapularis attachment to the lesser tuberosity can be

Figure 19-4. Viewing a right shoulder from the PP, frayed biceps (BT) is intra-articular, posterior to the torn upper-third of the subscapularis (arrows). G, glenoid; HH, humeral head.

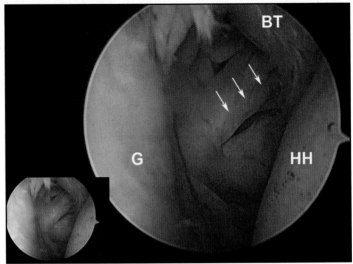

Figure 19-5. Viewing from a PP of a right shoulder, the superolateral border of the subscapularis (arrows) is identified by the position of the comma sign (C), which consists of the superior glenohumeral and coracohumeral ligaments forming the medial sling of the bicipital groove. HH, humeral head; SSc, subscapularis

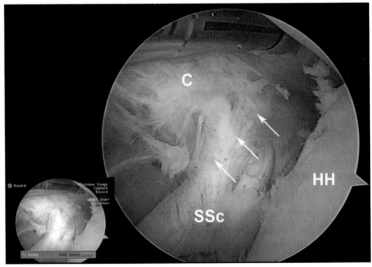

better visualized with a 70-degree arthroscope from this position. The position of the biceps is also carefully inspected. In cases of subscapularis detachment, the biceps can occupy an intra-articular position medial to the subscapularis attachment site (Figure 19-4). If not well seen, an AIP placed over the leading edge of the subscapularis can be established and a probe used to test the stability of the biceps within the groove. In chronic, retracted subscapularis tears, the "comma" sign[21] can be helpful as a landmark identifying the superolateral border of the subscapularis (Figure 19-5). The comma sign is composed of the superior glenohumeral and coracohumeral ligaments, forming the medial sling of the bicipital groove. Often, this tissue can be incorporated into the repair as it is stout; however, in those instances in which mobilization of the subscapularis is problematic, the comma sign tissue can be divided, allowing lateral mobilization of the subscapularis.

Step 2

If the biceps is dislocated medially or substantially frayed, a tenotomy or tenodesis can be performed. The authors' preference in the majority of cases is to proceed with a tenodesis. Spinal needles are placed percutaneously while viewing intra-articularly, straddling the biceps at the

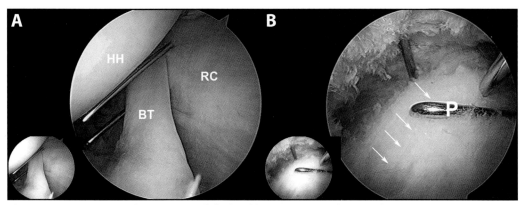

Figure 19-6. (A) Viewing from a PP in a left shoulder, 2 spinal needles are placed percutaneously, straddling the biceps tendon (BT) as it exits the joint. (B) Viewing from the ALP with a 70-degree arthroscope, the 2 spinal needles are identified. A probe (P) is placed on top of the bicipital groove (arrows), which can be unroofed to reveal a suprapectoral view of the biceps. HH, humeral head; RC, rotator cuff.

entrance into the bicipital groove (Figure 19-6). The arthroscope is introduced into the subacromial space and the 2 marking needles are identified. An ALP is established midway between a lateral portal and the anterolateral corner of the acromion. The arthroscope is then placed through this portal for viewing and a BP is subsequently created. This portal is midway between the coracoid tip and ALP, allowing direct access to the bicipital groove. Internal and external rotation facilitate palpation of the lesser and greater tuberosities with the groove easily identified as a soft spot between the needles. The tip of the coracoid can be palpated and the conjoint tendon visualized anterior to the tuberosities and bicipital groove. Great care should be taken to avoid the inadvertent inclusion of the conjoint tendon into the subscapularis repair. An ASP is now established at the edge of the anterolateral corner of the acromion. This accessory portal can be used to grasp and manipulate the subscapularis as well as handle sutures being passed from the AMP in a medial-to-lateral direction. The transverse ligament is then unroofed and the biceps identified. At the inferior extent of the bicipital groove, the biceps is tenodesed utilizing a suture anchor technique with the elbow in full extension to allow anatomic resting length. After tenodesis, the proximal biceps is released and the stump debrided. Choosing an inferior location for the tenodesis is critical because it places the tendon inferior to the lesser tuberosity and facilitates a panoramic view of the subscapularis footprint.

Step 3

Using the 70-degree arthroscope at this time promotes a direct view of the leading edge of the subscapularis and footprint (Figure 19-7). Its "rolled" up, thicker appearance is easily identified as it blends with the overlying rotator interval structure (Figure 19-8). Grasping instruments, placed through the BP, can facilitate manipulation of the soft tissues as well as tying sutures. The space between the coracoid process and the anterior border of the subscapularis should be evaluated for subcoracoid impingement anatomy. Less than 7 mm of clearance requires a decompression during which the posterolateral aspect of the coracoid is resected until 11 to 12 mm of clearance is achieved.

Step 4

A traction stitch consisting of #1 PDS can be placed through the lateral free edge of the subscapularis tear so that the cuff can be placed on tension and mobilization enhanced. This suture can be brought outside of the working cannula and clamped at the skin level, freeing up an extra

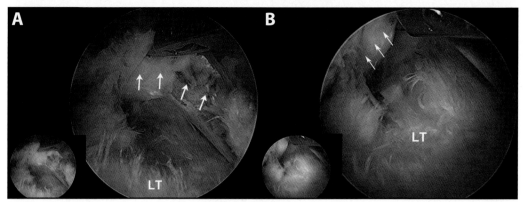

Figure 19-7. Viewing a right shoulder subscapularis tear from the ALP, (A) a 30-degree arthroscope allows visualization of the edge of the subscapularis tear (small arrows), while (B) using a 70-degree arthroscope facilitates a better view of the tear and the lesser tuberosity (LT).

Figure 19-8. Viewing from the ALP of a right shoulder, the bulky upper border (arrows) of the subscapularis is readily identified. HH, humeral head; LT, lesser tuberosity.

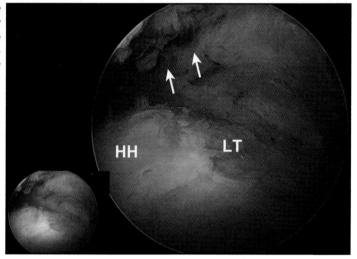

hand to handle instruments. While placing traction on the suture, a 15-degree angled elevator is used through the BP to liberate the subscapularis beginning on the articular side of the subscapularis, progressing to the superior surface underneath the coracoid arch, followed by mobilization of the anterior subscapularis. The 70-degree arthroscope facilitates viewing down the medial neck of the glenoid. Great care must be exercised during this last phase of liberation as the axillary nerve rests at the inferomedial border of the subscapularis. If desired, the arthroscope can be passed anterior and medial to the muscle belly until the axillary nerve is identified.

Step 5

With the 70-degree arthroscope in the ALP, the lesser tuberosity footprint is prepared to bleeding bone with a shaver and curette. If the lesser tuberosity is difficult to visualize, a posteriorly directed force on the proximal humerus can "open" up the subdeltoid space. In difficult exposure cases due to soft tissue swelling, a switching stick can be placed through the ASP and used to retract the deltoid muscle anteriorly to improve visualization (Figure 19-9). One triple-loaded anchor is placed for every 1 cm of the tear, and in most cases, 2 suture anchors are sufficient. For massive, retracted tears, medializing the footprint 5 to 6 mm[22] can help prevent overtensioning of the final construct without jeopardizing the healing process (Figure 19-10).

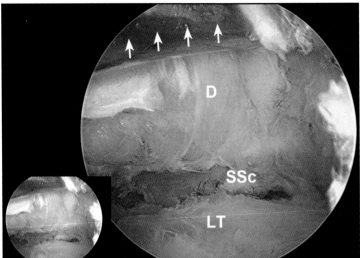

Figure 19-9. Viewing from the ALP of a right shoulder, a switching stick (arrows) is passed through the ASP and serves as a retractor for the deltoid (D), creating more extra-articular working space. LT, lesser tuberosity; SSc, anterior border of the subscapularis.

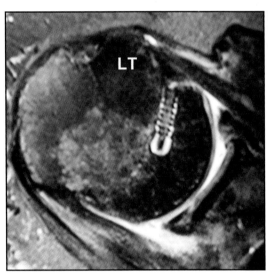

Figure 19-10. Axial MRI following repair of a chronic, retracted subscapularis tear (see Figure 19-3 as preoperative image) and medialization of the lesser tuberosity footprint. LT, lesser tuberosity.

Step 6

Once the anchors have been inserted, suturing is initiated at the inferior aspect of the torn tendon, working inferior to superior. Through the BP, a grasper is used to reduce the subscapularis to the footprint. One must ascertain that the superior border of the subscapularis is reduced to the superior-most portion of the lesser tuberosity footprint.[23] A crescent suture hook is introduced through the AMP perpendicular to the superior surface of the tendon, 5 to 6 mm medial to the leading edge (Figure 19-11). An absorbable #1 PDS suture is passed through the cuff as a suture shuttle for retrograde suture passage. The suture shuttle is grasped through the BP, loaded with a suture tail, and retrograded, exiting the AMP percutaneously.

Step 7

Vertical mattress sutures from the first anchor are placed and tied followed by insertion of the second anchor and creation of additional vertical mattress sutures with the same retrograde shuttling technique.

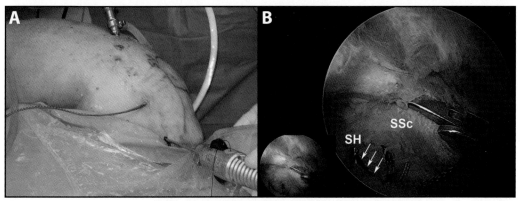

Figure 19-11. (A) Viewing the anterior aspect of a right shoulder, the suture hook (SH) is passed through the AMP medial to the coracoids (C). (B) Viewing from the ALP, the suture hook passes through the edge of the subscapularis tendon tear (SSc) and a suture shuttle consisting of #1 PDS is used to then retrograde a suture tail through the tendon (arrows).

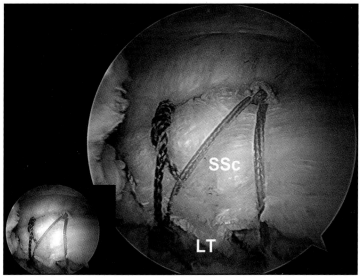

Figure 19-12. Viewing from the ALP of a right shoulder, the transosseous suturing pattern of the subscapularis tendon (SSc) tear provides for maximum coverage and compression of the lesser tuberosity (LT) footprint.

If adequate tissue is available, the repair is completed with the insertion of knotless lateral row anchors bordering on the bicipital groove laterally (Figure 19-12). Two knotless anchors usually suffice in creating a transosseous repair with optimum coverage of the footprint.

POSTOPERATIVE PROTOCOL

Rehabilitation is based on the pathology encountered, but for an isolated subscapularis repair, the postoperative protocol calls for avoiding external rotation beyond neutral rotation for 6 weeks. Passive forward flexion dangling exercises are permitted at 1 to 2 weeks postoperatively, while passive external rotation exercises are started 2 to 3 weeks following surgery. After 6 weeks, active forward flexion and external rotation are increased 10 to 15 degrees per week until a functional range of motion is achieved. Internal rotation should be delayed for 6 to 8 weeks postoperatively. Strengthening is not initiated until 3 months following surgery, while a complete return to activities is delayed for a minimum of 6 months.

POTENTIAL COMPLICATIONS

As with all surgical procedures, the risks of thrombosis, infection, and neurovascular injury must be considered. For an extra-articular subscapularis repair, the axillary nerve is vulnerable during the mobilization of adhesions along the anterior border of the muscle-tendon unit. The complications inherent to a rotator cuff repair include anchor pull-out, tissue-suture interface failure, suture breakage, as well as knot unraveling.

TOP TECHNICAL PEARLS FOR THE PROCEDURE

1. Be able to recognize the comma sign. In chronic, retracted tears, the leading border of the subscapularis can be difficult to identify. The comma sign identifies the superolateral border of the subscapularis and provides a definitive visual clue to the altered anatomy.

2. Lowering the handle of the suture anchor inserter and pointing the tip toward the jaw facilitates the proper angle of approach for anchors in relation to the lesser tuberosity. Externally rotating the humerus during anchor insertion can also provide a margin of safety for bony purchase. This angle accounts for the retroverted humeral head alignment. Insertion with the anchor perpendicular to the floor runs the risk of articular penetration.

3. Avoid debriding the fascia of the deltoid in the anterior subdeltoid space as muscle swelling will compromise the surgical exposure. Using a switching stick through the ASP to "retract" the deltoid anteriorly can significantly improve the operative exposure if swelling becomes problematic.

4. Sequencing for a 2- to 3-tendon tear that includes the subscapularis as well as the biceps should proceed as follows: biceps tenotomy vs tenodesis (possible coracoplasty), subscapularis repair, supra-infraspinatus repair, acromioplasty (if indicated), and distal clavicle excision last (if indicated). This repair sequence permits optimal visualization in a step-wise manner and accounts for fluid extravasation and its effect on operative space.

5. The ALP allows an extra-articular parallel approach to the coracoid tip. The posterolateral aspect of the coracoid can be removed without risk of detaching the conjoint tendon or neurovascular injury. An instrument tip of known diameter can be used to quantify the adequacy of the resection. Alternatively, access to the coracoid tip while viewing from the PP can be enhanced by creating a window in the rotator interval directly above the superior edge of the subscapularis.

REFERENCES

1. Warner JJP, Higgins L, Parsons IM, et al. Diagnosis and treatment of anterosuperior rotator cuff tears. *J Shoulder Elbow Surg.* 2001;10:37-46.
2. Lo IK, Burkhart SS. The etiology and assessment of subscapularis tendon tears: a case for subcoracoid impingement, the roller-wringer effect and TUFF lesions of the subscapularis. *Arthroscopy.* 2003;19:1142-1150.
3. Wellmann M, Wiebringhaus P, Lodde I, et al. Biomechanical evaluation of a single row versus double row repair for complete subscapularis tears. *Knee Surg Sports Traumatol Arthrosc.* 2009;17:1477-1484.

4. Grueninger P, Nikolic N, Schneider J, et al. Arthroscopic repair of traumatic isolated subscapularis tendon lesions (Lafosse type III or IV): a prospective magnetic resonance imaging-controlled case series with 1 year follow-up. *Arthroscopy.* 2014;30;665-672.

5. Denard PJ, Jiwani AZ, Ladermann A, et al. Long-term outcome of a consecutive series of subscapularis tears repaired arthroscopically. *Arthroscopy.* 2012;28:1587-1591.

6. Bartl C, Scheibel M, Magosch P, et al. Open repair of isolated traumatic subscapularis tendon tears. *Am J Sports Med.* 2011;39:490-496.

7. Lafosse L, Jost B, Reiland Y, et al. Structural integrity and clinical outcomes after arthroscopic repair of isolated subscapularis tears. *J Bone Joint Surg Am.* 2007;89;1184-1193.

8. Bartl C, Salzmann GM, Seppel G, et al. Subscapularis function and structural integrity after arthroscopic repair of isolated subscapularis tears. *Am J Sports Med.* 2011;39:1255-1262.

9. Heikenfeld R, Gigis I, Chytas A, et al. Arthroscopic reconstruction of isolated subscapularis tears: clinical results and structural integrity after 24 months. *Arthroscopy.* 2012;28:1805-1811.

10. Kim SH, Oh I, Park JS, et al. Intra-articular repair of an isolated partial articular-surface tear of the subscapularis tendon. *Am J Sports Med.* 2005;33:1825-1830.

11. Burkhart SS, Tehrany AM. Arthroscopic subscapularis repair: technique and preliminary results. *Arthroscopy.* 2002;18:454-463.

12. Burkhart SS, Nottage WM, Ogilvie-Harris DJ, et al. Partial repair of irreparable rotator cuff tears. *Arthroscopy.* 1994;10:363-370.

13. Goutallier D, Postel JM, Bernageau J, et al. Fatty muscle degeneration in cuff ruptures. Pre and postoperative evaluation by CT scan. *Clin Orthop Relat Res.* 1994;304:78-83.

14. Burkhart SS, Barth JS, Richards DP, et al. Arthroscopic repair of massive rotator cuff tears with stage 3-4 fatty degeneration. *Arthroscopy.* 2007;23:347-354.

15. Tokish JM, Decker MJ, Ellis HB, et al. The belly press test for the physical examination of the subscapularis muscle: electromyographic validation and comparison to the lift off test. *J Shoulder Elbow Surg.* 2003;5:427-430.

16. Barth JS, Burkhart SS, DeBeer JF. The bear hug sign: a new test for detecting subscapularis tendon tears. *Arthroscopy.* 2006;22:1076-1084.

17. Pfirrmann CW, Zanetti M, Weishaupt D, et al. Subscapularis tendon tears: detection and grading at MR arthrography. *Radiology.* 1999;213:709-714.

18. Adams CR, Schoolfield JD, Burkhart SS. Accuracy of preoperative magnetic resonance imaging in predicting a subscapularis tendon tear based on arthroscopy. *Arthroscopy.* 2010;26:1427-1433.

19. Adams CR, Brady PC, Koo SS, et al. A systematic approach for diagnosing subscapularis tears with preoperative magnetic resonance imaging. *Arthroscopy.* 2012;28:1592-1600.

20. Kim YK, Moon SH, Cho SH. Treatment outcomes of single versus double row repair for larger than medium sized rotator cuff tears: the effect of preoperative remnant tendon length. *Am J Sports Med.* 2013;41:2270-2277.

21. Lo IK, Burkhart SS. The comma sign: an arthroscopic guide to the torn subscapularis tendon. *Arthroscopy.* 2003;19:334-337

22. Denard PJ, Burkhart SS. Medialization of the subscapularis footprint does not affect functional outcome of arthroscopic repair. *Arthroscopy.* 2012;28:1608-1614.

23. Ryu RK, Bedi A. Arthroscopic subscapularis repair. In: David TS, Andrews JR, eds. *Arthroscopic Techniques of the Shoulder: A Visual Guide.* Thorofare, NJ: SLACK Incorporated; 2009:75-86.

Please see videos on the accompanying website at

www.ArthroscopicTechniques.com

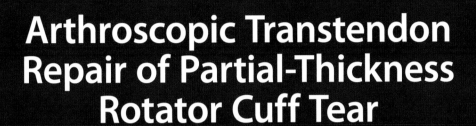

20

Arthroscopic Transtendon Repair of Partial-Thickness Rotator Cuff Tear

Richard L. Angelo, MD

INTRODUCTION

The etiology of partial articular-sided tears is likely multifactorial with overstress of the rotator cuff tissue a common feature. Partial-thickness rotator cuff tears (PTRCT) exhibit little evidence for spontaneous, natural healing. Several factors contribute to the occurrence of PTRCTs. The modulus of elasticity is greater (stiffer) on the articular compared to the bursal surface and may account, in part, for the greater incidence of articular compared with bursal surface tears.[1] Further, as the arm moves into abduction, stress in the rotator cuff moves from the rotator cable to the articular surface of the cuff.[2] Partly as a consequence of these biomechanical factors, articular-sided partial cuff tears primarily fail in tension. As articular-sided tears enlarge, strain increases in the remaining intact cuff tissue.[3] In patients with microinstability, overstretch may play a role as well. In patients with tears related to internal impingement, it is not clear whether tensile strain or mechanical impaction of the greater tuberosity onto the posterosuperior glenoid with abduction and external rotation is predominantly responsible. Tears due to internal impingement are not likely to be repairable, and it may be undesirable to do so as it can impair throwing and overhead athletic function. Debridement of articular-sided tears alone may result in reasonably good early pain relief and function, but the results tend to deteriorate with time.[4,5]

A transtendon repair for an articular-sided tear of the rotator cuff affords the opportunity to preserve the intact bursal surface layer when it is of acceptable integrity. This method only requires healing of the repaired layer rather than the full-thickness of the rotator cuff. In addition, the anatomic insertion of the cuff and the resting length of the corresponding muscle are preserved. In a cadaver model, a transtendon repair has been shown to result in a biomechanically stronger (less gap formation and greater load to failure) construct than completing and repairing partial articular tears with a defect of 50%.[6] The results of repairing these created tears, in which the bursal surface was relatively "normal," underscores the importance of the quality of the intact bursal surface for structural integrity. Good to excellent clinical outcomes have been reported for patients whom have undergone a transtendon repair for a partial articular-sided tears.[7-13] When the clinical results were compared with completing and repairing the full-thickness defect, a transtendon

Ryu RKN, Angelo RL, Abrams JS, eds. *The Shoulder:*
AANA Advanced Arthroscopic Surgical Techniques (pp 245-255).
© 2016 AANA.

repair may result in somewhat more pain and slower recovery, but with less of a tendency for post-operative cuff defects to be present.[14] A systematic review comparing the 2 techniques showed that both resulted in favorable outcomes with no clear distinction between the two.[15]

Physical examination findings are generally nonspecific for a partial cuff tear and are reflective of cuff pathology in general. Imaging studies are helpful but not consistently reliable. Magnetic resonance imaging (MRI) and MR arthrogram (MRA) studies are of variable help with the diagnosis of partial articular-sided cuff tears and are often interpreter-dependent.[16-18]

This chapter reviews the key steps of a transtendon rotator cuff technique employed to create an anatomic repair of an articular-sided cuff tear and to avoid a tension mismatch between the deep and superficial layers of the rotator cuff.

INDICATIONS

▶ An articular surface PTRCT with a 30% to 70% defect and acceptable integrity of the remaining bursal surface layer

▶ "Younger" patients (age < 50 years; greater healing potential and better integrity of the bursal layer)

Controversial Indications

▶ Poor quality remaining intact bursal cuff layer

▶ Deep layer of rotator cuff that is not reducible to the medial aspect of the footprint with the arm in an adducted position

▶ Restricted passive range of shoulder motion

PERTINENT PHYSICAL FINDINGS

▶ Tenderness at the greater tuberosity

▶ Positive impingement signs (Neer, Hawkins, simple shoulder test)

▶ Pain and/or weakness on resisted abduction, elevation, or external rotation of the arm

PERTINENT IMAGING

▶ MRI and MRA are only fair to good for detecting articular-sided PTRCTs

▶ Interobserver agreement on grading of partial cuff tears is relatively poor[19]

▶ Abduction and external rotation may improve the sensitivity to partial articular-sided tears, especially those with delamination[20]

▶ MRI reveals increased signal on T1 images without loss of continuity coupled with a corresponding defect on T2 images

▶ MRA may show a "filling defect" at the tear site[21]

EQUIPMENT

- ▶ 30-degree arthroscope
- ▶ Loop graspers/retrievers
- ▶ Full-radius synovial resector
- ▶ Barrel burr (if acromioplasty)
- ▶ Hook probe
- ▶ Obturated cannula (5.5 mm)
- ▶ 18-gauge spinal needle
- ▶ #11 blade scalpel (long handle preferred)
- ▶ Kirschner wire to pre-drill the anchor hole for nonmetallic anchor if desired (same or smaller than internal diameter of selected anchor)
- ▶ Punch/tap if nonmetallic anchor
- ▶ 0 or #1 monofilament suture
- ▶ Anchor of choice (double-loaded)
- ▶ Knot pusher
- ▶ Knot cutter

POSITIONING AND PORTALS

- ▶ Either the lateral decubitus or the beach chair positions for the patient work well
- ▶ The ability to abduct/adduct and to internally/externally rotate the shoulder is necessary
- ▶ Posterior portal (glenohumeral and subacromial): 2 cm inferior, 1 cm medial to the posterolateral corner of the acromion
- ▶ Anterior portal: midway between the anterolateral acromial corner and the coracoid tip
- ▶ Lateral acromial portal: defined using a spinal needle under direct visualization from the posterior glenohumeral portal; lies immediately adjacent to the lateral acromial margin (arm must be adducted)
- ▶ Spinal needle suture delivery: approximately 2 to 2.5 cm lateral to the acromion and roughly parallel to the greater tuberosity (arm abducted approximately 45-degrees)

STEP-BY-STEP DESCRIPTION OF THE PROCEDURE

Step 1

Confirmation of the surgical site and anticipated procedure is completed in the preoperative waiting area. Following a pause to again verify the site and operative procedure, induction of general anesthesia is performed and may be supplemented with an interscalene block. Some surgeons may prefer an interscalene block only. During an examination under anesthesia, confirm that acceptable range of motion is present. A routine skin prep and drape is completed.

The posterior portal is established 1.5 cm inferior and 1 cm medial to the posterolateral corner of the acromion. A spinal needle is then used to identify an anterior portal midway between the anterolateral corner of the acromion and the coracoid tip. An obturated cannula is introduced

Figure 20-1. Debridement of the partial articular-sided cuff tear.

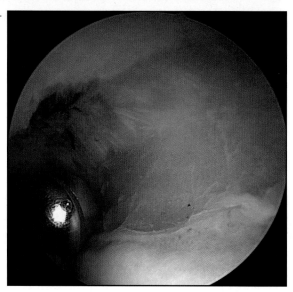

Figure 20-2. Exposure of the cuff footprint.

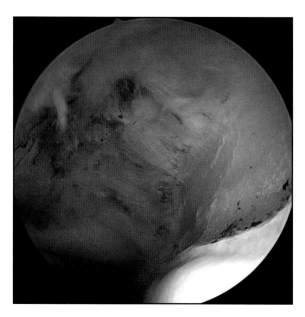

at this site. Assisted with a hook probe, a thorough diagnostic survey is performed viewing alternately from the posterior and then the anterior portal. A partial articular-sided tear of the supraspinatus is confirmed and may extend into the infraspinatus. Confirmation of a tear at the supraspinatus-infraspinatus junction, often seen in internal impingement, is best accomplished while viewing from the anterior portal.

Step 2

Debride the torn tendon tissue back to a healthy margin. A full-radius synovial resector is preferred and will not cut into healthy tendon tissue as a more aggressive shaver with teeth is prone to do (Figures 20-1 and 20-2). Resect the residual tendon fibers from the greater tuberosity. The width in millimeters of the exposed cuff footprint can be estimated using the known diameter of the shaver barrel (Figure 20-3). Given an average cuff footprint insertion of 12 to 14 mm,[22]

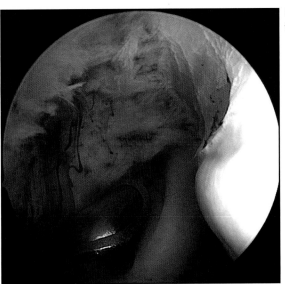

Figure 20-3. Bleeding articular surface of cuff following debridement.

a percentage of cuff thickness defect can be calculated. Repair of tears from 30% defect may be appropriate in higher-demand patients to a 70% thickness tear when the remaining bursal layer is of acceptable integrity. The anteroposterior dimension of the repair is measured with a calibrated hook probe.

Several methods can be used when assessing the quality of the remaining intact cuff tissue. Organized parallel tendon fibers, firm tension of the fibers on palpation, the lack of "billowing" of the remaining intact cuff on alternating the fluid inflow pressure, and an acceptably healthy appearance on the preoperative MRI are all suggestive that the intact bursal cuff tissue is reasonably healthy and that a transtendon repair can be expected to have a high degree of success. If the bursal layer of cuff is of marginal quality, the repair sutures may tend to cut through the tendon substance.

It is essential to verify that the cuff margin of the deep layer can be reduced to the tuberosity with the arm in an adducted position. If the cuff is not reducible, due either to the extent of deep layer tendon tissue loss or the presence of scarring and retraction, consideration should be given for completing the tear and repairing the full-thickness defect. An attempt to repair the deep layer of cuff with inadequate length will likely result in problematic postoperative stiffness, a tension mismatch with the superficial layer, poor healing, and a greater degree of postoperative pain. When the quality of the remaining intact bursal surface layer is unacceptable due to degeneration or partial bursal surface tearing, the tear should also be completed.

Step 3

When electing to proceed with a transtendon repair, re-establish the arthroscope in the subacromial space using the same skin entry as for the glenohumeral access. While viewing from posterior, a spinal needle enters the bursa 1 cm posterior and 2 cm lateral to the anterolateral corner of the acromion. If deemed an acceptable approach, a stab incision is created and the shaver and a radiofrequency device are alternately used from that lateral approach to resect enough bursal tissue to obtain an unobstructed view of the greater tuberosity and cuff insertion. Completing this step in advance facilitates suture identification and knot tying, both of which can be jeopardized if surrounding bursal tissue impedes visualization. Verifying reasonable cuff integrity on the bursal surface and the absence of a bursal-sided cuff defect is the final confirmation that a transtendon repair is a reasonable treatment option.

Figure 20-4. Incise the cuff to prepare for and insert the anchor.

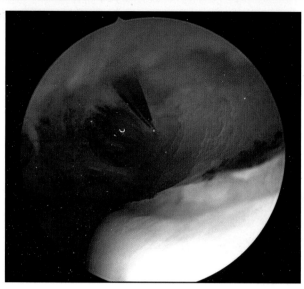

Step 4

The arthroscope is then re-established into the glenohumeral joint posteriorly. The region of exposed footprint should be excoriated with the shaver. With the arm in an adducted position, the spinal needle is introduced immediately adjacent to the lateral border and 1 cm posterior to the anterolateral border of the acromion. The needle is passed through the intact cuff to identify an acceptable approach to the medial aspect of the footprint. Without adequate humeral adduction, the approach to the footprint is generally too shallow and risks violation of the articular surface of the humeral head as instruments and anchors are inserted. If the use of 2 anchors is anticipated, internal or external rotation of the humerus will allow for an approach to both anchor insertion sites. At the selected site, a 3- or 4-mm stab incision is made through the skin and down through the bursal layer of the cuff parallel to the tendon fibers (Figure 20-4). If nonmetallic anchors are used and the bone is expected to be dense, a Kirschner wire equal to or smaller than the internal diameter of the anchors used will aid in preserving the integrity of the bone cortex. The appropriate punch and tap prepare for insertion of the anchor. Alternatively, metallic anchors generally require no special bone preparation.

While maintaining the same adducted orientation of the humerus, the posterior anchor is inserted if 2 are anticipated (Figure 20-5). A loop grasper retrieves all of the anchor suture limbs out of the anterior portal. It is critical that the margin of the rotator cuff be reduced to the cuff footprint during delivery of the repair sutures. The arm should be brought into approximately 45 degrees of abduction. This position will enable the introduction of the spinal needle used for suture delivery to be relatively parallel to the surface of the tuberosity and facilitate the creation of an anatomic repair. If the needle is brought in too far medial through the intact cuff, a tension mismatch will be created between the superficial and deep layers of the cuff as the sutures are tied, which results in buckling of the bursal layer (Figure 20-6). Once the cuff is reduced with a loop grasper, the spinal needle is introduced approximately 2 cm lateral to the acromion, through the intact bursal layer of the cuff, and into the deep layer approximately 3 mm from the margin. Begin with placement of the most posterior suture. A 0 or #1 monofilament suture is delivered through the needle. The monofilament suture and one limb of the anchor suture from the posterior aspect of the anchor are grasped simultaneously with a loop grasper and retrieved out of the anterior cannula. Grasping them together ensures that tangling with the other anchor suture limbs will be avoided. The spinal needle is then removed. A simple overhand knot is tied with the

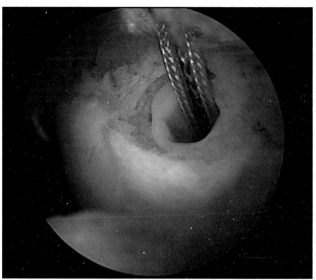

Figure 20-5. Insert the suture anchor of choice.

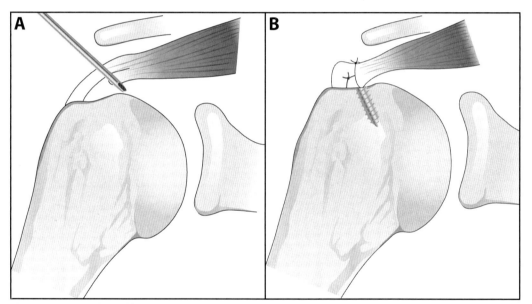

Figure 20-6. (A) The cuff is not reduced during passage of the spinal needle, which enters too far medial through the bursal surface layer, (B) creating a tension mismatch and buckling of the bursal layer.

monofilament suture around the anchor limb outside of the anterior cannula. The free lateral limb of monofilament suture is used to shuttle the anchor limb out through the deep layer of cuff tissue. This sequence of steps is repeated to pass each of the anchor sutures through the deep cuff layer, evenly spaced in a horizontal mattress configuration. If needed, the second anchor is inserted at the anterior site and the sutures are delivered in a similar manner (Figure 20-7).

Step 5

The arthroscope is then re-established into the subacromial space where the anchor suture limbs should be apparent laterally near the tuberosity (Figure 20-8). Beginning with the posterior matched pair of mattress sutures, the sliding knot of choice is tied, delivered, and secured by 3 or

Figure 20-7. All sutures delivered through articular tear margin.

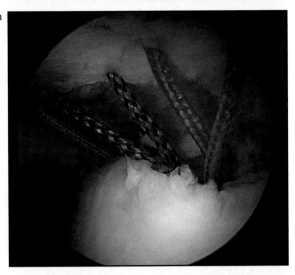

Figure 20-8. Sutures exiting from the bursal surface of the cuff.

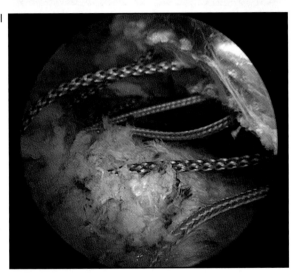

4 half-hitches (Figure 20-9). All pairs are tied in a similar manner. The arthroscope is returned to the glenohumeral joint and, using a hook probe, palpation and direct visualization confirm the security and integrity of the repair construct during flexion, extension, abduction, and adduction of the arm (Figure 20-10).

Remove the arthroscope and anterior cannula, irrigate the portals, and close in the manner of choice. After the dressing is placed on the shoulder wounds, secure the shoulder in a padded sling with mild abduction.

POSTOPERATIVE PROTOCOL

- ► Sling for 4 weeks
- ► Gentle pendulum exercises on postoperative day 2, performed 4 times per day
- ► Begin physical therapy for gentle passive range of motion exercises at 2 weeks; the goal is for 90% of full passive range of motion at 12 weeks postoperatively and complete range of motion by 4 months postoperatively

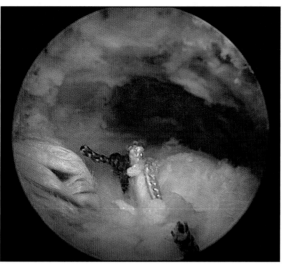

Figure 20-9. Bursal sutures are tied completing the repair.

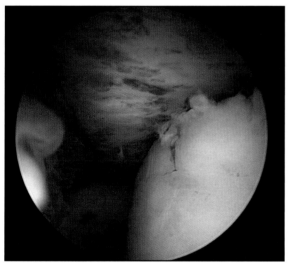

Figure 20-10. Final examination of the repaired cuff from the articular side.

► Begin light cuff isometrics/scapular strengthening at 6 weeks postoperatively

► Light progressive resistance exercises at 12 weeks postoperatively

► Graduated return to full activities at 6 months postoperatively

POTENTIAL COMPLICATIONS

► Stiffness

► Protracted pain

► Failure of the cuff to heal

► Cuff defect/tear at the mattress row of sutures

► Repair construct failure: anchor implant, sutures, suture knots

Management of postoperative stiffness must take into account the severity of the restriction, the time from repair, whether the patient is making any progress in restoration of motion, and the overall adverse impact on the patient's quality of life. Gradual improvement may occur months after the repair, and there is no specific "window of opportunity." That said, if the patient has clearly reached a plateau and is no longer realizing improvement in motion over a 1-month period of time, is a minimum of 5 to 6 months following repair, and is functionally impaired, consideration for an arthroscopic lysis of intra-articular and subacromial adhesions coupled with gentle manipulation should be considered. While early postoperative pain may be somewhat greater following a transtendon repair than a release and full-thickness repair, it is generally related to stiffness and should be expected to improve. Occasionally, inflammatory adhesive capsulitis can present in the postoperative period. A positive result with significant improvement following a diagnostic intra-articular injection of a short- or intermediate-term anesthetic agent supports the diagnosis. The use of injectable corticosteroid agents should be used judiciously. If the cuff repair fails to heal and either a symptomatic residual partial defect or a full-thickness defect are present, consideration can be given to a revision full-thickness repair. Should a type II failure occur at the medial margin of the footprint, a 5- to 7-mm medialization of the footprint during revision may help avoid undue cuff tension in the revision repair.

TOP TECHNICAL PEARLS FOR THE PROCEDURE

1. Confirm that the integrity of the intact bursal layer is acceptable (complete the partial articular-sided tear only when you expect the repair and potential healing to be superior to the bursal tissue that is being sacrificed).

2. Confirm that the deep margin of the rotator cuff can be reduced to the footprint on the greater tuberosity with the arm in an adducted position.

3. Using a loop grasper, reduce the deep layer of cuff to the tuberosity before passing the spinal needle through the deep layer for repair.

4. The spinal needle should be passed relatively parallel to the tuberosity before entering the cuff to avoid a tension mismatch between the superficial and deep cuff layers.

5. Retrieve the delivered monofilament suture and the selected anchor suture limb at the same time to avoid entanglement as the suture is shuttled from deep to superficial through the cuff.

REFERENCES

1. Yamanaka K, Matsumoto T. The joint side tear of the rotator cuff. *Clin Orthop Relat Res*. 1994:304;68-73.
2. Sano H, Wakabayashi I. Stress distribution in the supraspinatus tendon with partial-thickness tears: an analysis using a two-dimensional finite element model. *J Shoulder Elbow Surg*. 2006;15:100-105.
3. Mazzocca A, Rincon L, O'connor, et al. Intra-articular partial-thickness rotator cuff tears: analysis of injured and repaired strain behavior. *Am J Sports Med*. 2008;36:110-116.
4. Budoff JE, Nirschl RP, Guidi EJ. Debridement of partial-thickness tears of the rotator cuff without acromioplasty - long-term follow-up and review of the literature. *J Bone Joint Surg*. 1998;80;733-748.
5. Andrews, JR, Broussard TS, Carson WG. Arthroscopy of the shoulder in the management of partial tears of the rotator cuff: a preliminary report. *Arthroscopy*. 1985;1:117.
6. Gonzales-Lomas G, Kippe M, Brown G, et al. In situ transtendon repair outperforms tear completion and repair for partial articular-sided supraspinatus tendon tears. *J Shoulder Elbow Surg*. 2008;17:722-728.
7. Castagna A, Borroni M, Garofalo R, et al. Deep partial rotator cuff tear: transtendon repair of tear completion and repair? A randomized clinical trial. *Knee Surg Sports Traumatol Arthrosc*. 2015;23(2):460-463.

8. Castagna A, Eelle Rose G, Conti M, et al. Predictive factors of subtle, residual shoulder symptoms after transtendinous arthroscopic cuff repair: a clinical study. *Am J Sports Med.* 2009;37:103-108.

9. Ide J, Maeda S, Takagi K. Arthroscopic transtendon repair of partial-thickness articular-side tears of the rotator cuff: anatomical and clinical study. *Am J Sports Med.* 2005;33:1672-1679.

10. Duralde X, McClelland W, Jr. The clinical results of arthroscopic transtendinous repair of grade III partial articular-sided supraspinatus tendon repairs. *Arthroscopy.* 2012;28:160-168.

11. Franceschi F, Papalia R, Del Buono A, et al. Articular-sided rotator cuff tears: which is the best repair? A three-year prospective randomized controlled trial. *Int Orthop.* 2013;37:1487-1493.

12. Stuart K, Karzel R, Ganjianpour M, Snyder S. Long-term outcome for arthroscopic repair of partial articular-sided supraspinatus tendon avulsion. *Arthroscopy.* 2013;29:818-823.

13. Fukuda H, Craig EV, Yamanaka K. Surgical treatment of incomplete thickness tears of the rotator cuff: long-term follow-up. *Orthop Trans.* 1987;223:51-58.

14. Shin S. A comparison of 2 repair techniques for partial-thickness articular-sided rotator cuff tears. *Arthroscopy.* 2012;28:25-33.

15. Strauss EJ, Salata MJ, Kercher J, et al. Multimedia article. The arthroscopic management of partial-thickness rotator cuff tears: a systematic review of the literature. *Arthroscopy.* 2011;27:568-580.

16. Lenza M, Buchbinder R, Takwoingi Y, et al. Magnetic resonance imaging, magnetic resonance arthrography and ultrasonography for assessing rotator cuff tears in people with shoulder pain for whom surgery is being considered. *Cochrane Database Syst Rev.* 2013; 9:CD009020.

17. Bryant L, Shnier R, Bryant C, et al. A comparison of clinical estimation, ultrasonography, magnetic resonance imaging, and arthroscopy in determining the size of rotator cuff tears. *J Shoulder Elbow Surg.* 2002:11;219-224.

18. Teefey S, Rubin D, Middleton W, et al. Detection and quantification of rotator cuff tears. Comparison of ultrasonographic, magnetic resonance imaging, and arthroscopic findings n seventy-one consecutive cases. *J Bone Joint Surg.* 2004;86:708-716.

19. Spencer E Jr, Dunn W, Wright R, el al. Interobserver agreement in the classification of rotator cuff tears using magnetic resonance imaging. *Am J Sports Med.* 2008;36:99-103.

20. Herold T, Bachthaler M, Hamer O, et al. Indirect MR arthrography of the shoulder: use of abduction and external rotation to detect full- and partial-thickness tears of the supraspinatus tendon. *Radiology.* 2006;240:152-160.

21. Meister K, Thesing J, Montomery W, et al. MR arthrography of partial thickness tears of the rotator cuff: an arthroscopic correlation. *Skel Radiol.* 2004;33:136-141.

22. Curtis A, Burbank K, Tierney J, et al. The insertional footprint of the rotator cuff: an anatomic study. *Arthroscopy.* 2006;22:603-609.

Please see videos on the accompanying website at

www.ArthroscopicTechniques.com

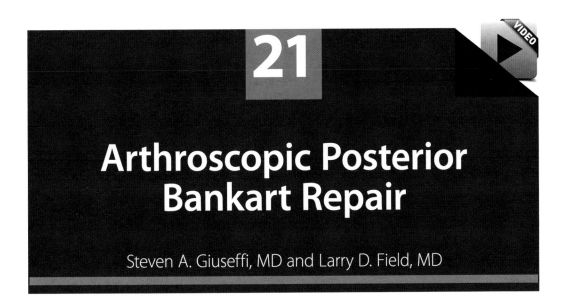

INTRODUCTION

Posterior glenohumeral instability is less common than anterior instability and occurs in only 2% to 10% of patients with shoulder instability.[1-3] The diagnosis can be challenging as symptoms may be vague and often do not localize posteriorly.[4,5] Frequently, patients complain of pain rather than instability episodes. Recurrent subluxation is more common than frank dislocation, and most patients do not recall a specific traumatic event.[6,7] Etiologies include acute trauma, chronic repetitive microtrauma, and atraumatic instability.[8] Posterior instability is more common in athletes who repetitively load their shoulders in a flexed and adducted position (weightlifters, football lineman, baseball batters, rowers, etc). Pathoanatomy is varied and can include injury to the posterior capsuloligamentous structures, bony glenoid or humerus, rotator interval, and rotator cuff.[9-13]

Operative intervention is indicated for patients with recurrent posterior instability who fail nonoperative management. While posterior shoulder instability was historically treated with open surgery, this required large surgical dissections and reported failure rates ranged from 30% to 70%.[14] This led to the increasing use of arthroscopy for the management of posterior glenohumeral instability in patients without significant osseous deficiency. Advantages of an arthroscopic approach include its minimally invasive nature as well as the ability to address the variety of pathoanatomy seen in posterior instability.[1,15,16] Various studies have shown that arthroscopic management of posterior glenohumeral instability can successfully restore shoulder stability.[9,17-22]

INDICATIONS

- ▶ Traumatic posterior glenohumeral dislocation with recurrent instability
- ▶ Recurrent posterior glenohumeral subluxation during activity

Ryu RKN, Angelo RL, Abrams JS, eds. *The Shoulder:*
AANA Advanced Arthroscopic Surgical Techniques (pp 257-267).
© 2016 AANA.

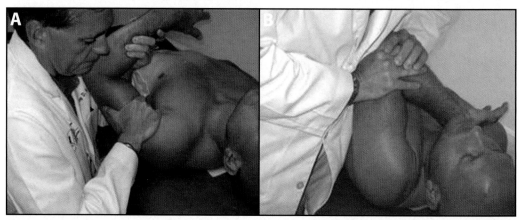

Figure 21-1. Senior author performing (A) a posterior load and shift test and (B) the jerk test. Note that in posterior instability, the patient may have apprehension but often complains of posterior pain or discomfort instead.

Controversial Indications

▶ Posteroinferior-dominant multidirectional instability

▶ Posterior glenohumeral instability with significant glenoid or humeral bone loss

PERTINENT PHYSICAL FINDINGS

▶ Posterior load and shift test: Patient is placed supine on the examining table to stabilize the scapula. The arm is positioned in approximately 20 degrees of abduction and forward flexion. A slight axial load is first applied to center the humeral head in the glenoid, and the examiner then attempts to translate the humeral head posteriorly. The examiner notes whether the humeral head can be translated beyond the glenoid rim and whether this reproduces the patient's posterior shoulder pain/discomfort (Figure 21-1A).

▶ Jerk test: Patient is placed supine on the examining table to stabilize the scapula. The patient's arm is placed in 90 degrees of forward flexion with the elbow bent and arm internally rotated across his or her body. The arm is then slightly adducted and a posterior axial load is applied along the axis of the humerus. A sudden clunk or jerk is indicative of posterior humeral head subluxation (Figure 21-1B).

▶ Sulcus sign: The patient's arm is placed at the side and an inferior traction force is applied. The examiner looks for a dimple or sulcus between the humeral head and acromion greater than 1 cm. If a sulcus is seen, the examiner then performs the test with the arm in external rotation to determine if the sulcus sign diminishes with rotator interval tensioning.

PERTINENT IMAGING

▶ Three-view radiographs of shoulder: These are closely evaluated for humeral head subluxation, reverse Hills-Sachs humeral head lesions, fractures or bony deficiency of the posterior glenoid, and glenoid retroversion.

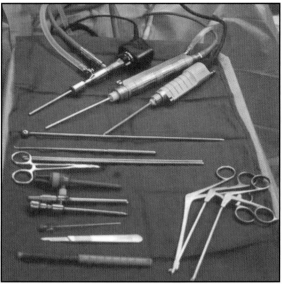

Figure 21-2. Standard arthroscopic instruments used: standard 4-mm, 30-degree arthroscope, arthroscopic shaver and burr, various trocars and switching sticks as well as plastic and metal cannulas, and arthroscopic graspers and suture retrievers. Not included in image is surgeon's choice of suture passer and labral anchors. It is helpful to have multiple suture passers with a variety of angles in both right- and left-facing orientations.

▶ Magnetic resonance imaging (MRI) or MR arthrography of the shoulder: MRI allows the surgeon to assess the integrity of the posterior labrum and capsule. Patients with posterior glenohumeral instability may not have obvious labral tears, and capsular redundancy or reverse humeral avulsion of the glenohumeral ligament (HAGL) lesions may be seen. Rotator cuff integrity is also evaluated, and glenoid rim fractures or excessive glenoid retroversion may be seen.

Equipment

▶ Traction apparatus for suspension of operative arm, axillary roll, inflatable bean bag for lateral decubitus positioning with the operative arm positioned in approximately 45 degrees of abduction and 10 degrees of forward flexion (Figure 21-2)

▶ Standard 30-degree, 4-mm arthroscope

▶ Various suture passers of different angles. The authors prefer to use a 60-degree retrograde, disposable suture retriever (IDEAL Suture Grasper [DePuy Mitek, Inc])

▶ Spinal needle for portal localization

▶ Arthroscopic probe, elevator, rasp, and shaver/burr

▶ Switching stick or long trocar

▶ Labral suture anchors, appropriate drill guide, and drill for suture anchor placement

Positioning and Portals

General anesthesia is induced. A complete examination under anesthesia is performed to evaluate glenohumeral instability. The patient is then placed in a lateral decubitus position. The patient's torso is rotated approximately 30 degrees posteriorly, bringing the glenoid parallel to the operating room floor. An axillary roll is placed, and all bony prominences are well padded. An inflatable bean bag is used to stabilize the patient in this position, and the nonoperative arm is placed on an arm board.

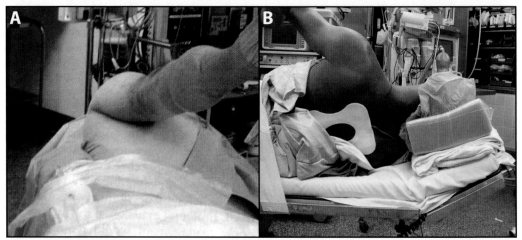

Figure 21-3. A posterior labral detachment viewed from the anterosuperior portal. Assessment of the posterior labral and capsular structures via this anterosuperior portal is helpful in identifying and accurately assessing pathology in the posteroinferior aspect of the glenohumeral joint.

STEP-BY-STEP DESCRIPTION OF THE PROCEDURE

Step 1

The patient's operative arm is prepped and draped. The operative arm is then placed in approximately 45 degrees of abduction and 10 degrees of flexion and attached to the traction apparatus. Ten lbs of traction is the standard, with 15 lbs reserved for larger patients when 10 lbs is insufficient.

A standard posterior portal is created in the posterior soft spot. The arthroscope is inserted into the posterior viewing portal and standard glenohumeral diagnostic arthroscopy is performed. An anterior portal is created in an outside-in fashion in the center of the rotator interval. A medium-sized (7 mm) plastic cannula is placed in the anterior portal.

The arthroscope is then switched to the anterior portal and a switching stick is placed into the posterior portal. While viewing from the anterior portal, the anterior humeral head is thoroughly evaluated for a reverse Hill-Sachs lesion. Attention is then turned to the posterior capsulolabral structures. A cannula is placed over the posterior switching stick under direct arthroscopic visualization. A probe is then placed through the posterior cannula, and the posterior labrum and capsule are thoroughly evaluated. It is important to note that posterior labral injury may be less dramatic than that commonly seen with anterior Bankart lesions. However, there is often associated posterior capsular injury or redundancy.

After posterior capsuloligamentous pathology is confirmed, the arthroscope is then placed back into the posterior portal. An accessory anterosuperior portal is then created in the rotator interval just anterior to the leading edge of supraspinatus. A 5.5-mm cannula is placed in the accessory anterosuperior portal and the arthroscope is then moved to this cannula.

Viewing from the anterosuperior portal allows complete visualization of the glenoid and associated capsuloligamentous structures. A probe is inserted into the posterior portal cannula and used to evaluate the posterior labrum and posterior capsule again from this viewing angle (Figure 21-3).

Not infrequently, the surgeon will note injury to both the labrum and the capsule (Figure 21-4). The labrum can be detached from the posterior glenoid rim with or without an associated bony lesion. The posterior capsule can be torn in its midsubstance, or it can be avulsed off the humerus (reverse HAGL).

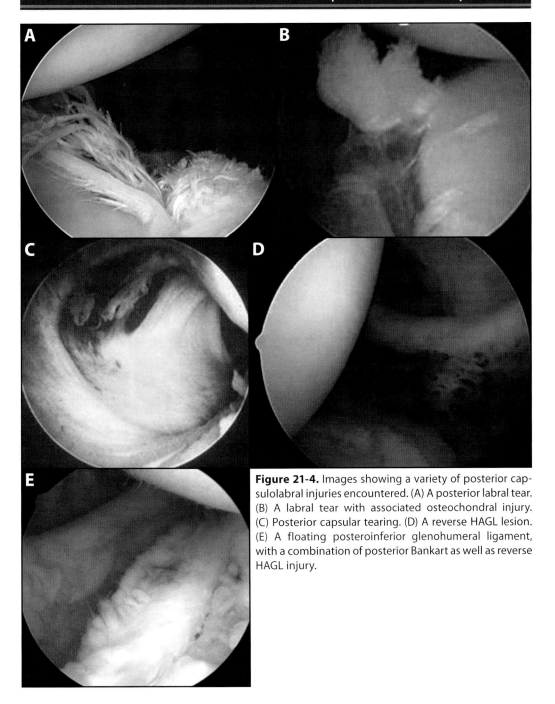

Figure 21-4. Images showing a variety of posterior capsulolabral injuries encountered. (A) A posterior labral tear. (B) A labral tear with associated osteochondral injury. (C) Posterior capsular tearing. (D) A reverse HAGL lesion. (E) A floating posteroinferior glenohumeral ligament, with a combination of posterior Bankart as well as reverse HAGL injury.

Step 2

Access to the posteroinferior glenoid is crucial for success during arthroscopic posterior labral repair. The standard posterior viewing portal is typically too medial for posterior labral elevation, glenoid preparation, and suture anchor insertion. Furthermore, the inferior capsule may be difficult to reach via the standard posterior portal. Therefore, an accessory inferior posterolateral working portal (posterior instability portal) is created. This portal is typically 1 to 2 cm lateral and distal to the standard posterior portal. As accurate positioning of this portal is critical, it is best

Figure 21-5. Arthroscopic portals typically used for posterior labral repair, as viewed from posterior with the patient's head to the left of the image. Plastic cannula anterosuperiorly is used primarily for viewing with an arthroscope but can also be used for labral preparation and suture management as necessary. The metal cannula is in standard posterior portal. The accessory posterolateral portal, shown here by the spinal needle with green cap, is distal and lateral to standard posterior portal. This portal is created under direct arthroscopic visualization and is instrumental to effective posterior labral repair. The accessory posterolateral portal provides the proper trajectory for posterior anchor placement and also allows the surgeon to more easily access the posteroinferior capsule for capsular shift and plication.

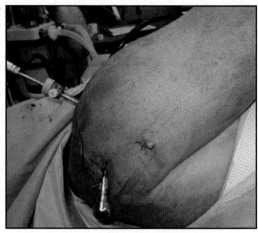

localized with a spinal needle while viewing with the arthroscope from the anterosuperior portal. The spinal needle position and trajectory should be critically evaluated prior to the creation of the accessory posterolateral portal. Portal location should allow the surgeon to easily reach the posteroinferior capsule and glenoid as well as provide optimal trajectory for posterior glenoid anchor placement. After localization of the accessory inferior posterolateral portal, a large (7 or 8.5 mm) plastic cannula is inserted over a switching stick into this portal (Figure 21-5).

Step 3

In cases of posterior shoulder instability without labral injury, the surgeon may choose to plicate the posterior capsule to the intact labrum. In the authors' experience, however, posterior labral injury is commonly seen and suture anchor fixation is preferred in that setting. In preparation for anchor placement, an elevator is inserted via one of the posterior portals to mobilize the posterior labrum off the glenoid. Alternatively, the elevator can be placed via the mid-glenoid anterior portal if this provides a better trajectory for labral mobilization. One should avoid capsular plication to a frayed and attenuated labrum, even if a complete Bankart lesion is not identified. The labrum should be freed and a suture anchor technique implemented.

After the posterior labrum and capsule have been sufficiently mobilized off the glenoid, a rasp is then used to gently abrade the labrum and capsule to encourage healing. An arthroscopic shaver or burr is then used to debride the glenoid rim to create a bleeding surface. Every attempt should be made to preserve bone.

Step 4

Anchors are then placed via the accessory inferior posterolateral portal while the arthroscope remains in the anterosuperior portal. The inferior-most anchor is placed first, typically in the 7 o'clock position for a right shoulder. Anchors are placed at the articular margin of the glenoid and are spaced about 5-mm apart. Typically, 2 to 4 anchors are used, depending on the extent of labral injury. Double-loaded anchors are preferable for their increased load to failure.

Step 5

After anchors have been placed, the surgeon prepares for suture passage. Determining the appropriate amount of capsular shift and plication is challenging and must be assessed on a case-by-case basis. To estimate the amount of capsular shift and plication needed, the surgeon can use

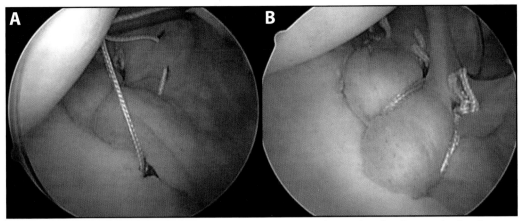

Figure 21-6. Arthroscopic images of posterior labral repair and capsular plication as viewing from an anterosuperior portal. (A) The capsular limb of the anchor suture is passed inferior and lateral to its respective anchor. When the sutures are subsequently tied, the capsule is shifted superiorly and the redundant capsule is plicated to form (B) a labral "bumper." Note that anchor placement and suture passage/tying proceeds in an inferior to superior fashion.

an arthroscopic grasper to provisionally reduce the labrum to the glenoid. The surgeon can then further tension the posterior capsule by pulling the capsule farther superiorly and/or anteriorly until sufficient capsular tension is obtained. The surgeon then attempts to replicate this capsular tension during suture passage and tying. If there is any evidence of inferior capsular laxity in addition to the labral pathology, the inferior capsule must be directly addressed with an inferiorly placed anchor.

Sutures will be passed through the capsule and labrum in an inferior-to-superior progression. In this manner, the more difficult inferior suture is passed first. Furthermore, the surgeon can more easily assess the posterior capsular plication achieved with each successive suture.

A suture retriever (or suture shuttle) is placed into the joint via the accessory inferior posterolateral portal. The suture retriever is then used to penetrate the posteroinferior capsule inferior and lateral to the respective glenoid anchor position, thus effecting capsular plication and superior capsular shift.

If the inferior capsule is difficult to reach with the suture passer, an arthroscopic grasper or a traction stitch can be used to pull the capsule superiorly. This facilitates suture shuttling while also tensioning the inferior capsule and providing a superior capsular shift. Care is taken to penetrate the posteroinferior capsule under control to avoid iatrogenic axillary nerve injury. Passing through the tissue with a suture hook and then rapidly supinating allows for penetration of the capsule without plunging, thus avoiding iatrogenic injury to surrounding neurovascular structures.

After the suture passer penetrates the lateral aspect of the posteroinferior capsule, it is then delivered under the torn labrum at the glenoid margin near the respective suture anchor. The suture retriever is deployed to shuttle one of the inferior anchor sutures through the posterior capsule. The suture shuttling steps are repeated to create a horizontal mattress suture if desired. If a simple suture configuration is used, the limb passing through the capsule is designated as the tying post. In this manner, the arthroscopic knot rests off of the glenoid and redundant capsule is pushed up against the glenoid to act as a "bumper" to limit posterior humeral head translation.

These steps are repeated as necessary for the more superior anchors. Capsular tension is evaluated after each successive knot is tied. The posteroinferior capsule is where the majority of capsular shift and plication should be performed (Figure 21-6).

Step 6: Management of Posterior Humeral Avulsion of Glenohumeral Ligaments

Posterior shoulder instability can be caused by a posterior Bankart lesion, capsular redundancy, and/or posterior HAGL (reverse HAGL).[11-12] Posterior HAGL lesions can occur in isolation or in combination with a posterior Bankart lesion.[10] Several additional surgical steps are needed to repair a posterior HAGL lesion. First, an arthroscopic shaver is used to debride the bone along the posterior humeral neck in the area of the posterior capsular insertion. Two suture anchors are then placed into the humeral neck at the anatomic insertion of the posterior inferior glenohumeral ligament and posterior capsule.

The posterior cannula is then backed up slightly so that it is superficial to the joint capsule but deep to the deltoid. A penetrating suture retriever is then used through the cannula to penetrate the posterior capsule and retrieve one of the suture limbs from a respective anchor. The penetrator is then used to pierce the capsule again and retrieve the other respective suture, taking care to retrieve this suture from a separate capsular window so that a mattress suture construct is created.

The shoulder is then placed in external rotation. The sutures are tensioned while still viewing from the glenohumeral joint so the surgeon can watch the ligament anatomically reduce to the humeral neck. The sutures are then tied extracapsularly in blind fashion.

Next, standard repair of the posterior Bankart lesion is completed. Note that the posterior HAGL is repaired before the posterior Bankart. If posterior Bankart repair and capsular plication were undertaken first, the surgeon could excessively plicate the posterior capsule. This would prevent subsequent reduction of the posteroinferior glenohumeral ligament to the humeral neck.

Step 7: Rotator Interval Plication

Rotator interval closure for posterior shoulder instability is a controversial topic. Some surgeons utilize rotator interval plication routinely for patients with posterior shoulder instability, while others use it rarely and underline that excellent results have been reported without rotator interval closure.[15,17,18,23] Selective rotator interval closure is reserved predominantly for those patients with very high or even extreme degrees of posterior instability. These patients often have hyperlaxity and a prominent sulcus sign on physical examination. Thin or poor capsular tissue and/or revision surgery are other potential indications for rotator interval plication to augment posterior labral repair.

When rotator interval plication is performed, the superior glenohumeral ligament (SGHL) is plicated to the middle glenohumeral ligament (MGHL). This is accomplished while viewing with the arthroscope in the standard posterior portal. The first step in performing the authors' preferred rotator interval closure technique begins by delivering one end of a free, braided suture into the glenohumeral joint via the anterosuperior portal. This suture is then grasped by a retrograde suture retriever placed percutaneously through the inferior rotator interval and MGHL. This retrograde retriever, now grasping the suture, is then backed out of the glenohumeral joint slightly, remaining immediately adjacent to the anterior (extra-articular) rotator interval capsule, and is then redirected superiorly back into the joint through the SGHL. This suture limb now spans the entire rotator interval capsule, enveloping not only the MGHL and SGHL, but also the coracohumeral ligament as well. This suture is then retrieved through the anterosuperior portal and tied with the arm positioned in approximately 45 degrees of abduction and 45 degrees of external rotation. This rotator interval closure technique offers the advantages of incorporating the coracohumeral ligament, important in limiting posterior humeral translation, into the rotator interval plication and accomplishing arthroscopic knot tying intra-articularly (without the necessity to tie the plication suture "blindly," as some techniques require; Figure 21-7).

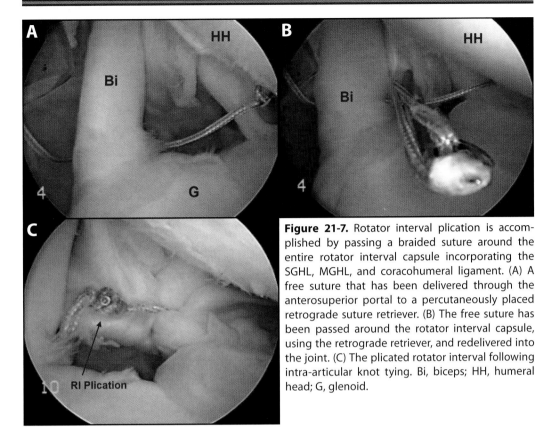

Figure 21-7. Rotator interval plication is accomplished by passing a braided suture around the entire rotator interval capsule incorporating the SGHL, MGHL, and coracohumeral ligament. (A) A free suture that has been delivered through the anterosuperior portal to a percutaneously placed retrograde suture retriever. (B) The free suture has been passed around the rotator interval capsule, using the retrograde retriever, and redelivered into the joint. (C) The plicated rotator interval following intra-articular knot tying. Bi, biceps; HH, humeral head; G, glenoid.

POSTOPERATIVE PROTOCOL

Patients are kept in a shoulder immobilizer with their operative arm in approximately 15 degrees of external rotation for 4 weeks postoperatively. The arm is maintained posterior to the patient's trunk to minimize stress on the repair. The patient participates in gentle elbow, wrist, and hand range of motion exercises.

After 4 weeks, patients begin active-assisted range of motion to include forward elevation in the scapular plane and external rotation with the arm at the side. Internal rotation behind the patient's back is also initiated, but internal rotation with the arm elevated is prohibited at this time. Limited strengthening exercises are also initiated.

At 8 weeks postoperatively, patients progress to more advanced rehabilitation with unrestricted range of motion and comprehensive shoulder and periscapular strengthening. Sport-specific training typically begins 3 to 4 months postoperatively, and return to collision sports and unrestricted weightlifting is usually allowed after 6 months.

POTENTIAL COMPLICATIONS

Recurrent instability is the most common complication, with reported recurrence rates after arthroscopic repair ranging from 3% to 20%.[7,9,13,15,19,23] Revision surgery after traumatic re-injury is typically more successful than revision for atraumatic instability.[6] Revision arthroscopic posterior Bankart repair and capsular shift can be successful for patients without posterior glenoid bone loss or excessive glenoid retroversion.[24]

Stiffness after posterior labral repair is likely underestimated in the literature and typically manifests as internal rotation loss.[6] This may be acceptable for many patients as a tradeoff for shoulder stability. However, shoulder stiffness may be particularly limiting for overhead athletes.

The axillary nerve is at risk during shoulder instability surgery and is particularly close to the inferior capsule at the level of the posteroinferior glenoid.[25] The surgeon must take care to minimally penetrate the capsule in controlled fashion when performing inferior capsular plication and shift.

TOP TECHNICAL PEARLS FOR THE PROCEDURE

1. Utilize lateral decubitus position. This facilitates access to the posteroinferior labrum and capsule.

2. View from the anterosuperior portal. This provides a circumferential view of the labrum and allows the posterior and mid-glenoid anterior portals to be used for instrumentation and suture management.

3. Thoroughly evaluate and treat all potential pathoanatomy. Posterior shoulder instability may occur in association with injury to the labrum, capsule, osseous glenoid or humerus, and/or rotator interval.

4. Use an accessory inferior posterolateral portal (posterior instability portal). This facilitates posterior glenoid preparation and anchor placement as well as capsular shift of the inferior capsule.

5. The elevator can be used through the anteroinferior or anterosuperior portal when liberating the posteroinferior labrum. Starting the labral elevation from an anterior portal and then completing the task via one of the posterior portals is recommended.

REFERENCES

1. Provencher MT, LeClere LE, King S, et al. Posterior instability of the shoulder: diagnosis and management. *Am J Sports Med*. 2011;39:874-886.

2. Owens BD, Campbell SE, Cameron KL. Risk factors for posterior shoulder instability in young athletes. *Am J Sports Med*. 2013;41:2645-2649.

3. Robinson CM, Seah M, Akhtar MA. The epidemiology, risk of recurrence, and functional outcome after an acute traumatic posterior dislocation of the shoulder. *J Bone Joint Surg Am*. 2011;93:1605-1613.

4. Van Tongel A, Karelse A, Berghs B, Verdonk R, De Wilde L. Posterior shoulder instability: current concepts review. *Knee Surg Sports Traumatol Arthrosc*. 2011;19:1547-1553.

5. Lenart BA, Sherman SL, Mall NA, Gochanour E, Twigg SL, Nicholson GP. Arthroscopic repair for posterior shoulder instability. *Arthroscopy*. 2012;28:1337-1343.

6. Millett PJ, Clavert P, Hatch GF, Warner JP. Recurrent posterior shoulder instability. *J Am Acad Orthop Surg*. 2006;14:464-476.

7. Bradley JP, Tejwani SG. Arthroscopic management of posterior instability. *Orthop Clin N Am*. 2010;41:339-356.

8. Tannenbaum EP, Sekiya JK. Posterior shoulder instability in the contact athlete. *Clin Sports Med*. 2013;32:781-796.

9. Savoie FH III, Holt MS, Field LD, Ramsey JR. Arthroscopic management of posterior instability: evolution of technique and results. *Arthroscopy*. 2008;24:389-396.

10. Pokabla C, Hobgood ER, Field LD. Identification and management of "floating" posterior inferior glenohumeral ligament lesions. *J Shoulder Elbow Surg*. 2010;19:314-317.

11. Shah AA, Butler RB, Fowler R, Higgins LD. Posterior capsular rupture causing posterior shoulder instability: a case report. *Arthroscopy.* 2011;27:1304-1307.

12. Hill JD, Lovejoy JF, Kelly RA. Combined posterior Bankart lesion and posterior humeral avulsion of the glenohumeral ligaments associated with recurrent posterior shoulder instability. *Arthroscopy.* 2007;23:327.e1-327.e3.

13. Kim SH, Kim HK, Sun J II, Park JS, Oh I. Arthroscopic capsulolabroplasty for posteroinferior multidirectional instability of the shoulder. *Am J Sports Med.* 2004;32:594-607.

14. Hawkins R, Koppert G, Johnston G. Recurrent posterior instability (subluxation) of the shoulder. *J Bone Joint Surg Am.* 1984;66:169-174.

15. Wolf EM, Eakin CL. Arthroscopic capsular plication for posterior shoulder instability. *Arthroscopy.* 1998;14:153-163.

16. Bottoni CR, Franks BR, Moore JH, DeBerardino TM, Taylor DC, Arciero RA. Operative stabilization of posterior shoulder instability. *Am J Sports Med.* 2005;33:996-1002.

17. Kim SH, Ha KI, Park JH, et al. Arthroscopic posterior labral repair and capsular shift for traumatic unidirectional recurrent posterior subluxation of the shoulder. *J Bone Joint Surg.* 2003;85-A:1479-1487.

18. Bradley JP, McClincy MP, Arner JW, Tejwani SG. Arthroscopic capsulolabral reconstruction for posterior instability of the shoulder: a prospective study of 200 shoulders. *Am J Sports Med.* 2013;41:2005-2014.

19. Bahk MS, Karzel RP, Synder SJ. Arthroscopic posterior stabilization and anterior capsular plication for recurrent posterior glenohumeral instability. *Arthroscopy.* 2010;26:1172-1180.

20. Williams RJ, Strickland S, Cohen M, Altcheck DW, Warren RF. Arthroscopic repair for traumatic posterior shoulder instability. *Am J Sports Med.* 2003;31:203-209.

21. Wanich T, Dines J, Dines D, Gambardella RA, Yocum LA. Batter's shoulder: can athletes return to play at the same level after operative management? *Clin Orthop Relat Res.* 2012:470:1565-1570.

22. Abrams JS, Bradley JP, Angelo RL, Burks R. Arthroscopic management of shoulder instabilities: anterior, posterior, and multidirectional. *AAOS Instr Course Lect.* 2010;59:141-155.

23. Provencher MT, Bell SJ, Menzel KA, Mologne TS. Arthroscopic treatment of posterior shoulder instability: results in 33 patients. *Am J Sports Med.* 2005;33:1463-1471.

24. Chalmers PN, Hammond J, Juhan T, Romeo AA. Revision posterior shoulder stabilization. *J Shoulder Elbow Surg.* 2013;22:1209-1220.

25. Scully WF, Wilson DJ, Parad SA, Arrington ED. Iatrogenic nerve injuries in shoulder surgery. *J Am Acad Orthop Surg.* 2013;21:717-726.

Please see videos on the accompanying website at

www.ArthroscopicTechniques.com

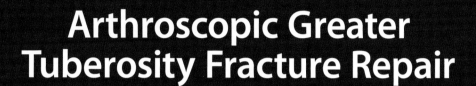

22

Arthroscopic Greater Tuberosity Fracture Repair

Brody A. Flanagin, MD; Joe Burns, MD; Connor Larose, MD;
Raffaele Garofalo, MD; MAJ Kelly Fitzpatrick, DO, MC, US Army;
and Sumant G. Krishnan, MD

INTRODUCTION

Fractures of the proximal humerus represent roughly 5% of all fractures and show a unimodal distribution in older patients.[1,2] The majority of these fractures are adequately managed nonoperatively with immobilization followed by early motion. Isolated fractures of the greater tuberosity proximal humerus fractures represent a small subset of all fractures of the proximal humerus.[2] These fractures typically occur as a result of either impaction, shearing, or avulsion; they are commonly seen in association with an anterior dislocation of the humeral head.[3]

Treatment of greater tuberosity fractures is in large part predicated on the associated attachments of the supraspinatus, infraspinatus, and teres minor tendons. The principal goal of treatment is to avoid significant displacement of the tuberosity in order to preserve rotator cuff function and avoid impingement with range of motion. Controversy exists within the literature regarding appropriate indications for surgical repair of isolated greater tuberosity fractures. Neer's criteria of > 1 cm of displacement has been traditionally used as an indication for surgical repair, but more recent studies suggest that 3 to 5 mm of displacement represents a relative indication for surgical repair in active patients and overhead athletes.[4-8] Failure to adequately reduce the greater tuberosity can lead to poor outcomes with limited salvage options in both younger and/or active patients.

Both open and percutaneous surgical approaches have been described in the past with satisfactory results.[9,10] Suture fixation has historically been preferred over screw fixation for comminuted greater tuberosity fractures.[11] More recently, both arthroscopic-assisted and all arthroscopic repair of isolated greater tuberosity fractures with suture anchors has been described with favorable outcomes.[12-16] This technique allows for improved visualization of the entire rotator cuff and any associated pathology while simultaneously avoiding the morbidity associated with more formal "open" surgical approaches.

Ryu RKN, Angelo RL, Abrams JS, eds. *The Shoulder:*
AANA Advanced Arthroscopic Surgical Techniques (pp 269-276).
© 2016 AANA.

Figure 22-1. (A) True anteroposterior view of the right shoulder in external rotation demonstrating a minimally displaced greater tuberosity fracture. (B) Representative modified axillary view of the left shoulder.

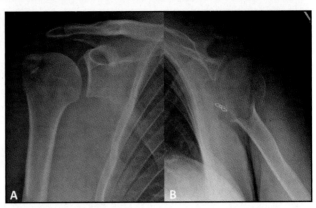

INDICATIONS

▶ Displacement greater than 10 mm
▶ Displacement greater than 3 to 5 mm in younger, active patients or overhead athletes

Controversial Indications

▶ Displaced and comminuted greater tuberosity fractures
▶ Advanced age/elderly patients with poor/insufficient bone stick
▶ Severe displacement and/or fixed retraction of the tuberosity

PERTINENT PHYSICAL FINDINGS

▶ Swelling/bruising affecting the ipsilateral shoulder and arm
▶ Pain and/or weakness with active elevation, external rotation, and internal rotation of the affected shoulder
▶ Presence of any associated trauma
▶ Presence of deltoid isometric contraction (to assess axillary nerve motor function)
▶ Sensory function in the lateral deltoid region (not always a reliable marker of axillary nerve injury)
▶ Neurovascular changes in the affected extremity (to assess for associated brachial plexus injury when the causative event is an anterior glenohumeral dislocation)

PERTINENT IMAGING

▶ True anteroposterior view of the shoulder in neutral or external rotation, scapular Y view, and axillary view of the affected shoulder. The authors prefer an anteroposterior view in neutral or external rotation, which allows for appropriate visualization of the profile of the greater tuberosity (Figure 22-1).
▶ A modified axillary view is routinely performed as previously described for patients with shoulder trauma who otherwise cannot lift their arm.[17] This is critical to rule out any subluxation or dislocation of the glenohumeral joint (see Figure 22-1).

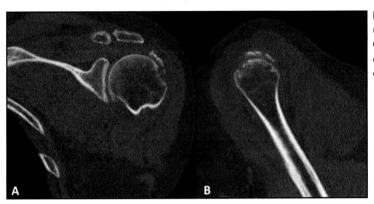

Figure 22-2. Representative (A) coronal and (B) sagittal CT images of a left shoulder demonstrating a displaced greater tuberosity fracture.

▶ Computed tomography (CT) imaging can be obtained in cases where further information is desired regarding the amount and/or direction of displacement of the tuberosity. This modality is often utilized if younger and/or more active patients with apparent minimally displaced fractures on plain radiographs. Posterior displacement of the tuberosity is best evaluated on the axial images and superior displacement on the coronal images. The sagittal images can be used to judge both superior and posterior displacement (Figure 22-2). Three-dimensional reconstructions can be incorporated with CT imaging for further information at the discretion of the treating physician.

▶ Magnetic resonance imaging is not routinely used in the evaluation of greater tuberosity fractures, but this modality may be helpful in determining the presence of any associated tearing of the rotator cuff.

EQUIPMENT

Preoperative planning before entering the operating room is critical to ensure the surgeon is appropriately prepared with all necessary equipment to ensure the procedure runs in as efficient a manner as possible. Given the limited indications for this procedure and resultant lack of widespread experience with arthroscopic treatment of greater tuberosity fractures, the authors feel all surgeons should be prepared to convert to an open technique if optimal fixation is not possible arthroscopically. Standard arthroscopic equipment is required for this technique, which may vary from surgeon to surgeon. A sterile, articulated arm holder/positioner is a helpful tool to place and hold the arm in space when trying to reduce the tuberosity and visualize the repair. A reduction tool such as a blunt/nonpenetrating awl or Kirschner wire may be helpful to place percutaneously through an accessory portal prior to assist in holding the tuberosity reduced before tying sutures. The authors strongly recommend passing sutures through the rotator cuff using either retrograde or shuttling techniques with the treating surgeon's preferred instruments. The authors also recommend against performing antegrade suture passing through the rotator cuff for these cases in order to avoid the potential for iatrogenic damage to the attached greater tuberosity fracture fragment. Any commercially available suture anchors may be utilized for performing the repair and is at the discretion of the treating surgeon. Both traditional double-row and double-row linked suture-bridge techniques have been described to perform arthroscopic repair of greater tuberosity fractures.[13-16] When utilizing suture anchors, the authors prefer the suture-bridge technique as they feel this provides more effective "tension band" stability of tuberosity than either a single-row or traditional double-row repair construct. In addition, arthroscopic repair of greater tuberosity fractures can be performed using arthroscopic transosseous techniques without the use of suture anchors as previously described.[18-20]

Positioning and Portals

Surgery is performed under general anesthesia in the beach chair position. Lateral decubitus positioning can be utilized as well depending on the surgeon's preference. A 4-portal (anterior, posterior, anterolateral, and posterolateral) technique is utilized and can be supplemented with accessory portals as needed for the introduction of instrumentation or implants.

Step-by-Step Description of the Procedure

The authors' preferred method for arthroscopic reduction and fixation of greater tuberosity fractures utilizes a transosseous technique with a commercially available device (ArthroTunneler [Tornier]) as previously described by Garofalo et al.[19]

Diagnostic arthroscopy is begun through a standard posterior portal in order to perform a complete intra-articular examination after removal of any residual hemarthrosis/blood clots caused by the fracture. Any associated intra-articular pathology (ie, biceps tendon tear and/or labral/superior labral anteroposterior tear) can be diagnosed and treated if necessary. The location of the fracture is assessed from the undersurface. A shaver is used to very gently debride any hematoma from the undersurface of the tuberosity fracture fragment. Careful attention is paid not to remove any bone from the tuberosity. The arthroscope is then placed into the subacromial space and any hemorrhagic bursa is removed for visualization of the fracture fragment and donor bed. The authors do not perform routine acromioplasty for these cases. The subacromial bursectomy is performed with extreme attention to detail while avoiding excessive removal of the bursa directly overlying the portion of the rotator cuff attached to the tuberosity fragment(s) in order to avoid iatrogenic damage to the intact rotator cuff and fractured tuberosity fragment. Intersecting transosseous bone tunnels are created using a modification of a previously described technique by Garofalo et al.[19] The medial tunnel is first made at the most medial and superior aspect of the fracture bed along the proximal humerus (generally right at the articular margin). Appropriate placement of the medial transosseous tunnel or medial row of suture anchors can be challenging as the fracture bed is oftentimes more vertical in orientation. Of note, whether utilizing either a transosseous repair technique or suture anchors, if the fractured tuberosity fragment provides an impediment to visualization of the fracture bed along the proximal humerus, then a traction suture can be placed through the attached rotator cuff in order to pull the tuberosity fracture fragment posterior for improved visibility. The number of transosseous tunnels is determined at the time of surgery based on the tuberosity fragment size. In general, the authors prefer to utilize one transosseous tunnel for each centimeter of the greater tuberosity fracture fragment. A lateral tunnel is drilled in the intact metaphysis of the humerus distal to the fracture fragment (one lateral tunnel for each corresponding medial tunnel) and 3 high-tensile strength sutures are shuttled through each tunnel (Figure 22-3). The authors routinely utilize 2 semi-permanent #2 Orthocord (Ethicon) sutures and one permanent #3-4 Force Fiber (Tornier) suture. The sutures are then passed sequentially through the rotator cuff at the bone-tendon junction. A retrograde suture-shuttling device is used to penetrate the rotator cuff at the bone-tendon junction and sequentially pass sutures through the rotator cuff. The authors find the execution of this step with a suture-shuttling device to be less challenging from a technical standpoint than using a direct retrograde retrieval device, especially when dealing with a larger or thicker tuberosity bone fragment, which can oftentimes impede visualization of the retrograde retrieval device. The authors strongly recommend against passing sutures through the rotator cuff with an antegrade suture passer in order to avoid further damage to the greater tuberosity fracture fragment.

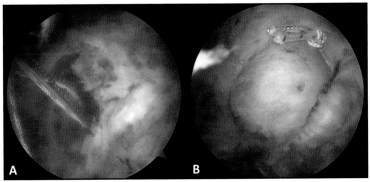

Figure 22-3. (A) Once the fragment has been properly mobilized, the transosseous tunnels are established and sutures shuttled through as described. Similar to arthroscopic rotator cuff repair, the medial tunnel is placed just lateral to the articular margin. It is important to remember to pass sutures through the rotator cuff at the bone-tendon junction in order to obtain adequate fixation and stability of the fragment to the fracture bed. (B) Placement of a mattress suture allows further compression of the fragment as well as adding additional security of the simple sutures by forming a "rip-stop" suture, which may prevent suture "cut-out" medially.

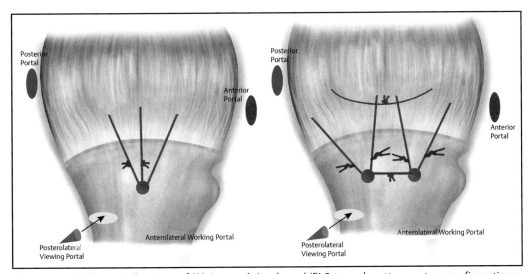

Figure 22-4. Schematic drawings of (A) 1-tunnel simple and (B) 2-tunnel mattress suture configurations.

After all sutures are passed through the rotator cuff, a direct reduction of the greater tuberosity to its donor bed is performed and held in position with the assistance of a 2-mm nonpenetrating awl. The sutures are then tied in either a simple (ie, one tunnel) or mattress (ie, 2 or more tunnels) configuration to complete the repair (see Figure 22-3). The authors prefer a mattress suture configuration when utilizing 2 or more tunnels in order to provide further compression/stability of the fracture fragment as well as to create a "rip-stop" effect, which may help reduce the chance of suture "cut-out" medially (Figure 22-4).

Figure 22-5. Anteroposterior radiograph preoperatively and at 1 year postoperatively after arthroscopic greater tuberosity repair.

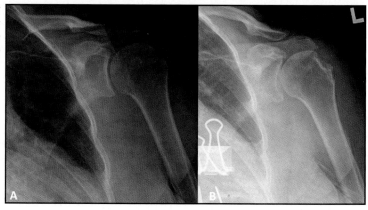

POSTOPERATIVE PROTOCOL

Postoperatively, all patients are placed into a sling with the arm at the side and an additional strap around the waist for 6 weeks. Abduction pillows may or may not be used depending on the preference of the surgeon. The authors start immediate passive and active-assisted elbow/wrist/hand motion and scapular kinetic exercises the day after surgery. They recommend supervised physical therapy be initiated within the first 7 to 10 days after surgery, but this can be altered on an individual case-by-case basis depending on the size of the fracture fragment and overall stability of the construct. The authors perform supine passive anterior elevation and external rotation for the first 6 weeks and advance accordingly during this time based on the size of the fracture fragment and cuff involvement. Initiation of passive internal rotation is added at 6 weeks postoperatively. Radiographs are taken at 2 weeks, 6 weeks, and 3 months postoperatively (Figure 22-5). Active range of motion is initiated once there is radiographic evidence of healing of the tuberosity. Gentle strengthening is typically added at 12 weeks and full release to all activities is patient specific but generally allowed by 6 months after surgery.

POTENTIAL COMPLICATIONS

Arthroscopic repair of greater tuberosity fractures is a challenging procedure to perform and should only be performed by advanced arthroscopic shoulder surgeons with adequate experience and technical skill. Inadequate construct stability with loss of reduction remains the most likely complication following this technique. Delayed range of motion is an option in patients where there is a concern for loss of reduction with early range of motion. Suture cut-out and suture anchor pull-out are additional complications that can lead to early or late displacement of the tuberosity. With the transosseous repair technique described in this chapter, there is the option of utilizing a polyetheretherketone implant (TunnelPro [Tornier]) for the lateral tunnel along the metaphysis to reduce the likelihood of either suture cut out through bone or suture breakage as a result of abrasion. Furthermore, there is a high risk of overtensioning/over-reduction of the tuberosity and rotator cuff with this technique; intraoperative fluoroscopy can be utilized to verify satisfactory reduction prior to final repair.

TOP TECHNICAL PEARLS FOR THE PROCEDURE

1. Arthroscopic repair using either suture anchors or a transosseous technique allows for secure fixation of the fragment down to the fracture bed while minimizing the morbidity of formal "open" approaches.

2. The medial sutures should exit at the bone-tendon junction to allow for adequate stability/fixation of the fracture fragment.

3. One tunnel (or suture anchor) should be placed per 1 cm of anteroposterior width of the greater tuberosity fragment. Maximize the number of sutures per tunnel/suture anchor for passage through the rotator cuff.

4. The suture should "bridge" the fragment to essentially form a tension-band repair.

5. Provisional reduction with either a Kirschner wire or nonpenetrating awl may be helpful prior to securing the repair.

REFERENCES

1. Court-Brown CM, Caesar B. Epidemiology of adult fractures: a review. *Injury.* 2006;37(8):691-697.

2. Kristiansen B, Barfod G, Bredesen J, et al. Epidemiology of proximal humeral fractures. *Acta Orthop Scand.* 1987;58(1):75-77.

3. Bahrs C, Lingenfelter E, Fischer F, Walters EM, Schnabel M. Mechanism of injury and morphology of the greater tuberosity fracture. *J Shoulder Elbow Surg.* 2006;15(2):140-147.

4. Neer CS II. Displaced proximal humeral fractures: Part 1. Classification and evaluation. *J Bone Joint Surg Am.* 1970;52(6):1077-1089.

5. McLaughlin HL. Dislocation of the shoulder with tuberosity fracture. *Surg Clin North Am.* 1963;43:1615-1620.

6. Platzer P, Thalhammer G, Oberleitner G, et al. Displaced fractures of the greater tuberosity: a comparison of operative and nonoperative treatment. *J Trauma.* 2008;65(4):843-848.

7. Park TS, Choi IY, Kim YH, Park MR, Shon JH, Kim SI. A new suggestion for the treatment of minimally displaced fractures of the greater tuberosity of the proximal humerus. *Bull Hosp Jt Dis.* 1997;56(3):171-176.

8. Yin B, Moen TC, Thompson SA, Bigliani LU, Ahmad CS, Levine WN. Operative treatment of isolated greater tuberosity fractures: retrospective review of clinical and functional outcomes. *Orthopedics.* 2012;35(6):e807-e814.

9. Flatow EL, Cuomo F, Maday MG, Miller SR, McIlveen SJ, Bigliani LU. Open reduction and internal fixation of two-part displaced fractures of the greater tuberosity of the proximal part of the humerus. *J Bone Joint Surg Am.* 1991;73(8):1213-1218.

10. Herscovici D Jr, Saunders DT, Johnson MP, Sanders R, DiPasquale T. Percutaneous fixation of proximal humeral fractures. *Clin Orthop Relat Res.* 2000;375:97-104.

11. George, MS. Fractures of the greater tuberosity of the humerus. *J Am Acad Orthop Surg.* 2007;15(10):607-613.

12. Gartsman GM, Taverna E, Hammerman SM. Arthroscopic treatment of acute traumatic anterior glenohumeral dislocation and greater tuberosity fracture. *Arthroscopy.* 1999;15(6):648-650.

13. Ji JH, Kim WY, Ra KH. Arthroscopic double-row suture anchor fixation of minimally displaced greater tuberosity fractures. *Arthroscopy.* 2007;23(10):1133.e1-e4.

14. Song HS, Williams GR Jr. Arthroscopic reduction and fixation with suture-bridge technique for displaced or comminuted greater tuberosity fractures. *Arthroscopy*. 2008;24(8):956-960.

15. Kim KC1, Rhee KJ, Shin HD, Kim YM. Arthroscopic fixation for displaced greater tuberosity fracture using the suture-bridge technique. *Arthroscopy*. 2008;24(1):120.e1-e3.

16. Ji JH, Shafi M, Song IS, Kim YY, McFarland EG, Moon CY. Arthroscopic fixation technique for comminuted, displaced greater tuberosity fracture. *Arthroscopy*. 2010;26(5):600-609.

17. Geusens E1, Pans S, Verhulst D, Brys P. The modified axillary view of the shoulder, a painless alternative. *Emerg Radiol*. 2006;12(5):227-230.

18. Baudi P, Rasia Dani E, Campochiaro G, Rebuzzi M, Serafini F, Catani F. The rotator cuff tear repair with a new arthroscopic transosseous system: the Sharc-FT®. *Musculoskelet Surg*. 2013;97(Suppl 1):57-61.

19. Garofalo R, Castagna A, Borroni M, Krishnan SG. Arthroscopic transosseous (anchorless) rotator cuff repair. *Knee Surg Sports Traumatol Arthrosc*. 2012;20(6):1031-1035.

20. Kuroda S, Ishige N, Mikasa M. Advantages of arthroscopic transosseous suture repair of the rotator cuff without the use of anchors. *Clin Orthop Relat Res*. 2013;471(11):3514-3522.

Please see videos on the accompanying website at

www.ArthroscopicTechniques.com

23

Arthroscopic Bursectomy and Superomedial Angle Resection for the Treatment of Scapulothoracic Bursitis and Snapping Scapula Syndrome

Simon A. Euler, MD; Ryan J. Warth, MD; and Peter J. Millett, MD, MSc

INTRODUCTION

The shoulder complex is composed of 4 complementary articulations assembled in a manner that allows maximal range of motion across the glenohumeral joint. Dynamic, coordinated contraction of surrounding musculature is necessary to adequately position the glenoid in 3-dimensional space, which maximizes the area of contact between the glenoid and the humeral head. More specifically, glenoid positioning is determined by the position of the scapular body, which is controlled by the synchronous action of the periscapular musculature. When glenohumeral motion is initiated, the scapula must tilt, rotate, protract, and/or retract to compensate for the position of the humeral head. To achieve these motions, the concave scapular body must glide smoothly over the convex posterior thorax with the aid of strategically placed muscular tissue and interposed bursae. Therefore, anatomic derangements within the scapulothoracic space can produce disordered glenohumeral kinematics, leading to painful bursitis with or without mechanical crepitus. These conditions are often collectively referred to as *snapping scapula syndrome* and/or *scapulothoracic bursitis*.

The wide range of possible symptoms associated with these conditions can be classified according to the most likely etiology. For example, scapulothoracic incongruence as a result of space-occupying skeletal or soft-tissue lesions, kyphoscoliotic posture,[1] or predisposing anatomic variation, such as hyperangulation of the superomedial scapular angle or the presence of a so-called *Luschka tubercle*,[2-4] are more likely to generate symptoms related to mechanical crepitation. In contrast, patients who complain of pain in the absence of mechanical symptoms are more likely to have symptomatic bursitis, often as a result of chronic overuse. However, although this basic classification can be helpful, it is important to recognize that symptomatic bursitis can lead to mechanical crepitation (via bursal fibrosis[5-8]), while mechanical crepitation can lead to symptomatic bursitis (via disordered scapular motion).[9]

Although the etiology is often unknown in the clinical setting, symptoms related to scapulothoracic bursitis and/or crepitus are most often associated with adventitial (pathologic) infraserratus or supraserratus bursal tissue located deep to the superomedial angle of the scapula.

Ryu RKN, Angelo RL, Abrams JS, eds. *The Shoulder: AANA Advanced Arthroscopic Surgical Techniques* (pp 277-284). © 2016 AANA.

Figure 23-1. This axial magnetic resonance imaging slice demonstrates a prominent superomedial angle (yellow arrow) in a patient with recalcitrant scapulothoracic bursitis and mechanical crepitus.

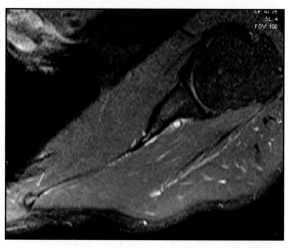

Arthroscopic excision of pathologic bursal tissue and bony resection of the superomedial scapular angle have each been found to provide significant improvements in pain and function in the majority of patients.[10-13] The purpose of this chapter and corresponding video is to demonstrate a reliable technique for arthroscopic scapulothoracic bursectomy with additional bony resection of the superomedial scapular angle.

Indications

▸ Symptoms persist despite 3 to 6 months of appropriate nonoperative treatment.

▸ Diagnostic imaging reveals a clinically relevant prominence or anterior hyperangulation of the superomedial angle (Figure 23-1).

▸ Mechanical crepitus is persistent during intraoperative dynamic examination despite removal of pathologic bursal tissue.

Controversial Indications

▸ Diagnostic or therapeutic injection results in symptomatic relief[14-16]

▸ Symptoms related to kyphoscoliosis

Pertinent Physical Findings

▸ Scapular dyskinesis

▸ Scapular malposition, inferomedial border prominence, anterior coracoid pain, scapular dyskinesis; glenohumeral internal rotation deficit; posterosuperior glenoid impingement; and SLAP tears in overhead athletes[17,18]

▸ Scapular winging (neuromuscular etiology) or pseudowinging (mechanical etiology, such as the presence of a mass within the scapulothoracic space)

▸ Localized tenderness on superficial and/or deep palpation

▸ Periscapular muscle weakness or imbalance

PERTINENT IMAGING

- Plain radiographs
  - ▷ Anteroposterior
  - ▷ Tangential Y
  - ▷ Axillary
- Computed tomography (CT)
  - ▷ Indicated when a relevant skeletal lesion is apparent on plain radiographs
- Magnetic resonance imaging
  - ▷ Identification of soft-tissue structures within the scapulothoracic space that may contribute to symptoms
  - ▷ Evaluation of potentially predisposing anatomy
- Ultrasound
  - ▷ Mostly used to guide diagnostic or therapeutic injections
- Electromyograms
  - ▷ Used to evaluate patients with unexplained periscapular muscle weakness or winging

EQUIPMENT

- Fully equipped arthroscopic tower
- Basic arthroscopic instrumentation
  - ▷ Arthroscopic shaver
  - ▷ Radiofrequency ablator
  - ▷ Arthroscopic burr
  - ▷ Arthroscopic rasp
- 4-mm 30- and 70-degree arthroscopes
- Basic surgical set in the event of conversion to an open procedure

POSITIONING AND PORTALS

After the induction of general anesthesia, the patient is placed prone on the operating table (see video). The operative extremity and posterior thorax are widely prepared and draped using a sterile technique. The humerus is then extended and internally rotated such that the dorsum of the forearm is positioned over the lumbar spine (Figure 23-2). This so-called *chicken wing position* induces a physiologic posterior scapular tilt, which enlarges the operative field and aids in arthroscopic visualization. "Bayonet apposition" of the scapular body can also increase this potential space by applying a medially directed force over the humeral head.[10]

The medial scapular border is palpated and a sterile marking pen is used to outline its most medial margin. Typically, 2 arthroscopic portals are established inferior to the level of the scapular spine and at least 3 cm medial to the medial scapular border to prevent injury to underlying neurovascular structures (Figure 23-3). In addition, medial portal positioning mitigates the risk for intrathoracic penetration, which can occur when arthroscopic instruments are inserted into the scapulothoracic space at an acute angle.[19] An accessory superior portal may also be helpful when

Figure 23-2. This preoperative photograph demonstrates the "chicken wing" position in which the dorsum of the forearm is placed over the lumbar spine. This position subjects the humerus to nearly maximal internal rotation, which forces the scapula to tilt posteriorly, thus increasing the available operating space between the anterior scapula and the posterior chest wall. When additional space is needed for visualization during the procedure, application of a medially directed pressure on the proximal humerus may help increase the volume of the scapulothoracic space via "bayonet apposition."

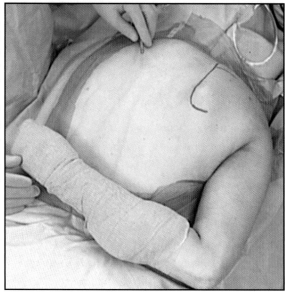

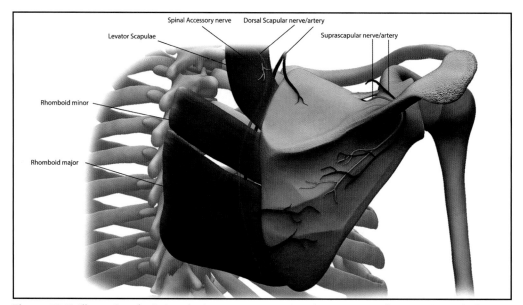

Figure 23-3. Illustration depicting the important neurovascular anatomy relevant to scapulothoracic bursectomy and superomedial angle resection. Arthroscopic portals should be established at least 3 cm medial to the medial scapular border to avoid iatrogenic injury to the dorsal scapular nerve and artery, which run together beneath the rhomboid major, rhomboid minor, and levator scapulae muscles. In addition, risk of injury to the spinal accessory nerve can be minimized by establishing portals inferior to the level of the scapular spine. The suprascapular nerve and artery are rarely at risk unless an accessory superior portal is needed to complete the procedure or excessive lateral dissection is undertaken.

bony resection of the superomedial angle is indicated[20,21]; however, there is an increased risk for iatrogenic injury using this portal site and it is not used on a routine basis.

Prior to the insertion of arthroscopic instruments, approximately 100 mL of saline mixed with local anesthetic and epinephrine is injected deep to the superomedial angle to both expand the infraserratus bursa for adequate visualization and to provide hemostasis during the procedure.

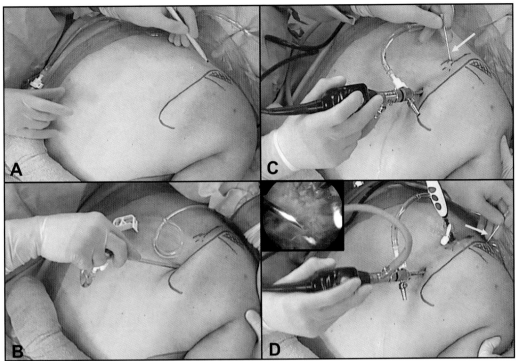

Figure 23-4. (A) A sterile marking pen is used to outline the margins of the medial scapula and the area of possible bony resection. (B) A small stab incision is made approximately 3 cm medial to the inferomedial scapular angle and a 30-degree arthroscope is inserted, thus establishing the inferior viewing portal. (C) A spinal needle is inserted at the site of the medial working portal and, under direct visualization, arthroscopic instruments are introduced into the scapulothoracic space (yellow arrow). (D) Following diagnostic arthroscopy, a second spinal needle is inserted at the most superior aspect of the superomedial angle to guide bony resection and to provide orientation during the procedure (yellow arrow). The image inset is an arthroscopic view of the spinal needle placed at the superomedial angle.

STEP-BY-STEP DESCRIPTION OF THE PROCEDURE

A small stab incision is made approximately 3 cm medial to the inferomedial angle and a 30-degree arthroscope is inserted, taking care to remain as parallel to the chest wall as possible. Care should be taken to maintain a fluid pump pressure of less than 50 mm Hg throughout the procedure to avoid excessive fluid extravasation into surrounding tissues. A spinal needle is inserted approximately 3 cm medial to the medial scapular border at a point just inferior to the level of the scapular spine, marking the location of the medial working portal. Once this portal is established, diagnostic arthroscopy is performed using both the 30- and 70-degree arthroscopes to accurately localize the superomedial scapular angle. Another spinal needle is inserted at the location of the superomedial angle for orientation during arthroscopy and to confirm adequate bony resection at the conclusion of the procedure (Figure 23-4).

Debridement and resection of the infraserratus bursa is then performed using an arthroscopic radiofrequency ablator or shaver (Figure 23-5). Using the previously placed spinal needle for orientation, debridement is continued until the superomedial scapular angle is completely exposed. When necessary, access to the supraserratus bursa can be achieved by bluntly penetrating the laterally positioned serratus anterior muscle.[10] At this point, dynamic examination is performed to identify the location and extent of osseous impingement between the superomedial scapular angle and the posterior thorax. If mechanical crepitus is still present and skeletal impingement is still visible following complete bursectomy, superomedial angle resection is then performed.

Figure 23-5. Arthroscopic view of the anterior scapula from the scapulothoracic space. The asterisk (*) represents the bony margin of the superomedial angle. The red arrow points to the area of the infraserratus bursa. The yellow arrow points to the tendinous insertion of the subscapularis muscle.

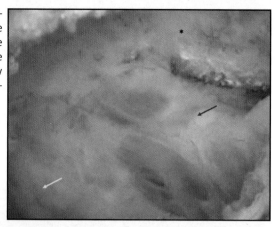

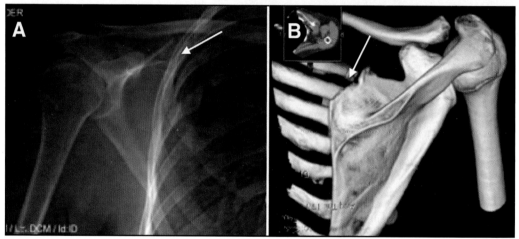

Figure 23-6. (A) An anteroposterior radiograph of a right shoulder demonstrating previous resection of the superomedial scapular angle (arrow) in a patient who initially presented with scapulothoracic pain and crepitus. (B) CT scan with 3-dimensional reconstruction of the right shoulder in the same patient. Note that a triangular section of the superomedial scapular angle has previously been resected (arrow). (Reprinted with permission from Millett PJ, Gaskill TR, Horan MP, van der Meijden OA. Technique and outcomes of arthroscopic scapulothoracic bursectomy and partial scapulectomy. *Arthroscopy.* 2012;28(12):1776-1783.

Although a triangular section of bone is typically removed approximately 2 cm superoinferiorly and 3 cm mediolaterally, it is important to mark the extent of the planned resection in every case using several spinal needles, depending on the degree and location of scapulothoracic impingement. This method facilitates complete, accurate bony resection of the superomedial angle without increasing the risk to nearby vascular structures.[20] Resection is typically performed using a high-speed arthroscopic burr until the deep surface of the supraspinatus muscle is identified. A rasp is typically used to smooth the edges of the resection. The operative extremity is again placed through a range of motion while directly visualizing the scapulothoracic space through both portals to confirm both adequate resection and the presence of a smooth articulating surface. The portal sites are closed using a standard technique, a simple sling is applied, and the patient is transferred to the post-anesthesia care unit. Because the scapulothoracic articulation is not surrounded by a joint capsule, some patients may experience significant swelling that can extend down the arm or around the torso within the immediate postoperative period; however, this side effect typically resolves over a period of days. Postoperative radiographs or CT scans may be obtained in some cases to evaluate the adequacy of superomedial angle resection (Figure 23-6).

POSTOPERATIVE PROTOCOL

Active and passive range of motion exercises, such as scapular protraction, retraction, and rotation, are begun immediately postoperatively with a progression toward glenohumeral strengthening at approximately 4 weeks followed by periscapular strengthening at approximately 8 weeks. Most patients return to sports after 3 months of structured and supervised rehabilitation. In all cases, physical therapy protocols should be individualized according to patient tolerance and progress.

POTENTIAL COMPLICATIONS

Although uncommon, there are several important surgical complications unique to this procedure that can be prevented by using appropriate arthroscopic techniques. Injury to the dorsal scapular artery and/or nerve can occur when arthroscopic portals are placed < 3 cm medial to the medial scapular border. The spinal accessory nerve is also in danger when an arthroscopic portal is placed superior to the level of the scapular spine. Puncture of pleural tissue can be avoided by maintaining the arthroscopic instruments at an angle that is approximately parallel with the thoracic cage.[19] Other complications include incomplete bursectomy and/or scapulectomy that may result in recurrent symptomatology and inferior outcomes.

TOP TECHNICAL PEARLS FOR THE PROCEDURE

1. Placing the operative limb in the "chicken wing" position increases the potential space between the scapula and the posterior chest wall, which improves arthroscopic visualization.

2. Always establish arthroscopic portals at least 3 cm medial to the medial scapular border and inferior to the level of the scapular spine to prevent injury to important neurovascular structures, such as the dorsal scapular nerve and artery and the spinal accessory nerve.

3. Always use spinal needles to facilitate arthroscopic orientation to avoid excessive bony resection and to prevent neurovascular injuries as a result of excessive superior or lateral dissection.

4. To avoid becoming "lost" in the subscapularis and serratus anterior muscle bellies, it is important to ensure that the arthroscope is advanced down to the posterior thorax.

5. Avoid resection of red muscle fibers, such as those of the subscapularis, as this may produce increased postoperative pain and lengthen rehabilitation.

REFERENCES

1. Manske RC, Reiman MP, Stovak ML. Nonoperative and operative management of snapping scapula. *Am J Sports Med.* 2004;32(6):1554-1565.
2. Aggarwal A, Wahee P, Harjeet, Aggarwal AK, Sahni D. Variable osseous anatomy of costal surface of scapula and its implications in relation to snapping scapula syndrome. *Surg Radiol Anat.* 2011;33(2):135-140.

3. Totlis T, Konstantinidis GA, Karanassos MT, Sofidis G, Anasasopoulos N, Natsis K. Bony structures related to snapping scapula: correlation to gender, side and age. *Surg Radiol Anat.* 2014;36(1):3-9.

4. Edelson JG. Variations in the anatomy of the scapula with reference to the snapping scapulas. *Clin Orthop Relat Res.* 1996;(322):111-115.

5. Percy EC, Birbrager D, Pitt MJ. Snapping scapula: a review of the literature and presentation of 14 patients. *Can J Surg.* 1988;31(4):248-250.

6. Sisto DJ, Jobe FW. The operative treatment of scapulothoracic bursitis in professional baseball pitchers. *Am J Sports Med.* 1986;14(3):192-194.

7. Milch H. Partial scapulectomy for snapping of the scapula. *J Bone Joint Surg Am.* 1950;32-A(3):561-566.

8. Milch H. Snapping scapula. *Clin Orthop.* 1961;20:139-150.

9. Warth RJ, Spiegl UJ, Millett PJ. Scapulothoracic bursitis and snapping scapula syndrome: a critical review of current evidence. *Am J Sports Med.* 2015;43(1):236-245.

10. Millett PJ, Gaskill TR, Horan MP, van der Meijden OA. Technique and outcomes of arthroscopic scapulothoracic bursectomy and partial scapulectomy. *Arthroscopy.* 2012;28(12):1776-1783.

11. Tashjian RZ, Granger EK, Barney JK, Partridge DR. Functional outcomes after arthroscopic scapulothoracic bursectomy and partial superomedial angle scapulectomy. *Orthop J Sports Med.* 2013;1(5):1-5.

12. Blønd L, Rechter S. Arthroscopic treatment for snapping scapula: a prospective case series. *Eur J Orthop Surg Traumatol.* 2014;24(2):159-164.

13. Pearse EO. Bruguera J, Massoud SN, Sforza G, Copeland SA, Levy O. Arthroscopic management of the painful snapping scapula. *Arthroscopy.* 2006;22(7):755-761.

14. Harper GD, McIlroy S, Bayley JI, Calvert PT. Arthroscopic partial resection of the scapula for snapping scapula: a new technique. *J Shoulder Elbow Surg.* 1999;8:53-57.

15. Lehtinen JT, Macy JC, Cassinelli E, Warner JJ. The painful scapulothoracic articulation: surgical management. *Clin Orthop Relat Res.* 2004;423:99-105.

16. Nicholson GP, Duckworth MA. Scapulothoracic bursectomy for snapping scapula syndrome. *J Shoulder Elbow Surg.* 2002;11:80-85.

17. Burkhart SS, Morgan CD, Kibler WB. The disabled throwing shoulder: spectrum of pathology. Part I: pathoanatomy and biomechanics. *Arthroscopy.* 2003;19(4):404-420.

18. Burkhart SS, Morgan CD, Kibler WB. The disabled throwing shoulder: spectrum of pathology. Part III: the SICK scapula, scapular dyskinesis, the kinetic chain, and rehabilitation. *Arthroscopy.* 2003;19:641-661.

19. Ruland LJ III, Ruland CM, Matthews LS. Scapulothoracic anatomy for the arthroscopist. *Arthroscopy.* 1995;11:52-56.

20. Bell SN, van Riet RP. Safe zone for arthroscopic resection of the superomedial scapular border in the treatment of snapping scapular syndrome. *J Shoulder Elbow Surg.* 2008;17:647-649.

21. Chan BK, Chakrabarti AJ, Bell SN. An alternative portal for scapulothoracic arthroscopy. *J Shoulder Elbow Surg.* 2002;11:235-238.

Please see videos on the accompanying website at

www.ArthroscopicTechniques.com

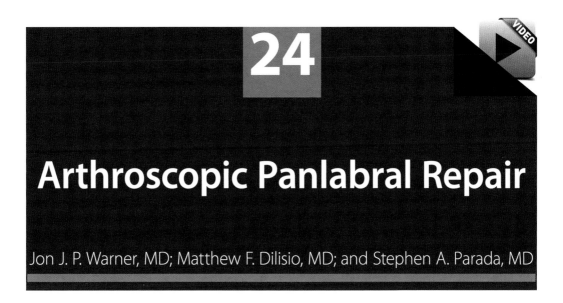

INTRODUCTION

Anterior, posterior, and superior labral lesions are well-described causes of shoulder pain and disability, and arthroscopic repair of labral pathology has been the mainstay of treatment over the last 10 to 20 years.[1-3] While there are hundreds of reports of the diagnosis and treatment of focal tears of the glenoid labrum dating back to at least 1938,[4] there are surprisingly few published reports of circumferential (ie, panlabral) labral tears.

The senior author described that successful treatment combined anterior and superior labral lesions in 1994.[5] The first published report of a panlabral tear was described in 2004 as a variant of a superior labral anteroposterior (SLAP) tear[6] almost 15 years after SLAP tears were first described, coined, and classified.[7,8] Lo and Burkhart described their experience in 7 patients with "triple labral lesions" consisting of anterior, posterior, and SLAP tears.[9] In 2009, Tokish et al described the results of 41 military patients with arthroscopic repair of circumferential labral lesions.[10] All patients returned to their pre-injury activity level, and the authors found significant improvement in pain, stability, and function. Ricchetti et al reported similar findings in 44 patients who had undergone a panlabral repair.[11]

This chapter provides an overview of the authors' approach to the evaluation and arthroscopic management of circumferential tears of the glenoid labrum. The authors highlight the surgical indications, physical findings, pertinent preoperative imaging, technique, postoperative protocol, and common complications. An excellent surgical result can be achieved if the principles outlined in this chapter are followed.

INDICATIONS

► Circumferential labral tears with associated instability symptoms and/or pain that have not responded to conservative care[10]

Ryu RKN, Angelo RL, Abrams JS, eds. *The Shoulder:*
AANA Advanced Arthroscopic Surgical Techniques (pp 285-295).
© 2016 AANA.

Controversial Indications

► Glenoid bone loss[12]

► Poor quality tissue

► Glenohumeral arthritis

► Rotator cuff tear

► Tendinopathy of the long head of the biceps (Note: The authors recommend a biceps tenodesis in this scenario instead of a superior labral repair.)

PERTINENT PHYSICAL FINDINGS

► Multiple exam maneuvers have been described for anterior instability, posterior instability, and SLAP tears, but the extent of the labral pathology in panlabral tears can produce a positive result with nearly all provocative maneuvers making the diagnosis by only the physical exam difficult. This is especially true when patient guarding is present, which is common in acute, traumatic injuries.

► Most patients present after several unidirectional dislocations, have positive provocative instability tests in all directions, and have significantly more pain for longer periods of time than patients with focal labral tears.[10]

► There are several key exam elements of the shoulder that can provide useful information to guide surgical decision making: anterior instability, posterior instability, superior labral/biceps pathology, ligamentous laxity, rotator cuff pathology, and scapular function.

► Anterior instability: The anterior apprehension and relocation tests are accurate methods to assess anterior labral pathology.[13] The anterior load and shift test can provide the clinician with a sense of ligamentous laxity, but this is more useful with the patient under general anesthesia. Complaints of instability within midranges of motion may be indicative of significant glenoid bone loss,[14] which often suggests that the patient's pathology is not amendable to a soft tissue repair.[12]

► Posterior instability: The posterior load and shift, jerk, and push-pull tests are effective tests for posterior labral pathology and instability. These are often performed best with the patient supine and the scapula stabilized. Patients are often more tolerant of posterior instability testing than anterior instability testing. Most shoulders have a moderate amount of physiologic laxity, so it is useful to examine the contralateral shoulder in order to delineate discrepancies between sides in regard to pain and laxity with posterior instability testing.

► Superior labrum/biceps pathology: O'Brien's sign/active compression test can be useful to diagnose SLAP tears, but it is relatively nonspecific. Bicipital groove tenderness/Speed's sign/Yergason's sign are also indicative of biceps pathology.

► Ligamentous laxity should be assessed and compared with the contralateral shoulder to delineate benign laxity from instability.

► Range of motion and rotator cuff strength must be assessed to rule out concomitant pathology.

► Patients with scapular dyskinesia and winging commonly present with complaints of an unstable shoulder,[15] and it is essential to confirm that the periscapular muscles are functioning appropriately.

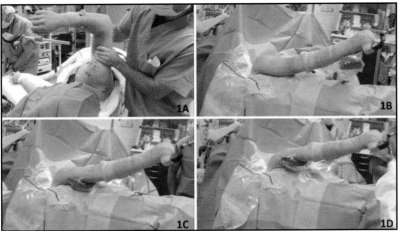

Figure 24-1. (A) A thorough exam under general anesthesia is performed on bilateral shoulders once the patient is anesthetized in order to assess physiologic and/or pathologic laxity. (B through D) The authors utilize a pneumatic arm holder in the lateral decubitus position with an axillary traction device that optimizes glenohumeral visualization.

Pertinent Imaging

▶ Grashey anteroposterior, scapular Y, and axillary lateral radiographic views are utilized in the initial assessment of most patients with shoulder pain. A Hill-Sachs lesion can often be accentuated on an internal rotation Grashey anteroposterior, and an osseous Bankart lesion or anterior glenoid erosion can be visualized on an axillary lateral in patients with a history of traumatic anterior instability.

▶ Alternatively, in patients with a history of anterior glenohumeral instability, a Stryker notch view can be utilized to screen for a Hill-Sachs lesion, and a West Point view can be utilized to screen for an osseous Bankart lesion or glenoid deficiency.[16]

▶ Advanced imaging modalities such as computed tomography and magnetic resonance imaging (MRI) with and without intra-articular contrast are often utilized in cases of instability. The authors' preferred modality is a computed tomography arthrogram in order to best assess glenoid bone and labral anatomy.[17] Alternatively, an MR arthrogram is also an accurate method of assessing glenoid labral lesions[18] and is the best modality to assess associated soft tissue pathology such as rotator cuff tears.

Equipment

The authors' preferred technique is to perform the procedure in the lateral decubitus position with a full-length bean bag. The authors utilized a pneumatic arm holder (SPIDER Limb Positioner [Smith & Nephew]) that allows both distal and lateral traction to enhance visualization and working space (Figure 24-1). A standard 30-degree arthroscope is all that is required if the trans-cuff portal is utilized, which provides excellent visualization of all aspects of the labrum. Seventy-degree cameras are useful when performing labral repairs without the use of this portal.

A variety of commercially available tissue elevators are available to free the labrum and prepare the glenoid surface. The authors utilized a radiofrequency blade device (CoVator [Arthrocare]) in order to thoroughly free the labrum and capsule to perform an anatomic repair.

Many glenoid-specific suture anchors can be utilized to perform a panlabral repair that usually range from 2.5 to 3.5 mm. There is no clear evidence of the superiority of one type of anchor over another. It is the authors' preference to not routinely utilized knotless fixation when performing labral repairs. The authors use an average of 5 double-loaded anchors for panlabral repairs (2 posterior, 2 anterior, and 1 superior).

Many tissue penetrators are available to shuttle suture through the labral tissue. Patient anatomy and portal location dictates the optimal device geometry in order to pass the suture, so select the device that allows the optimal angle of attach. This is often a curved device between 45 and 90 degrees for anterior repairs and a straight device for posterior repairs.

While well-placed cannulas can be helpful, they can often restrict the surgeon's freedom to manipulate and access glenohumeral tissue. The authors generally utilized a 5.5-mm threaded cannula to shuttle suture, a smooth 5.2-mm cannula for the trans-cuff portal, and an 8.5-mm cannula in order to accommodate larger tissue penetrators, if necessary.

POSITIONING AND PORTALS

A panlabral repair can be performed in both the beach chair and lateral decubitus position. It is the senior author's preference to utilize the lateral decubitus position with a pneumatic arm holder that assists in both distal and lateral traction in order to maximize glenohumeral space and optimize visualization and working space to perform the repair (see Figure 24-1). It is paramount to identify and pad all bony prominences and areas of potential nerve compression during the procedure. Specifically, the brachial plexus and the common peroneal nerve are at risk of compression during procedures performed in the lateral decubitus position. An axillary roll must be used to protect the axillary structures and the lateral knee must be free of compression throughout the procedure.

Prior to sterile preparation and draping, a thorough instability exam is performed once the patient is anesthetized and the airway is protected. Glenohumeral range of motion, translation, and laxity are assessed relative to the contralateral shoulder. Often, ligamentously lax patients have similar exam findings on the nonsymptomatic side, so any discrepancies are useful to note as the surgeon attempts to recreate the patient's own "normal" anatomy.

While an exam under anesthesia can provide useful information, this exam serves mainly to confirm the preoperative diagnosis and surgical plan. The patient's preoperative history and physical are significantly more important than this exam, and the decision to perform surgery and the choice of the surgical procedure should be made preoperatively since the difference between physiologic laxity and pathologic instability is mainly determined by the patient's perception of his or her shoulder function.

The superficial surface anatomy of the shoulder is marked in order to optimize portal placement. The glenohumeral joint is first insufflated with 60 mL of normal saline in order to distend the capsule and optimize safe trocar entry. This is especially useful in these cases since the posterior viewing portal is created slightly more lateral than normal, which facilitates posterior anchor placement at the expense of ease of intra-articular trocar entry.

A posterior viewing portal is established approximately 1 cm medial and 3 cm distal to the posterolateral border of the acromion, with the trocar aimed at the tip of the coracoid. The authors tend to make this portal slightly more lateral than normal in posterior instability cases because posterior anchors can often be placed through this portal. However, a surgeon should not hesitate to make additional portals in order to obtain optimal visualization, anchor placement, and suture passage. The morbidity of an additional portal is far less than a poorly done labral repair that was not appropriately executed due to unfavorable portal placement.

Once intra-articular placement of the camera is confirmed, an anterosuperior portal is established with 18-gauge spinal needle localization just anterior to the biceps tendon and just lateral to the coracoid. More medial placement of this portal will facilitate the surgeon's ability to get past the humerus to access the posterior glenohumeral joint in order to perform the posterior repair. The authors utilize a 5-mm cannula for this portal.

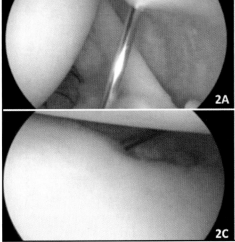
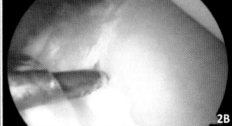

Figure 24-2. (A) A trans-cuff superior portal is established at the musculotendinous junction of the supraspinatus just medial to the rotator cable with spinal needle localization visualized from the posterior viewing portal in the lateral decubitus position. The arthroscope is switched to the trans-cuff portal and provides an excellent global view of both the (B) posterior and (C) anterior labrum.

A probe is introduced and a thorough diagnostic arthroscopy then performed to quantify the extent of the capsulolabral pathology, identify and quantify glenoid bone loss, and identify any additional intra-articular pathology such as a rotator cuff tear or biceps tendon lesion.

Once a panlabral tear is confirmed, a trans-cuff superior portal is established at the musculotendinous junction of the supraspinatus just medial to the rotator cable with spinal needle localization (Figure 24-2).[19,20] If appropriately placed, the trans-cuff portal does not need to be repaired at the conclusion of the procedure. An 11-blade scalpel is then used to pierce the superficial skin, deltoid, and supraspinatus in line with its fibers, and a blunt switching stick is then introduced followed by an additional 5-mm cannula over the switching stick. The camera is then switched to the trans-cuff portal, which provides an excellent global view of the glenoid and labrum, and an 8-mm cannula is replaced over a switching stick in the original posterior viewing portal.

An accessory posterolateral portal (7 o'clock portal) is often created using a spinal needle. This portal is usually in line with the posterolateral border of the acromion and 2 to 3 cm distal to the original posterior viewing portal. This portal is purposely more lateral and distal than a traditional posterior portal in order to optimize appropriate placement of the posterior glenoid anchors.[21,22] No cannula is utilized in this portal. Care must be taken not to injure the axillary nerve during portal placement and manipulation.

Finally, a mid-glenoid portal is created just superior to the subscapularis and as lateral as necessary in order to optimize anterior glenoid anchor placement. This portal is created after the posterior repair is completed since the glenoid and humeral relationship changes after the posterior repair/plication is performed.

STEP-BY-STEP DESCRIPTION OF THE PROCEDURE

The procedure begins with the arthroscope in the trans-cuff portal and a complete release of the torn labrum from the glenoid (Figure 24-3). This is likely the most important aspect of the repair and should be done carefully and completely. A radiofrequency blade device is used to exploit the interval between the labrum and glenoid neck until the rotator cuff muscle is visualized. Care must be taken to keep the radiofrequency device on the glenoid neck and proceed medially on bone. If the dissection is not maintained between the glenoid and labrum, then significant iatrogenic injury could occur to the labrum, rotator cuff tendon, or axillary nerve. However, an

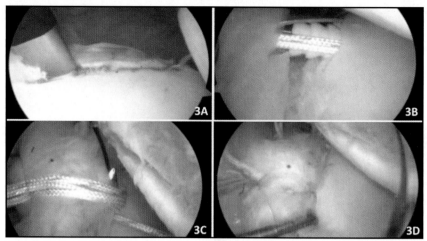

Figure 24-3. (A) The posterior labrum is addressed first by using a radiofrequency blade device to free the labrum from the posterior glenoid neck, as visualized from the trans-cuff portal in the lateral decubitus position. (B) An anchor is then inserted at the 7 o'clock position on the peripheral glenoid face utilizing a percutaneous posteroinferior portal in order to optimize the trajectory of anchor insertion. (C) A curved suture-shuttling device is then used to grab the torn inferior labrum at the 6 o'clock position. The second suture in the double-loaded anchor is passed slightly superior to the first pass at the 8 o'clock position, and then a second anchor is placed and the sutures are passed in a similar fashion. (D) A sliding, locking knot is tied while care is taken to keep the knot away from the articular surface in order to complete the posterior repair.

inadequate release will not allow an anatomic restoration of the labrum and failure will occur. Once the tissues are free, a shaver is used to lightly debride the glenoid neck free of all soft tissue and down to bleeding bone.

The posterior labrum is addressed first from inferior to superior since this area of the shoulder is usually the most difficult to access, and the shoulder becomes progressively tighter as the sutures are tied down. A percutaneous posteroinferior portal is usually created as noted previously if the original posterior portal does not provide the optimal trajectory for portal placement (Figure 24-4). This is done through spinal needle localization. The skin only is then incised, and the introducer for the anchor is used to pierce the capsule. A double-loaded anchor is then placed in the 7 o'clock position on the peripheral glenoid face. A single suture limb is retrieved through the posterior portal. A curved suture shuttling device is then used to grab the torn inferior labrum at the 6 o'clock position (Spectrum II [ConMed Linvatec]). The amount of capsule captured with the labrum is dependent on the amount of capsular laxity that the surgeon believes is present, which is usually 5 to 10 mm of capsule from the capsulolabral junction. Care must be taken only to capture capsulolabral tissue with the suture shuttle since the axillary nerve is immediately adjacent to the inferior capsule. The anchor suture is then shuttled and a limb of the second suture is then retrieved and placed through the capsulolabral tissue at the 8 o'clock position.

A second anchor is again placed through the percutaneous posteroinferior portal at the 9 o'clock position. A straight suture-shuttling device often provides an optimal angle of attack to capture the capsulolabral tissue at 8 and 10 o'clock. The sutures are then retrieved through the posterior portal and then tied after traction is removed from the arm. A sliding, locking knot is utilized with 3 alternating half-hitches, ensuring that the knot is as far away from the chondral surface as possible. A 2-anchor, 4-simple suture construct is completed. More aggressive bites of capsule are taken with the inferior suture limb of each of the anchors as opposed to the superior limb to effectively create an inferior capsular shift.

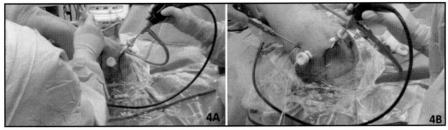

Figure 24-4. Posterior anchor placement in a left shoulder in the lateral decubitus position. (A) Due to the orientation of the scapula on the chest wall, the optimal trajectory of the posterior anchor is very lateral relative to the torso, which differs significantly from anterior glenoid anchor placement. (B) A percutaneous posteroinferior portal is useful both for anchor placement and suture passing in order to capture the posterior, inferior labrum.

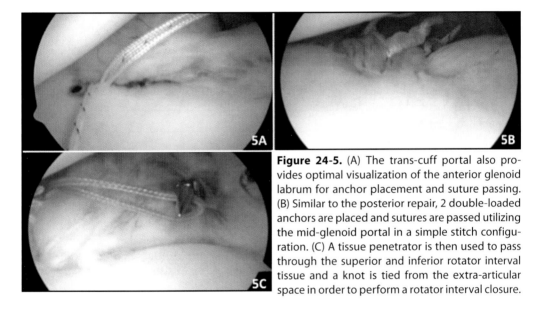

Figure 24-5. (A) The trans-cuff portal also provides optimal visualization of the anterior glenoid labrum for anchor placement and suture passing. (B) Similar to the posterior repair, 2 double-loaded anchors are placed and sutures are passed utilizing the mid-glenoid portal in a simple stitch configuration. (C) A tissue penetrator is then used to pass through the superior and inferior rotator interval tissue and a knot is tied from the extra-articular space in order to perform a rotator interval closure.

If there is any residual posterior capsular laxity, an independent plication stitch is passed using a curved tissue penetrator through the posterior portal and tied in a similar fashion.

The arthroscope remains in the trans-cuff portal for the anterior repair (Figure 24-5). A standard Bankart repair is performed after the capsulolabral tissue is completely mobilized until subscapularis muscle belly is visualized as noted previously. The mid-glenoid portal is utilized to place the anchors and pass the suture, which is as distal and lateral as possible just above the upper border of the subscapularis in order to optimize anchor placement. The first double-loaded anchor is placed at the 5 o'clock position at the lateral margin of the glenoid face. Three of the 4 suture limbs are retrieved out of the anterosuperior portal. Similar to the posterior repair, a curved tissue penetrator is used to grasp approximately 5 mm of capsule and labrum. The goal of this first pass is to capture inferior capsular tissue. The second suture limb is retrieved through the mid-glenoid portal and then shuttled after the tissue penetrator grasps the anteroinferior glenohumeral ligament in order to create the 1-anchor, 2-simple suture configuration. The sutures are retrieved through the posterior portal in order to avoid entanglement as the second anchor is passed. A second anterior anchor is placed in the 3 o'clock position and the sutures are passed in a similar position at the 4 and 3 o'clock positions, incorporating capsule, labrum, and the middle glenohumeral ligament. The sutures are then sequentially retrieved anteriorly from inferior to superior using a sliding, locking knot with alternating half-hitches keeping the knot away from the articular surface.

The arthroscope is then moved to the anterosuperior portal in order to address the superior labral tear, which most commonly acts like an extension of the posterior labral tear. A fifth double-loaded anchor is placed through the trans-cuff portal. The trans-cuff portal provides an optimal angle for superior glenoid anchor placement. A curved tissue penetrator is then used through the posterior portal to pass 2 simple sutures just posterior to the biceps origin, then tied. If the patient is physiologically older or significant biceps tendinopathy exists, a tenodesis will be performed instead of a SLAP repair.[23]

No tissue is usually captured at the anterosuperior glenoid position in order to prevent over-constraining the glenohumeral joint and to avoid excessive postoperative stiffness. Depending on the degree of capsular laxity inherent to the patient's anatomy, a rotator interval closure may be performed. This is performed with the arthroscope in the posterior viewing portal. A nonabsorbable suture is grasped by a straight tissue penetrator, and the superior interval tissue adjacent to the leading edge of the supraspinatus is pierced utilizing the anterosuperior portal approximately 1 cm medial from the biceps pulley. Care is taken not to incarcerate the biceps tendon. The suture is "parked" within the joint, the penetrator is withdrawn from the tissue, inferior interval tissue is penetrated just above the subscapularis, and the suture is retrieved from the joint. The suture is then tied blindly, but the interval closure is visualized as the suture is cinched down.

A complete evaluation of the labral repair with a probe is performed to confirm anatomic restoration of the labrum and appropriate capsular tension. The arm may be removed from the arm holder to gently range the shoulder. The wounds are closed and dressed, and a shoulder immobilizer is applied.

POSTOPERATIVE PROTOCOL

Regional anesthesia is encouraged for acute postoperative pain control. Patients are routinely placed in a shoulder immobilizer in external rotation for 6 weeks in order to protect the labral repair anteriorly and posteriorly. Full elbow, wrist, and hand range of motion are permitted immediately. Patients may remove the sling only for hygiene and are instructed on how to keep the shoulder in external rotation and the elbow fixed on the iliac crest while showering.

After 6 weeks of immobilization, the external rotation brace is discontinued, and supervised physical therapy begins. Full active and passive range of motion are permitted. Strengthening is usually permitted at 12 weeks postoperatively but can be deferred until full range of motion is achieved. Return to competitive sports is allowed at 4 to 6 months postoperatively depending on the type of sport and patient progress with therapy.

POTENTIAL COMPLICATIONS

The results of arthroscopic panlabral repairs are generally good,[10,11] although there are few reports in the literature and limited long-term follow-up. The main 2 complications of these extensive labral repairs are stiffness and recurrent instability. The incidence of postoperative stiffness requiring surgery ranges from 2% to 5%.[10,11] However, this is an unreliable estimate of overall stiffness since the decision to proceed with a capsular release postoperatively is often a subjective and personal patient decision. Ricchetti et al estimated the rate of overall stiffness to be 14%.[11] The incidence of recurrent instability ranges from 5% to 11%.[10,11] The recurrent instability rate 10 years after arthroscopic Bankart repair alone has been estimated to be between 3.4% to 35%,[24] so it is difficult to compare the recurrent instability rate after panlabral repairs to Bankarts alone because of the small numbers and lack of long-term follow-up in the panlabral repair population.

The decision to repair SLAP tears has become a controversial topic in the orthopedic community over the last 10 years[25] as more literature becomes available about patient prognostic factors for failure after SLAP repair. Specifically, age greater than 36 years is associated with failure of a SLAP repair.[23] Tokish et al reported a 5% revision rate after a panlabral repair due to biceps disease requiring a tenodesis.[10] However, the effect of repairing the labrum and subsequent potential stiffness may be a more important determinant of patient outcomes than postoperative biceps tendonitis. There is currently no compelling literature that provides worthwhile recommendations in the management of the superior labrum-biceps anchor complex in panlabral tears. It is the authors' practice to repair the superior labrum in younger patients with a panlabral tear, especially because it often very clearly appears to be an extension of the posterior labral tear that can anatomically be repaired. The authors will generally place their anchors posterior to the biceps root, and avoid placing anchors from the 12 o'clock to 2:30 position anteriorly. Older patients may benefit from a tenodesis, tenotomy, or SLAP debridement as opposed to a SLAP repair due to the theoretical risk of postoperative pain and stiffness.

There is always the risk of infection, but this incidence of postoperative infection requiring further surgery following arthroscopic shoulder surgery in general is extremely low. The rate of nerve injury is also low following arthroscopic Bankart repair,[26] but the risk may be higher in panlabral repairs due to more extensive pathology and distorted anatomy.

Cartilage injury can occur either during anchor placement or postoperatively with prominent anchor placement. The exact etiology of chondrolysis is still unknown, but this can be a devastating complication of arthroscopic shoulder surgery.[27] Intra-articular pain pumps should be avoided for this reason. Post-stabilization arthritis can also occur,[11] but the incidence or risk following panlabral repair is unknown.

TOP TECHNICAL PEARLS FOR THE PROCEDURE

1. While an exam under anesthesia can provide useful information, it is vital that this exam serves mainly to confirm the preoperative diagnosis and surgical plan. The patient's preoperative history and physical are significantly more important than this exam, and the decision to perform surgery and the choice of the surgical procedure should be made preoperatively since the difference between physiologic laxity and pathologic instability is mainly determined by the patient's perception of his or her shoulder function.

2. A surgeon should not hesitate to make additional portals in order to obtain optimal visualization, anchor placement, and suture passage. The morbidity of an additional portal is far less than a poorly done labral repair that was not appropriately executed due to unfavorable portal placement.

3. Utilizing a trans-cuff portal is a safe and effective method that provides global visualization of the glenoid and labrum in order to accurately and efficiently perform the repair.

4. The release of the scarred labrum from the glenoid neck is likely the most important aspect of the repair and should be done carefully and completely. If the dissection is not maintained between the glenoid and labrum, then significant iatrogenic injury could occur to the labrum, rotator cuff tendon, or axillary nerve. However, an inadequate release will not allow an anatomic restoration of the labrum and failure will occur.

5. No tissue is usually captured at the anterosuperior glenoid position in order to prevent overconstraining the glenohumeral joint and to avoid excessive postoperative stiffness.

REFERENCES

1. Harris JD, Gupta AK, Mall NA, et al. Long-term outcomes after Bankart shoulder stabilization. *Arthroscopy.* 2013;29(5):920-933.

2. Savoie FH 3rd, Holt MS, Field LD, Ramsey JR. Arthroscopic management of posterior instability: evolution of technique and results. *Arthroscopy.* 2008;24(4):389-396.

3. McCormick F, Bhatia S, Chalmers P, Gupta A, Verma N, Romeo AA. The Management of Type II Superior Labral Anterior to Posterior Injuries. *Orthop Clin North Am.* 2014;45(1):121-128.

4. Bankart ASB. The pathology and treatment of recurrent dislocation of the shoulder joint. *Br J Surg.* 1938;26:23-29.

5. Warner JJ, Kann S, Marks P. Arthroscopic repair of combined Bankart and superior labral detachment anterior and posterior lesions: technique and preliminary results. *Arthroscopy.* 1994;10:383-391.

6. Powell SE, Nord KD, Ryu RKN. The diagnosis, classification, and treatment of SLAP lesions. *Op Tech Sports Med.* 2004;12:99-110.

7. Andrews JR, Carson WG Jr, McLeod WD. Glenoid labrum tears related to the long head of the biceps. *Am J Sports Med.* 1985;13:337-341.

8. Snyder SJ, Karzel RP, Del Pizzo W, Ferkel RD, Friedman MJ. SLAP lesions of the shoulder. *Arthroscopy.* 1990;6:274-279.

9. Lo IK, Burkhart SS. Triple labral lesions: pathology and surgical repair technique—report of seven cases. *Arthroscopy.* 2005;21:186-193.

10. Tokish JM, McBratney CM, Solomon DJ, Leclere L, Dewing CB, Provencher MT. Arthroscopic repair of circumferential lesions of the glenoid labrum. *J Bone Joint Surg Am.* 2009;91(12):2795-2802.

11. Ricchetti ET, Ciccotti MC, O'Brien DF, et al. Outcomes of arthroscopic repair of panlabral tears of the glenohumeral joint. *Am J Sports Med.* 2012;40(11):2561-2568.

12. Burkhart SS, De Beer JF. Traumatic glenohumeral bone defects and their relationship to failure of arthroscopic Bankart repairs: significance of the inverted-pear glenoid and the humeral engaging Hill-Sachs lesion. *Arthroscopy.* 2000;16(7):677-694.

13. van Kampen DA, van den Berg T, van der Woude HJ, Castelein RM, Terwee CB, Willems WJ. Diagnostic value of patient characteristics, history, and six clinical tests for traumatic anterior shoulder instability. *J Shoulder Elbow Surg.* 2013;22(10):1310-1319.

14. Bhatia S, Ghodadra NS, Romeo AA, et al. The importance of the recognition and treatment of glenoid bone loss in an athletic population. *Sports Health.* 2011;3(5):435-440.

15. Post M. Pectoralis major transfer for winging of the scapula. *J Shoulder Elbow Surg.* 1995;4(1 Pt 1):1-9.

16. Engebretsen L, Craig EV. Radiologic features of shoulder instability. *Clin Orthop Relat Res.* 1993;(291):29-44.

17. Moroder P, Resch H, Schnaitmann S, Hoffelner T, Tauber M. The importance of CT for the preoperative surgical planning in recurrent anterior shoulder instability. *Arch Orthop Trauma Surg.* 2013;133(2):219-226.

18. Smith TO, Drew BT, Toms AP. A meta-analysis of the diagnostic test accuracy of MRA and MRI for the detection of glenoid labral injury. *Arch Orthop Trauma Surg.* 2012;132(7):905-919.

19. Costouros JG, Clavert P, Warner JJ. Trans-cuff portal for arthroscopic posterior capsulorrhaphy. *Arthroscopy.* 2006;22(10):1138.e1-5.

20. Oh JH, Kim SH, Lee HK, Jo KH, Bae KJ. Trans-rotator cuff portal is safe for arthroscopic superior labral anterior and posterior lesion repair: clinical and radiological analysis of 58 SLAP lesions. *Am J Sports Med.* 2008;36(10):1913-1921.

21. Tokish JM, McBratney CM, Solomon DJ, Leclere L, Dewing CB, Provencher MT. Arthroscopic repair of circumferential lesions of the glenoid labrum: surgical technique. *J Bone Joint Surg Am.* 2010;92(Suppl 1 Pt 2):130-144.

22. Cvetanovich GL, McCormick F, Erickson BJ, et al. The posterolateral portal: optimizing anchor placement and labral repair at the inferior glenoid. *Arthrosc Tech.* 2013;2(3):e201-e204.

23. Provencher MT, McCormick F, Dewing C, McIntire S, Solomon D. A prospective analysis of 179 type 2 superior labrum anterior and posterior repairs: outcomes and factors associated with success and failure. *Am J Sports Med.* 2013;41(4):880-886.

24. Randelli P, Ragone V, Carminati S, Cabitza P. Risk factors for recurrence after Bankart repair a systematic review. *Knee Surg Sports Traumatol Arthrosc.* 2012;20(11):2129-2138.

25. Weber SC, Martin DF, Seiler JG 3rd, Harrast JJ. Superior labrum anterior and posterior lesions of the shoulder: incidence rates, complications, and outcomes as reported by American Board of Orthopedic Surgery. Part II candidates. *Am J Sports Med.* 2012;40(7):1538-1543.

26. Owens BD, Harrast JJ, Hurwitz SR, Thompson TL, Wolf JM. Surgical trends in Bankart repair: an analysis of data from the American Board of Orthopaedic Surgery certification examination. *Am J Sports Med.* 2011;39(9):1865-1869.

27. Hasan SS, Fleckenstein CM. Glenohumeral chondrolysis: part I—clinical presentation and predictors of disease progression. *Arthroscopy.* 2013;29(7):1135-1141.

Please see videos on the accompanying website at

www.ArthroscopicTechniques.com

25

Arthroscopic Superior Labral Anteroposterior Repair

Anthony A. Romeo, MD; Peter N. Chalmers, MD; and Chris R. Mellano, MD

INTRODUCTION

Crossing both the shoulder and elbow joints and attaching proximally at the superior labrum and supraglenoid tubercle, the long head of the biceps is a unique anatomical structure.[1,2] At the proximal attachment point, this tendon and the labrum are susceptible to injury.[3] Tears of the superior labrum with involvement of the biceps anchor are called superior labral anteroposterior (SLAP) tears.[1] These tears occur in young overhead athletes and manual laborers and less commonly in older individuals.[1-3] SLAP tears most commonly present with a prodromal period of discomfort in the young overhead-throwing athlete or repetitive overhead laborer.[4] Conversely, a SLAP tear can present acutely after a traumatic mechanism of injury such as a fall with an attempt to grasp an object for support, causing a sudden eccentric biceps load. Snyder and colleagues classified SLAP lesions into 4 types: type I injuries have fraying at the superior labrum and biceps anchor; type II lesions have detachment of the superior labrum and biceps anchor from the superior glenoid; type III injuries have detachment of the superior labrum with displacement of the labrum in a "bucket-handle" configuration, but with continued attachment of the biceps anchor to the superior glenoid; and type IV lesions have detachment of the superior labrum and biceps anchor with extension of the tear into the biceps tendon.[1] Type II tears are the most common reported.[3] The Snyder classification has since been modified to include 4 additional types: type V tear have an anteroinferior labral tear that extends into the superior labrum; type VI tears have biceps tendon avulsion with associated unstable flap tear of labrum; type VII tears extend laterally inferior to the middle glenohumeral ligament; and type VIII tears have posterior extension.[5]

The optimal treatment of these injuries remains controversial. Regardless of age, onset of acuity, or mechanism of injury, most surgeons agree that first-line treatment includes cessation of provocative activity and supervised physiotherapy focused on rotator cuff rehabilitation and improved scapular kinesis and rhythm. For young patients (age < 30 years) who remain symptomatic and are unable to return to play or activity, arthroscopic SLAP repair utilizing suture anchors is the current gold standard.[6-9] Outcomes for arthroscopic repair with suture anchors can be unpredictable. In several series of elite athletes, approximately two-thirds are able to return to play at the same level and associated rotator cuff injuries are often a negative prognostic indicator.[8,10,11]

Ryu RKN, Angelo RL, Abrams JS, eds. *The Shoulder:*
AANA Advanced Arthroscopic Surgical Techniques (pp 297-311).
© 2016 AANA.

INDICATIONS

- ▶ Type II SLAP lesions that cause mechanical symptoms
- ▶ Type II SLAP lesions that have failed all nonoperative measures. In these cases, the history, physical examination, and imaging findings must all be concordant and the surgeon must have ruled out all other potential pain generators.

Relative Indications

- ▶ Patients aged 30 to 40 years
- ▶ Type III and IV[12] lesions with a large bucket-handle tear that has adequate vascular supply

Relative Contraindications

- ▶ Glenohumeral osteoarthritis
- ▶ Chronic or massive rotator cuff tears
- ▶ Bicipital tendon instability
- ▶ Biceps tendinitis
- ▶ Complex regional pain syndrome
- ▶ Unrealistic patient expectations
- ▶ Type I and III SLAP tears
- ▶ Degenerative tears. Recent literature has highlighted high failure rates of SLAP repair, especially in the older patients. For this reason, SLAP repair should be approached with caution and consideration should be given to bicep tenodesis in this patient population.[13,14]
- ▶ Tears found on magnetic resonance imaging (MRI) alone without corroborating history and exam

PERTINENT PHYSICAL FINDINGS

- ▶ An accurate diagnosis of a SLAP tear can be difficult to obtain with certainty because of the variable sensitivity and specificity of the available physical examination maneuvers and the frequency of concomitant pathology.[15]
- ▶ Examination begins with inspection, range of motion testing, strength testing, and palpation.
- ▶ Strength testing is crucial—SLAP tears have been associated with paralabral cyst formation, which can compress the suprascapular nerve at the spinoglenoid notch and lead to weakness of the infraspinatus.
- ▶ In Speed's test, the patient elevates the shoulder against resistance with the elbow extended and the forearm supinated with resultant anterior shoulder pain, denoting a positive test.[16] Of note, Speed's test is sensitive for all forms of biceps tendon disorders, such as bicep tendonitis, but Speed's test is not specific to SLAP tears.
- ▶ In Yergason's test, the patient supinates the forearm against resistance with the shoulder in adduction and neutral rotation and the elbow at 90 degrees of flexion.[16] Similar to Speed's test, a positive Yergason's test can be helpful to identify biceps tendon disorders but not necessarily SLAP tears specifically.
- ▶ During O'Brien's active compression test, the shoulder is held at 90 degrees of flexion and 10 degrees of adduction with the elbow extended. The patient performs active resisted

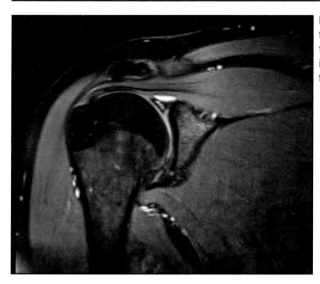

Figure 25-1. This coronal, T2-weighted, fat-suppressed MRI demonstrates a SLAP tear with associated intralabral signal intensity and associated paralabral cyst formation.

shoulder flexion. A positive test is denoted by pain in maximal shoulder internal rotation that is relieved when the test is repeated in maximal shoulder external rotation.[17] Although reports of diagnostic accuracy vary widely in the literature, the active compression test consistently has the highest sensitivity (47% to 78%) and specificity (11% to 73%) of available tests.[15,18]

▶ In the passive compression test, the shoulder is placed in an externally rotated and abducted position, then passively extended and axially loaded with resultant pain or painful clunk, denoting a positive test.[19]

▶ In the Mayo dynamic shear test, the examiner passively externally rotates the shoulder and then abducts the shoulder, producing pain or a clunk between 60 and 120 degrees of flexion, indicating a positive test.[16]

▶ Finally, the patient should be assessed for biceps tendinitis by examining for pain and tenderness localizable to the intertubercular groove, 5 to 7 cm distal to the anterolateral acromion. If symptoms and signs are most consistent with bicep tendonitis, such as primarily anterior shoulder pain, and there is tenderness with bicipital groove palpation, then consideration should be given to treating the bicep tendonitis primarily, regardless of imaging findings of the superior labrum.

▶ When in doubt, diagnostic injections of local anesthetic either in the glenohumeral joint or bicipital groove may aid in decision making. Ultrasound guidance may improve the accuracy of a biceps groove injection.

PERTINENT IMAGING

▶ The following radiographs should be obtained to evaluate for acromioclavicular or glenohumeral joint arthrosis as possible contributors to the patient's pain: Grashey anteroposterior, scapular-Y lateral, and axillary lateral views.

▶ MRI may be helpful to make the diagnosis of a SLAP tear (Figure 25-1). However, a closed MRI scanner with a magnet of at least 1.5 T is needed to discern the anatomic detail necessary to adequately visualize the biceps anchor.

▶ The addition of intra-articular gadolinium also improves diagnostic accuracy to a specificity of 89%, a sensitivity of 91%, and an accuracy of 90%.[20] In the authors' experience, even with an MR arthrogram, it can remain very difficult to differentiate an anatomic cleft from a pathologic SLAP tear. Signal defects in the superior labrum that follow the contour of the superior glenoid articular cartilage tend to be anatomic variants.

▶ Arthroscopy remains the gold standard for the diagnosis of SLAP tears.

Equipment

▶ 30-degree sheathed arthroscope with trocar

▶ Arthroscopic pump or set-up for gravity inflow depending on the surgeon's preference

▶ A motorized arthroscopic shaver and hooded burr

▶ A rasp, a full complement of labral elevators, and a probe

▶ A curved suture passing instrument

▶ A suture-retrieving hook or looped grasper, an arthroscopic knot pusher, and an arthroscopic suture cutter

▶ Standard-sized cannulas for the working portals—either the anterior or posterior portal depending on tear pattern. A smaller cannula (5 mm) is preferred if a trans-cuff portal is utilized.

▶ Suture anchors of surgeon preference. The authors' preference is to use knotless suture anchors with broad suture for superior labral fixation whenever possible to avoid knot irritation of the chondral surfaces.

Positioning and Portals

Although SLAP repair can be performed in both the beach chair and lateral decubitus positions, the senior author prefers the lateral decubitus position with weighted arm suspension. Use a suction beanbag to stabilize the patient, a gel axillary roll to take pressure off of the contralateral brachial plexus, and a folded blanket or pillow under the dependent leg and between the legs to pad bony prominences and the common peroneal nerve. The arm is then positioned at 30 to 40 degrees of abduction and 20 degrees of forward flexion. The authors prefer to apply 10 lbs of both longitudinal and abduction force for balanced traction. One advantage of the lateral decubitus position is that it avoids issues with cerebral hypoperfusion that have been associated with the beach chair position and may discourage anesthesiologists from utilizing hypotensive anesthesia. The authors prefer to utilize both an ultrasound-guided interscalene or supraclavicular block and general anesthesia.

Examination Under Anesthesia and Arthroscopic Evaluation of the Superior Labrum

First, perform an examination under anesthesia to document passive range of motion, anterior and posterior laxity, and the magnitude of the sulcus sign. A standard posterior arthroscopic portal should then be established 2 cm medial and 1 cm distal to the posterolateral acromion. The exact position varies from patient to patient and the surgeon must palpate the joint line during anterior and posterior "shuck" of the joint to accurately locate the ideal position for this portal (Figure 25-2). If the SLAP tear is known to extend posterior to the mid-glenoid level, adjust the portal 1 cm lateral to optimize the trajectory for anchor preparation and insertion. After entering the joint with the arthroscope, remove the shoulder from weighted suspension and evaluate the

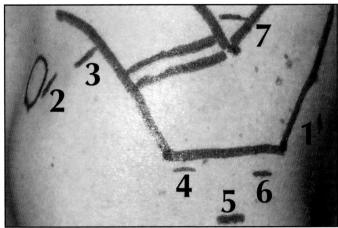

Figure 25-2. Clinical photograph of portal placement. The coracoid, clavicle, acromion, and scapular spine are outlined. 1 = posterior portal; 2 = midanterior portal within the rotator interval; 3 = anterosuperior portal within the rotator interval; 4 = usual placement for a trans-rotator cuff SLAP portal; 5 = lateral portal for subacromial work; 6 = Portal of Wilmington; 7 = Neviaser portal.

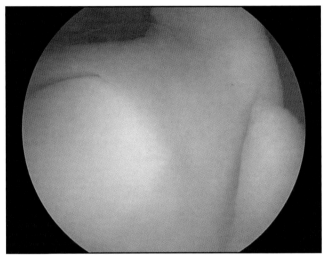

Figure 25-3. SLAP tear with posterior extension.

labrum by taking the shoulder through a full passive range of motion to assess for labral instability, labral peel-back, and findings suggestive of internal impingement (ie, direct contact between the greater tuberosity and adjacent cuff and the posterosuperior glenoid). An arthroscopic passive compression test or Mayo shear test can also be performed to evaluate for superior labrum instability. The arm is then returned to weighted suspension. Next, an anterior portal is created with an outside-in technique within the rotator interval, slightly more superior than during Bankart repair to facilitate the use of suture-passing instruments. Insert a cannula large enough to allow for delivery of suture-passing instruments. A probe introduced into this portal can then be used to further assess the superior labrum for stability as well as to manipulate the bicep tendon to assess for long head of biceps tendinopathy. At this juncture, the surgeon must also determine whether the superior labrum is pathologic or physiologic, processes that can be difficult to differentiate. Experience and knowledge of the spectrum of anatomic variations within the superior and anterosuperior labrum are critical.[21] Generally, if the superior labrum can be displaced from the superior glenoid with a probe and there is evidence of tearing at the labral attachment to the supraglenoid tubercle, a pathologic SLAP tear is suggested (Figures 25-3 and 25-4). However, regardless of the arthroscopic appearance, the surgical decision making is always based on the arthroscopic findings within the context of the history and physical exam findings. It is the opinion of the senior author that a type II SLAP tear found incidentally during routine arthroscopy should be left untreated if the history and physical exam are not supportive.

Figure 25-4. Displacement of the labrum from the glenoid using the shaver.

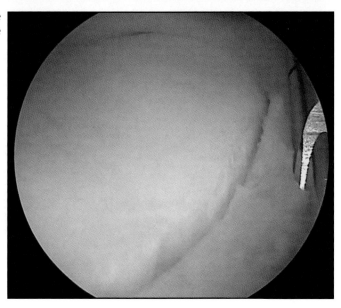

Understand the SLAP Tear Pattern and Plan the Repair Sequence

Once the surgeon has determined that a SLAP tear is present (see Figures 25-3 and 25-4) and that repair is clinically indicated, place the scope in the anterior cannula and probe the posterior labrum through the posterior portal to assess for posterior extension of the SLAP tear. This extent of posterior extension will determine the repair sequence. If the labral tear is isolated to the superior labrum under the bicep root and slightly posterior, then it is typically amenable to completing the repair with 1 or 2 anchors as described in the sequence presented next. If the SLAP tear is found to extend posteriorly down to the mid-glenoid region (as depicted in the arthroscopic video of a Type VIII SLAP tear pattern), then the repair sequence will require that the posterior repair be performed first, then the superior repair. The location and number of the suture anchors should be planned.

Labral Preparation and Accessory Portal Placement Options

The anterior cannula typically serves as the working cannula for labral preparation and the passing of sutures. The surgeon should start by preparing the superior glenoid bone with a hooded burr or shaver introduced through the anterior portal (Figure 25-5). To avoid causing iatrogenic chondral injury to the glenoid, the surgeon should start the burr off of bone with the teeth facing slightly medial. A cylindrical-shaped burr is typically easier to control compared to an acorn-shaped burr. If the posterior extent of the tear cannot be prepared safely with the burr from the anterior cannula, then the surgeon can switch to viewing from the anterior cannula and insert the burr in the posterior portal. The bony bed is prepared over the width of the labral footprint.

Once the superior glenoid bone preparation is complete, the surgeon must create an accessory portal for anchor insertion and possible suture shuttling. Accessory portals are needed as the trajectory from the anterior cannula does not allow for proper anchor insertion into the superior glenoid. Several accessory portal options exist. A portal can be established at the superior aspect of the rotator interval just off of the leading edge of the supraspinatus to provide anterosuperior and midanterior portals within the rotator interval. If 2 rotator interval portals are used, ensure that maximal distance separates the portals to avoid crowding. The more superior of these portals may

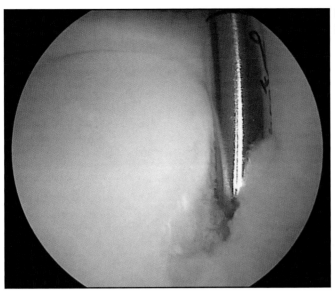

Figure 25-5. Preparation of the glenoid bony bed prior to labral repair.

or may not provide the optimal position or angulation 45 degrees relative to the articular surface of the superior glenoid. The advantage of using 2 cannulas within the interval is that damage to the rotator cuff is minimized.

A second option, and the senior author's preference, is to create a trans-rotator cuff portal. While viewing from either the posterior or anterior portal, a spinal needle is used for localization. The trans-rotator cuff portal skin incision is usually just off of the lateral acromion just posterior to the anterolateral corner. Confirm with the spinal needle that this portal is at the "deadman's angle" (ie, 45 degrees relative to the superior glenoid). To perform the knotless suture anchor fixation, the authors prefer to insert a small 5-mm metal cannula in this trans-rotator cuff portal to minimize rotator cuff injury. If traditional knotted suture anchor fixation is used, then this trans-rotator cuff portal can be percutaneous and does not require a cannula. Care should be taken to ensure that this portal passes medial to the rotator cable.[22]

A third option, which can be combined with the previous options for SLAP tears with posterior extension, is to use the portal of Wilmington. This portal lies 1 cm anterior and 1 cm lateral to the posterolateral corner of the acromion.

Knotted Suture Anchor Fixation vs Knotless Suture Anchor Fixation

The surgeon then has 2 options for suture anchor labral fixation: a knotless or a knotted suture anchor technique. In traditional knotted suture anchor fixation, the sequence of events include the following:

▶ Step 1: Anchor drilling and insertion

▶ Step 2: Suture shuttling under the labrum

▶ Step 3: Arthroscopic knot tying

In a knotless fixation technique, the sequence of events is different and includes the following:

▶ Step 1: Suture shuttling under the labrum

▶ Step 2: Anchor drilling

▶ Step 3: Suture passage through the anchor outside the body

▶ Step 4: Anchor insertion

Figure 25-6. Passage of a shuttling suture through the chondrolabral junction from the anterosuperior portal (cannula can be seen behind the biceps).

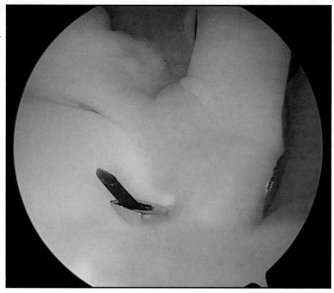

After experience with suture anchor chondral abrasion with knotted suture anchor SLAP repair, the senior author's preference is to perform a knotless anchor fixation for SLAP repair using broad suture (Labral tape [Arthrex]).[23]

STEP-BY-STEP DESCRIPTION: KNOTLESS ANCHOR FIXATION SUPERIOR LABRAL ANTEROPOSTERIOR REPAIR

Step 1: Shuttle Suture Passage Under the Labrum

In the knotless technique, a curved, cannulated suture passing device, such as the Spectrum (Conmed Linvatec), is first introduced via the anterior cannula located in the rotator interval. The curved suture passer is passed under the labrum at the capsulolabral junction at the site of the SLAP tear and the shuttle suture is advanced under the labrum (Figure 25-6).

At this point, suture management can be performed with 1 or 2 cannulas. For instance, a trans-rotator cuff portal with a 5-mm metal cannula can be used. The suture shuttle passed from the anterior cannula through the labrum can be retrieved from the trans-cuff portal using a suture-retrieving device. A broad free suture (Labral tape) is tied to the shuttling suture and delivered back under the labrum in a retrograde fashion by pulling the shuttling suture back out the anterior portal. Alternatively, to use a single anterior cannula for suture shuttling, the curved suture-passing device is passed under the labrum and the shuttling suture is advanced so that an abundant amount of suture is collected within the joint. Next, the curved suture passer handle is removed carefully from the anterior cannula without removing the shuttling suture from under the labrum. A suture retriever is then placed into the anterior cannula to retrieve the shuttling suture so that both suture ends are collected out of the anterior cannula (Figure 25-7). The broad labral tape is tied to one end of the shuttling suture and then passed under the labrum by retrieving the shuttling suture in a retrograde fashion to create a simple suture configuration (Figure 25-8). Both limbs of the suture are now retrieved and parked out of the anterior cannula. This process can be repeated to create a mattress configuration (Figures 25-9 and 25-10).

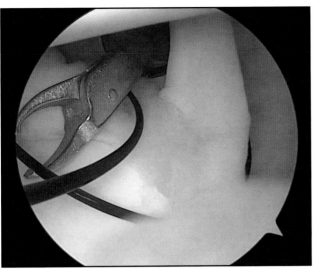

Figure 25-7. Retrieval of the shuttling suture through the same anterosuperior portal.

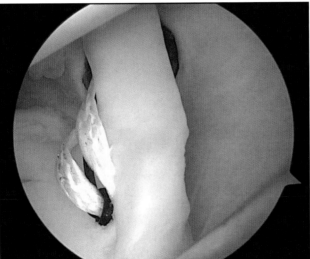

Figure 25-8. Use of the shuttling stitch to retrograde past labral tape.

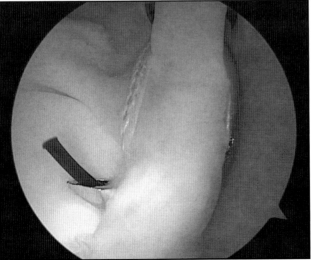

Figure 25-9. Passage of a second shuttling suture for creation of a mattress.

Figure 25-10. Retrograde passage of the labral side of the labral tape through the labral side of the shuttling suture such that both free ends of the labral tape lie at the articular surface.

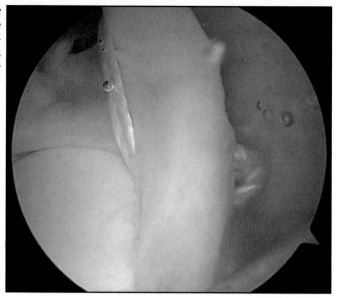

Figure 25-11. Use of a port of Wilmington portal for drilling for the arthroscopic anchor.

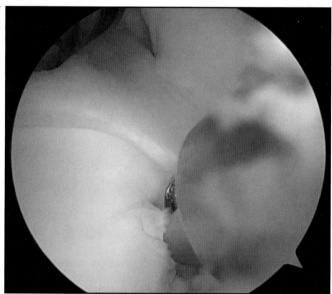

Step 2: Drill the Anchor Hole in the Glenoid

The drill and drill sleeve for the anchor is now inserted through the trans-rotator cuff cannula (Figure 25-11). Unlike Bankart repair, during SLAP repair, the drill sleeve is placed off of the articular margin to avoid leaving a prominent anchor and creating chondral injury. The drill is angled 45 degrees to the glenoid surface and introduced to the predetermined depth. Avoid shallow drilling as this will result in a prominent anchor position and possible chondral damage to the humeral head.

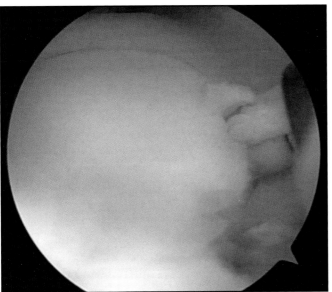

Figure 25-12. Use of the port of Wilmington portal for anchor insertion.

Step 3: Pass the Suture Through the Anchor

Using a suture retriever through the trans-rotator cuff cannula, the 2 suture ends are retrieved out of the trans-rotator cuff cannula. Care is taken that both suture limbs are on the same side of the bicep tendon to avoid incorporation of the tendon into the anchor repair. Both suture limbs are passed through the anchor outside of the cannula.

Step 4: Insert the Anchor Into the Predrilled Hole in the Glenoid

The anchor is brought through the trans-rotator cuff cannula and seated into the predrilled hole (Figure 25-12). Tensioning the broad suture is necessary while inserting the anchor into the hole to avoid "slack" in the suture fixation of the labrum. However, too much tension on the sutures during anchor insertion will prevent full seating of the anchor. Confirm that the anchor is fully seated to avoid possible chondral injury to the humeral head. The suture can then be cut (Figure 25-13) and the repair inspected (Figure 25-14). Note that the authors have described this technique using a trans-cuff portal. This technique can also be performed with anterior and anterosuperior portals with the anterior portal used for suture retrieval and the anterosuperior portal used for anchor drilling and insertion if the correct angle can be achieved.

Depending on the size of the tear and the surgeon's preference, multiple sutures may be necessary to achieve a stable repair. Generally, anchor placement is dictated by the tear configuration. If more than one anchor is planned, begin with the posterior anchor and suture placement. The same technique can be used to place sutures in a mattress configuration with the second passage of the Spectrum in a reversed orientation to the first (ie, from the chondrolabral junction to the capsulolabral junction or visa-versa; see Figures 25-9 and 25-10). The benefit of the mattress technique is that it may create a more anatomic labral "bumper" and does not leave any suture material exposed to the chondral surfaces. There is no evidence, however, that a mattress repair is stronger than a simple repair.[24]

Figure 25-13. Suture cutting.

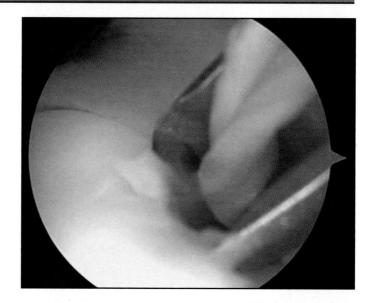

Figure 25-14. Completed SLAP repair. Please note that additional posterior simple sutures have been placed in addition to the knotless mattress placed in Figures 25-4 through 25-13.

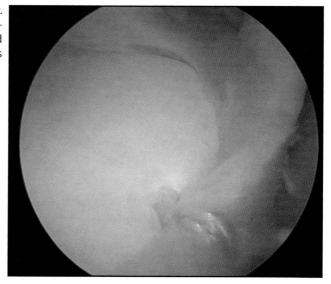

STEP-BY-STEP DESCRIPTION: KNOTTED ANCHOR FIXATION SUPERIOR LABRAL ANTEROPOSTERIOR REPAIR

The knotted repair is conceptually similar except that the steps are reversed as follows:

▶ Step 1: The anchor is placed first, either through the trans-rotator cuff portal or percutaneously.

▶ Step 2: The more medial of the suture limbs is then brought out of the anterior cannula.

▶ Step 3: A suture-passing device is then used to pierce the labrocapsular junction, exiting at the labrochondral junction in line with the anchor.

▶ Step 4: The suture is then shuttled using the anterosuperior portal similar to the previous description for the knotless repair.

► Step 5: Sutures can then be tied with a sliding knot of the surgeon's choice and backed up by 3 reversed half-hitches on alternating posts. During knot tying, all efforts must be made to ensure that the knot stack is as far medial and away from the articular surface as possible.

If a simple suture configuration is desired, then a suture retriever is inserted and used to retrieve the other limb of the suture on the same side of the bicep tendon. An arthroscopic knot is tied in a standard manner with the post limb being the more medial limb to prevent the knot from becoming entrapped within the joint. If a horizontal mattress configuration is desired, then suture passage and retrieval is repeated with the second limb on the same side of the bicep tendon. This process is repeated as many times as necessary to achieve a stable labral repair. When using a knotted repair, some surgeons prefer only to tie after all sutures have been passed because tying can obscure the labrochondral junction and hinder subsequent anchor placement and suture passage. In general, the surgeon should avoid anchor placement or even suture placement anterior to the bicep insertion. This will invariably lead to rotator interval tightening and limit external rotation.

Superior Labral Anteroposterior Repair With Posterior Extension

If the SLAP tear extends far posterior from the biceps root down to the mid-glenoid level, then it is best to start with posterior labral fixation and work anterosuperior toward the bicep root. In this case, a working cannula should be placed in the posterior portal and the scope placed in the anterior cannula. Under spinal needle guidance, a port of Wilmington approach is created using a small 5-mm smooth cannula inserted medial to the musculotendinous junction. This approach provides an appropriate orientation to the 11 o'clock position on the superior glenoid for a right shoulder (see Figure 25-11). The posterior labrum can be secured with knotless fixation using either the posterior or port of Wilmington cannulas for suture management (see Figures 25-11 and 25-12). Once delivered, the posterior labral sutures can be retrieved out of the port of Wilmington cannula and loaded into the knotless anchor. Anchor delivery and insertion completes the posterosuperior repair. Once the posterior labrum is repaired, the arthroscope can be moved to the posterior portal and the superior labrum can be repaired with the techniques described previously.

POSTOPERATIVE PROTOCOL

Postoperatively, patients are immobilized in a sling for the first 4 weeks, but they begin limited range of motion immediately in supervised physiotherapy. Initially, patients are instructed to avoid internal rotation to their back, external rotation behind their head, and resisted forward flexion. At 4 weeks postoperatively, the patient's range of motion goals include 90 degrees of forward flexion and 20 degrees of external rotation. At 8 weeks postoperatively, the range of motion goals include 140 degrees of forward flexion, 40 degrees of external rotation, 60 degrees of abduction, and internal rotation to the waist. Strengthening begins at 6 weeks postoperatively, beginning with isometric exercises for the rotator cuff and periscapular musculature. Light weights are incorporated at 8 weeks, followed by eccentric strengthening at 12 weeks. Pitchers begin a throwing program at 4.5 months and progress to throwing from the mound at 6 months.

POTENTIAL COMPLICATIONS

Although infrequent, complications can occur after SLAP repair, including persistent pain within the shoulder or biceps tendon precluding return to full preoperative function, arthrofibrosis, complex regional pain syndrome, and infection. The former has led some authors to suggest biceps tenodesis as an alternative treatment for SLAP tears, which remains controversial.[13]

TOP TECHNICAL PEARLS FOR THE PROCEDURE

1. Perform a thorough diagnostic arthroscopy, which includes a direct view while moving the shoulder through a full range of motion to evaluate for labral peel-back; thorough probing of the labrum to differentiate an anatomic labrochondral cleft from a pathologic SLAP tear is essential—an understanding of anatomic variants is crucial.

2. Assess the posterior labrum while viewing from the anterior cannula. If the tear extends to the mid-glenoid level, then repair the posterior labrum first and proceed superiorly and anteriorly.

3. Place anchors percutaneously or use an accessory trans-cuff portal to ensure that anchors are appropriately oriented relative to the glenoid articular surface.

4. Avoid placing anchors or suture anterior to the biceps root; this may lead to loss of motion.

5. An alternative to traditional knot fixation is knotless fixation, which can avoid chondral irritation and/or mechanical symptoms.

REFERENCES

1. Snyder SJ, Karzel RP, Del Pizzo W, Ferkel RD, Friedman MJ. SLAP lesions of the shoulder. *Arthroscopy*. 1990;6(4):274-279.
2. Kim TK, Queale WS, Cosgarea AJ, McFarland EG. Clinical features of the different types of SLAP lesions: an analysis of one hundred and thirty-nine cases. *J Bone Joint Surg Am*. 2003;85-A(1):66-71.
3. Snyder SJ, Banas MP, Karzel RP. An analysis of 140 injuries to the superior glenoid labrum. *J Shoulder Elbow Surg*. 1995;4(4):243-248.
4. Dun S, Kingsley D, Fleisig GS, Loftice J, Andrews JR. Biomechanical comparison of the fastball from wind-up and the fastball from stretch in professional baseball pitchers. *Am J Sports Med*. 2007;36(1):137-141.
5. Maffet MW, Gartsman GM, Moseley B. Superior labrum-biceps tendon complex lesions of the shoulder. *Am J Sports Med*. 1995;23(1):93-98.
6. Burkhart S. Shoulder injuries in overhead athletes: the "dead arm" revisited. *Clin Sports Med*. 2000;19(1):125-158.
7. Enad JG, Gaines RJ, White SM, Kurtz CA. Arthroscopic superior labrum anterior-posterior repair in military patients. *J Shoulder Elbow Surg*. 2007;16(3):300-305.
8. Ide J. Sports activity after arthroscopic superior labral repair using suture anchors in overhead-throwing athletes. *Am J Sports Med*. 2005;33(4):507-514.
9. Keener JD, Brophy RH. Superior labral tears of the shoulder: pathogenesis, evaluation, and treatment. *J Am Acad Orthop Surg*. 2009;17(10):627-637.
10. Paxinos A, Walton J, Rütten S, Müller M, Murrell GAC. Arthroscopic stabilization of superior labral (SLAP) tears with biodegradable tack: outcomes to 2 years. *Arthroscopy*. 2006;22(6):627-634.
11. Morgan CD, Burkhart SS, Palmeri M, Gillespie M. Type II SLAP lesions: three subtypes and their relationships to superior instability and rotator cuff tears. *Arthroscopy*. 1998;14(6):553-565.
12. Nho SJ, Strauss EJ, Lenart BA, et al. Long head of the biceps tendinopathy: diagnosis and management. *J Am Acad Orthop Surg*. 2010;18(11):645-656.
13. Boileau P, Parratte S, Chuinard C, Roussanne Y, Shia D, Bicknell R. Arthroscopic treatment of isolated type II SLAP lesions: biceps tenodesis as an alternative to reinsertion. *Am J Sports Med*. 2009;37(5):929-936.

14. McCormick F, Nwachukwu B, Solomon D, et al. The efficacy of biceps tenodesis in the treatment of failed superior labral anterior posterior repairs. *Am J Sports Med.* 2014;42(4):820-825.

15. Meserve BB, Cleland JA, Boucher TR. A meta-analysis examining clinical test utility for assessing superior labral anterior posterior lesions. *Am J Sports Med.* 2009;37(11):2252-2258.

16. Parentis MA. An evaluation of the provocative tests for superior labral anterior posterior lesions. *Am J Sports Med.* 2006;34(2):265-268.

17. O'Brien SJ, Pagnani MJ, Fealy S, McGlynn SR, Wilson JB. The active compression test: a new and effective test for diagnosing labral tears and acromioclavicular joint abnormality. *Am J Sports Med.* 1998;26(5):610-613.

18. Ben Kibler W, Sciascia AD, Hester P, Dome D, Jacobs C. Clinical utility of traditional and new tests in the diagnosis of biceps tendon injuries and superior labrum anterior and posterior lesions in the shoulder. *Am J Sports Med.* 2009;37(9):1840-1847.

19. Kim YS, Kim JM, Ha KY, Choy S, Joo MW, Chung YG. The passive compression test: a new clinical test for superior labral tears of the shoulder. *Am J Sports Med.* 2007;35(9):1489-1494.

20. Murray PJ, Shaffer BS. Clinical update: MR imaging of the shoulder. *Sports Med Arthrosc.* 2009;17(1):40-48.

21. Williams MM, Snyder SJ, Buford D. The Buford complex--the "cord-like" middle glenohumeral ligament and absent anterosuperior labrum complex: a normal anatomic capsulolabral variant. *Arthroscopy.* 1994;10(3):241-247.

22. Burkhart SS, Esch JC, Jolson RS. The rotator crescent and rotator cable: an anatomic description of the shoulder's "suspension bridge". *Arthroscopy.* 1993;9(6):611-616.

23. Rhee YG, Ha JH. Knot-induced glenoid erosion after arthroscopic fixation for unstable superior labrum anterior-posterior lesion: case report. *J Shoulder Elbow Surg.* 2006;15(3), 391-393

24. Boddula MR, Adamson GJ, Gupta A, McGarry MH, Lee TQ. Restoration of labral anatomy and biomechanics after superior labral anterior-posterior repair: comparison of mattress versus simple technique. *Am J Sports Med.* 2012;40(4):875-881.

Please see videos on the accompanying website at

www.ArthroscopicTechniques.com

Financial Disclosures

Dr. Jeffery S. Abrams is a consultant for Conmed Linvatec, Arthrocare Medical, DePuy Mitek, and Rotation Medical. He has stock options in KFx Medical, Cayenne Medical, Rotation Medical, and Ingen Medical and he receives royalties from Arthrocare Medical, Springer Publication, and SLACK Incorporated.

Dr. James R. Andrews has not disclosed any relevant financial relationships.

Dr. Richard L. Angelo is a consultant for DePuy/Mitek.

Dr. Guillermo Arce is a paid consultant for and receives research support from Mitek and Storz. He is on the *Arthroscopy* Journal Board of Trustees. He is also on the Executive Committee for the International Society of Arthroscopy, Knee Surgery and Orthopaedic Sports Medicine.

Dr. Craig R. Bottoni receives research support from Arthrex and the Musculoskeletal Transplant Foundation. He is also on the Board of Directors for the Musculoskeletal Transplant Foundation and is a consultant for Arthrex.

Dr. Stephen S. Burkhart is a consultant for and receives inventor's royalties from Arthrex, Inc. He also receives book royalties from Wolters Kluwer, Inc.

Dr. Robert T. Burks is a consultant for Virta Med and Mitek. He also receives royalties from Arthrex.

Dr. Joe Burns receives consulting income from Conmed and Mitek, research support from Conmed, and textbook royalties from Wolters Kluwer Health.

Dr. Peter N. Chalmers has no financial or proprietary interest in the materials presented herein.

Dr. Brian J. Cole is a consultant for Arthrex, Zimmer, Regentis, and DJ Ortho. He receives research support from Zimmer, Johnson & Johnson, and Medipost. He also receives royalties from Arthrex and DJ Ortho.

Dr. Alan Curtis is a teaching consultant for Stryker, Arthrex, and Donjoy. He has investments in Parcus Inc and receives royalties from Arthrex. He is also on the board of directors for AANA.

Dr. Patrick J. Denard is a consultant for Arthrex, receives book royalties from Wolters Kluwer, and is on the Editorial Board for *Arthroscopy* journal.

Dr. Matthew F. Dilisio has no financial or proprietary interest in the materials presented herein.

Matthew Doran has no financial or proprietary interest in the materials presented herein.

Dr. Matthew D. Driscoll is a consultant for DePuy Mitek.

Dr. James Esch is a consultant for Smith & Nephew Endoscopy and he has stock options in KFX Medical.

Dr. Simon A. Euler has a fellowship sponsored by Arthrex, AGA. He also receives research support from SPRI.

Dr. Nathan D. Faulkner has no financial or proprietary interest in the materials presented herein.

Dr. Eric Ferkel has no financial or proprietary interest in the materials presented herein.

Dr. Larry D. Field has no financial or proprietary interest in the materials presented herein.

Dr. MAJ Kelly Fitzpatrick has no financial or proprietary interest in the materials presented herein.

Dr. Brody A. Flanagin has no financial or proprietary interest in the materials presented herein.

Dr. Rachel M. Frank has no financial or proprietary interest in the materials presented herein.

Dr. Raffaele Garofalo has no financial or proprietary interest in the materials presented herein.

Dr. Mark H. Getelman is a consultant for DePuy Synthes Mitek Sports Medicine and a committee chairman and member of the BOD of AANA. He also receives fellowship support from Smith Nephew, DePuy Synthes Mitek Sports Medicine, and DJO.

Dr. Steven A. Giuseffi has no financial or proprietary interest in the materials presented herein.

Petar Golijanin has no financial or proprietary interest in the materials presented herein.

Dr. Ashish Gupta has no financial or proprietary interest in the materials presented herein.

Dr. Richard J. Hawkins has no financial or proprietary interest in the materials presented herein.

Dr. Sumant G. Krishnan receives royalties from Tornier, TAG Medical, Össur, and Wolters Kluwer; is a member of a speakers' bureau or has made paid presentations on behalf of Tornier; is a paid consultant to or is an employee of Tornier; has stock or stock options held in Johnson & Johnson and Tornier; has received non-income support (such as equipment or services), commercially derived honoraria, or other non-research–related funding (such as paid travel) from Tornier and Wolters Kluwer; and is a board member, owner, officer, or committee member of the Arthroscopy Association of North America, the *American Journal of Sports Medicine*, the American Shoulder and Elbow Surgeons, the *Journal of Bone and Joint Surgery*, and the *Journal of Shoulder and Elbow Surgeons*.

Dr. Kevin P. Krul has no financial or proprietary interest in the materials presented herein.

Dr. Laurent LaFosse receives royalties from DePuy.

Dr. Connor Larose has no financial or proprietary interest in the materials presented herein.

Dr. Ian Lo receives royalties from Smith & Nephew, Arthrex, and Lippincott Williams and Wilkins. He is also a consultant for Smith & Nephew and a paid speaker for Smith & Nephew and Arthrex.

Dr. Gregory C. Mallo has no financial or proprietary interest in the materials presented herein.

Dr. Matthew Mantell has no financial or proprietary interest in the materials presented herein.

Dr. Nolan R. May has no financial or proprietary interest in the materials presented herein.

Dr. Chris R. Mellano has no financial or proprietary interest in the materials presented herein.

Dr. Suzanne Miller is a consultant for Stryker and has a small ownership in Parcus medical.

Dr. Peter J. Millett is a consultant for and receives royalties from Arthrex. He also has stock options in Game Ready and Vumedi and receives research support from SPRI.

Dr. Katy Morris has no financial or proprietary interest in the materials presented herein.

Dr. Michael J. O'Brien is on the board/is a committee member of Arthroscopy Association of North America: Board and Association of American Medical Colleges. He is a paid consultant and receives research or other financial or material support from DePuy, A Johnson & Johnson Company, Mitek, and Smith & Nephew.

Dr. Stephen A. Parada has no financial or proprietary interest in the materials presented herein.

Dr. Robert A. Pedowitz is the chair of the Fundamentals of Arthroscopic Surgery Training (FAST) Program, a collaborative project sponsored by AANA/AAOS/ABOS.

Dr. Stephanie C. Petterson has no financial or proprietary interest in the materials presented herein.

Dr. Kevin D. Plancher has no financial or proprietary interest in the materials presented herein.

Dr. Matthew T. Provencher is a consultant for Arthrex and Joint Restoration Foundation. He also receives royalties from *Arthroscopy*, Elsevier, and SLACK Incorporated. Dr. Provencher is on the Board/Committee for AAOS; American Orthopaedic Society for Sports Medicine; American Shoulder and Elbow Surgeons; Arthroscopy Association of North America; International Society of Arthroscopy, Knee Surgery, and Orthopaedic Sports Medicine; San Diego Shoulder Institute; and Society of Military Orthopaedic Surgeons. He is also on the Editorial/Governing Board for *Arthroscopy*, *Knee*, and *Orthopedics*.

Dr. Andrew J. Riff has no financial or proprietary interest in the materials presented herein.

Dr. R. Judd Robins received an indirect donation from Zimmer, Inc and Smith & Nephew for travel and housing arrangements in non-CME training courses.

Dr. Anthony A. Romeo receives royalties from, is on the speaker's bureau for, is a paid consultant for, and receives other financial support from Arthrex Inc; receives research support from DJO Surgical, Smith & Nephew, and Ossur; and receives publishing royalties from Saunders/Mosby-Elsevier. He also serves on the boards of SLACK Incorporated, *Orthopedics Today*, *Orthopedics*, American Orthopaedic Society for Sports Medicine, American Shoulder and Elbow Surgeons, SAGE, and Wolters Kluwer Health.

Dr. Lane N. Rush has no financial or proprietary interest in the materials presented herein.

Dr. Richard K. N. Ryu is a paid consultant for MedBridge, receives honoraria for lectures from Mitek, and is on the advisory board for Rotation Medical. He has editorial affiliations with *Orthopedics Today* and *Operative Techniques in Sports Medicine*. He is also Chair of AANA Education Foundation and Journal Board of Trustees and a delegate of AOSSM Council of Delegates.

Dr. Felix H. Savoie III is on the board/is a committee member of American Shoulder and Elbow Surgeons: and Arthroscopy Association of North America. He is on the editorial or governing board for *Arthroscopy* and *Journal of Wrist Surgery*. He is an unpaid consultant for Biomet, Exactech, Inc, Mitek, Rotation Medical, and Smith & Nephew. He receives IP royalties from Exactech, Inc; is a paid presenter or speaker for Smith & Nephew; and is a paid presenter or speaker for and receives research support from Mitek.

Dr. Stephen J. Snyder receives royalties from Arthrex, ConMed Linvatec, DJO Global, Sawbones, Wolters Kluwer, and Wright Medical. He is also a consultant for DePuy Mitek, Smith & Nephew, and Wright Medical; is a speaker for ConMed Linvatec; and receives institutional support from DJO Global, DePuy Mitek, and Smith & Nephew.

Dr. Frederick S. Song is a consultant for DePuy Mitek.

Dr. Hiroyuki Sugaya is on the speakers bureau; receives paid presentations; and is a consultant, evaluator, and reviewer for DePuy Synthes and Smith & Nephew.

Dr. Jon J. P. Warner receives fellowship grant support from Smith & Nephew, Arthrex, Mitek, Johnson & Johnson, Breg, and DJ Ortho.

Dr. Ryan J. Warth, MD has no financial or proprietary interest in the materials presented herein.

Index

acromioclavicular joint
   anatomy of, 81-82
   biomechanics of, 82
   dislocation of, classification of, 71, 82-83
   repair of
      for acute injury, 71-80
      for reconstruction, 81-93
   suprascapular nerve branch to, 220-221
acromioclavicular ligaments, anatomy of, 81-82
ACUFEX Shoulder Positioner, 152
adhesive capsulitis
   pancapsular release for, 181-188
   after partial-thickness rotator cuff transendon repair, 254
allografts, for acromioclavicular joint repair, 86-90
"all-suture" anchors, 55
AMBRI classification, of multidirectional instability, 123
anesthesia. *See specific procedures*
anterior Bankart repair, 13-29
   complications of, 26-27
   equipment for, 16
   failure of, 26-27
   imaging for, 15
   indications for, 14
   physical findings and, 14-15
   postoperative protocol for, 25-26
   procedure for, 16-25
   revision of, 39-48

anterior drawer test, 15
anterior glenoid bone block stabilization, 189-197
   bone graft fixation for, 193-194
   bone graft introduction for, 193
   complications of, 195
   equipment for, 190-191
   imaging for, 190
   indications for, 190
   physical findings and, 190
   positioning and portals for, 192
   postoperative protocol for, 195
anterior interval slide, for rotator cuff repair, 67-68
apprehension test, 14
   for Hill-Sachs lesions, 108, 113
   for instability, 149
   for labral pathology, 286
ArthroTunneler, for greater tuberosity fracture repair, 272-273
athletes, Latarjet stabilization for, 203
autografts, for acromioclavicular joint repair, 86-90
axillary lateral view, for suprascapular nerve compression, 221
axillary nerve, protection and injury of
   in Bankart repair, 17
   in capsular plication, 129
   in HAGL repair, 36
   in instability, 149
   in Latarjet stabilization, 213-214

in pancapsular release, 186

in posterior Bankart repair, 266

axillary view, for greater tuberosity fractures, 270

Bankart repair

anterior, 13-29

bony, 147-167

for Hill-Sachs lesions, 111-112, 117

for labral pathology, 291

posterior, 257-267

"bayonet apposition," for scapular access, 279

beach chair position

for acromioclavicular joint repair, 75

for suprapectoral biceps tenodesis, 169-170

bear hug test, for subscapularis injury, 235

belly press test, for subscapularis injury, 149, 235

Bernageau view

for Bankart lesions, 15

for Latarjet stabilization, 200, 203

biceps

anatomy of, 297

dislocation of, 238-239

suprapectoral tenodesis of, 165-179

Biceps SwiveLock, 169

biceps tendinitis, 299

BioComposite SwiveLock C suture anchors, 137-138, 141

biologic augmentation

for acromioclavicular joint repair, 86

for rotator cuff repair, 57

biomechanics

of acromioclavicular joint, 82

of suture healing, 3

BioPushlock anchor, 160-161

BioSuturetac anchor, 158

"blind" instrument insertion, for rotator cuff repair, 64

bone bed preparation, for rotator cuff repair, 138

bone block, glenoid, stabilization of, 189-197

bone grafts, for anterior glenoid bone block stabilization, 192-194

bone loss

in HAGL, 34

revision shoulder stabilization for, 39-48

bone socket, reaming of, for suprapectoral biceps tenodesis, 172

Bone Stitcher, 152

bony Bankart repair, 147-167

complications of, 162

equipment for, 149-151

evolution of, 147-148

imaging for, 151-152

indications for, 148

pathology involved in, 154-155

physical findings and, 149

positioning and portals for, 152-153

postoperative protocol for, 162

procedure for, 154-162

braided sutures, 5

bursal debridement, for glenoid bone block stabilization, 193

bursectomy

for greater tuberosity fracture repair, 272-273

for rotator cuff repair, 52, 138

bursitis, scapulothoracic, treatment of, 277-284

buttons, for acromioclavicular joint repair, 77, 89-90

cable-crescent complex, of rotator cuff, 140-141

Calandra classification, for Hill-Sachs lesions, 109

capsular injury, posterior Bankart repair for, 257-267

capsular mobilization, for Bankart repair, 18-19

capsular plication, 123-131

capsular sling augmentation, 44-45

capsulolabral structures, Latarjet stabilization and, 203

capsulotomy, for Latarjet stabilization, 207

Caspari Suture Punch, 151-152

chicken wing position, for scapular access, 279

chondrolysis, after panlabral repair, 293

cinch-loop stitch, 141

clavicular fractures, after acromioclavicular joint repair, 78

"comma" sign, in subscapularis injury, 238

complex regional pain syndrome, after SLAP tear repair, 309

computed tomography

for acromioclavicular joint dislocation, 74

for bony Bankart repair, 149-150

for greater tuberosity fractures, 271

for Hill-Sachs lesions, 108-109

for labral pathology, 287

for Latarjet stabilization, 200, 203

for multidirectional instability, 125

for scapulothoracic bursitis, 279

for snapping scapula syndrome, 279

Connolly procedure, 107

coracoacromial ligament, suprascapular nerve release at, 224-225

coracoclavicular ligament

anatomy of, 81-82

reconstruction of, 86-87, 89-90

suprascapular nerve release at, 224-225

coracohumeral ligament, release of, in pancapsular release, 184-186

coracoid
fractures of, after acromioclavicular joint repair, 78
release of, in Latarjet stabilization, 207-212

cortical fixation buttons, for acromioclavicular joint repair, 89-90

corticosteroids
for adhesive capsulitis, 182
after partial-thickness rotator cuff transtendon repair, 254

"critical gap," for healing, 2-3

cross arm adduction test, for suprascapular nerve compression, 220-221

debridement, in partial-thickness rotator cuff transtendon repair, 247-248

diagnostic arthroscopy. *See specific procedures*

Dogbone button, 74,77

double-loaded suture, for multidirectional instability, 126

double-row "bridge" construct, in bony Bankart repair, 158-161

double-row rotator cuff repair, 133-145

drilling
for bone graft fixation, 194
for Latarjet stabilization, 211
for SLAP tear repair, 306
for suprapectoral biceps tenodesis, 172

Duncan loop, 5

electrocautery, for Latarjet stabilization, 207-208, 210

electromyography
for scapulothoracic bursitis, 279
for snapping scapula syndrome, 279
for suprascapular nerve compression, 220-221, 229

engaging Hill-Sachs lesions, 202

extracellular matrix grafts, for rotator cuff repair, 95-105

FAST knot tester, 4, 7-9

FiberTape and FiberWire, for rotator cuff repair, 74, 77, 137-142

"fish mouth" drill sleeve, 157

Flatow and Warner classification, for Hill-Sachs lesions, 109

fluid inflow pump, for rotator cuff repair, 57

fractures
clavicular, after acromioclavicular joint repair, 78

coracoid, after acromioclavicular joint repair, 78
greater tuberosity, repair of, 269-276
humeral. *See* Hill-Sachs lesions

fragment mobilization, in bony Bankart repair, 155

fragment repair, in bony Bankart repair, 157

fraying, of subscapularis, 234

frozen shoulder, pancapsular release for, 181-188

Gagey sign
for multidirectional instability, 124
for revision arthroscopy planning, 41

glenohumeral dislocation
Bankart repair for, 13-29
humeral fractures in, 107. *See also* Hill-Sachs lesions

glenohumeral instability
bony Bankart repair for, 147-167
posterior Bankart repair for, 257-267

glenohumeral ligaments
humeral avulsion of, repair of, 31-37
plication of, 264

glenoid bone block stabilization, 189-197

glenoid dislocation, Latarjet stabilization for, 199-217

glenoid rim fractures, in Bankart repair, 27

glenoid track, calculation of, 109

Goutallier changes, in subscapularis tears, 234

grafts
for acromioclavicular joint repair, 86-90
for Hill-Sachs lesions, 111-112
for rotator cuff repair, 95-105

granulomas, after acromioclavicular joint repair, 91

Grashey view
for labral pathology, 287
for suprascapular nerve compression, 221

graspers
for posterior Bankart repair, 263
for rotator cuff repair, 139

grasping sutures, 6-7

greater tuberosity fractures, repair of, 269-276

guide pins, for acromioclavicular joint repair, 76-77

guide wires
for glenoid bone block stabilization, 193-195
for Latarjet stabilization, 211

HAGL (humeral avulsion of the glenohumeral ligament) repair, 31-37, 257-267

half-hitch knots, 6

healing, "critical gap" for, 2-3

hematoma, in Latarjet stabilization, 213

Hill-Sachs lesions
    Bankart repair for, 13-29
    bony Bankart repair for, 148
    Latarjet stabilization for, 199-217
    remplissage for, 107-121
        complications of, 118-119
        equipment for, 113
        imaging for, 113
        indications for, 112
        physical findings and, 113
        positioning and portals for, 113-114
        postoperative protocol for, 118
        procedure for, 114-118
    revision surgery for, 39-48
hook plate fixation, for acromioclavicular joint repair, 90-91
humeral avulsion of the glenohumeral ligament (HAGL) repair, 31-37, 257-267
humeral ligament, release of, 171-172
humerus, greater tuberosity fracture of, repair of, 269-276
hyperabduction test, 15
hyperlaxity, in multidirectional instability, 123

Ideal Suture Grasper, 160, 259
iliac bone graft, for anterior glenoid bone block stabilization, 192-194
impingement signs, in partial-thickness rotator cuff tears, 246
infections
    after Latarjet stabilization, 213
    after panlabral repair, 293
    after subscapularis repair, 242
inferior glenohumeral ligament instability, Bankart repair for, 13-29
infraspinatus muscle, atrophy of, in suprascapular nerve compression, 219-231
injections, for suprascapular nerve compression detection, 221
instability severity index score, 40
interference screw fixation
    for coracoclavicular reconstruction, 89
    for suprapectoral biceps tenodesis, 168-169, 174-175
interval slides, in rotator cuff repair, 66-67
intra-articular release, for rotator cuff repair, 64-66
"inverted pear glenoid," Latarjet stabilization for, 199-217

jerk test
    for Hill-Sachs lesions, 108
    for labral pathology, 286

    for posterior glenohumeral instability, 258
    for revision arthroscopy planning, 41

Kirschner wires
    for acromioclavicular joint repair, 88
    for greater tuberosity fracture repair, 271
    for partial-thickness rotator cuff transtendon repair, 250
knot pushers, 4
knotless fixation devices, 2
    for bony Bankart repair, 160-161
    for SLAP tear repair, 303-304
    for subscapularis repair, 242
knotted sutures, 99-100, 303-304, 308-309
knot-tying, 1-11
    cannulas for, 4
    complications of, 7-10
    equipment for, 4-5
    importance of, 1
    indications for, 1-2
    knot pushers for, 4
    vs. knotless fixation devices, 2
    nonsliding, 5-7
    principles of, 2-5
    sliding, 5-7
    slippage after, 10
    suture materials for, 5
    training aids for, 7

labral injury
    in Hill-Sachs lesions, 34-35
    panlabral repair of, 285-295
    posterior Bankart repair for, 257-267
    superior labral anteroposterior repair of, 285-295
Labral Scorpion instrument, 151, 156-157
Lambotte osteotome, 223, 227
Latarjet stabilization, 199-217
    complications of, 213-214
    equipment for, 204
    history of, 199-200
    imaging for, 203
    indications for, 200-203
    physical findings and, 203
    portals for, 204-205
    positioning and portals for, 204-205
    postoperative protocol for, 213
    procedure for, 206-213
    results of, 214-215
lift off test, for subscapularis injury, 235
load and shift test
    for Bankart lesions, 15

for Hill-Sachs lesions, 108, 113
for labral pathology, 286
for multidirectional instability, 124
for posterior glenohumeral instability, 258
locking knots, 6
loop grabbers, 10
Luschka tubercle, 277

magnetic resonance arthrography
for HAGL, 32
for labral pathology, 287
for multidirectional instability, 125
for partial-thickness rotator cuff transtendon repair, 246
for posterior Bankart repair, 259
for SLAP tears, 300
magnetic resonance imaging
for acromioclavicular joint dislocation, 84
for Bankart lesions, 15
for bony Bankart repair, 149-150
for greater tuberosity fractures, 271
for Hill-Sachs lesions, 109
for labral pathology, 287
for multidirectional instability, 125
for partial-thickness rotator cuff transtendon repair, 246
for posterior Bankart repair, 259
for rotator cuff injury, 97
for scapulothoracic bursitis, 279
for SLAP tears, 299
for snapping scapula syndrome, 279
for subscapularis injury, 236
for subscapularis tears, 233
for suprapectoral biceps tenodesis, 167
for suprascapular nerve compression, 220-222
manipulation under anesthesia, for adhesive capsulitis, 182, 184
Mason-Allen sutures, modified, 6-7
massive cuff stitch, 7, 56
Matsen classification, for multidirectional instability, 123
mattress sutures, 143
for Bankart repair, 20-21
for greater tuberosity fracture repair, 273
for partial-thickness rotator cuff transtendon repair, 251-252
for SLAP tear repair, 307
for subscapularis repair, 241-242
Mayo dynamic shear test, for SLAP tears, 299, 301
middle glenohumeral ligament, plication of, 264
MILAGRO BR Biceps Tendonesis System, 169

mobilization techniques, for rotator cuff repair, 61-69
multidirectional instability, capsular plication for, 123-131
musculocutaneous nerve, injury of, in Latarjet stabilization, 213-214

"Needle Punch" device, 151
nerve conduction studies, for suprascapular nerve compression, 221
nerve injury. *See also* axillary nerve, protection and injury of
in rotator cuff repair, 57
in subscapularis repair, 242
nonlocking knots, 6
nonsliding knots, 5-7
nonsteroidal anti-inflammatory drugs, for adhesive capsulitis, 181
nonunion, after Latarjet stabilization, 214

O'Brien test
for biceps disorders, 167
for labral pathology, 286
for SLAP tears, 298-299
one-finger pain test, for biceps disorders, 167
opaque dome, for knot tying practice, 9
osteoarthritis, after acromioclavicular joint repair, 91
osteolysis, after Latarjet stabilization, 214
osteotomy
coracoid, for Latarjet stabilization, 209-211
for Hill-Sachs lesions, 111
Oxford Shoulder Score, 181

pancapsular release, 181-188
panlabral repair, 285-295
complications of, 292-293
equipment for, 287-288
failure of, 292-293
imaging for, 287
indications for, 285-286
physical findings and, 286
positioning and portals for, 288-289
postoperative protocol for, 292
procedure for, 289-292
partial-thickness rotator cuff tears, transtendon repair of, 245-255
complications of, 253-254
equipment for, 247
failure of, 253-254
imaging for, 246
indications for, 246

pathologic considerations in, 245

physical findings and, 246

positioning and portals for, 247

postoperative protocol for, 252-253

procedure for, 247-252

passive compression test, for SLAP tears, 299, 301

Penetrator devices, for bony Bankart repair, 151-152

Percutaneous Pinning Set, 148, 151-152

plate fixation, for acromioclavicular joint repair, 90-91

pleural tissue penetration, in scapulothoracic bursitis treatment, 283

plication

capsular, 123-131

of glenohumeral ligaments, 264

"Popeye sign," in suprapectoral biceps tenodesis, 175

portals. *See individual procedures*

posterior Bankart repair, 257-267

complications of, 265-266

equipment for, 259

failure of, 265-266

imaging for, 258-259

indications for, 257-258

physical findings and, 258

positioning and portals for, 259

postoperative protocol for, 265

procedure for, 260-264

posterior interval slide, for rotator cuff repair, 66-67

practice boards, for knot-tying, 7, 9

push-pull test, for labral pathology, 286

radiofrequency devices

for panlabral repair, 287, 289

for partial-thickness rotator cuff transtendon repair, 249-250

for scapulothoracic bursitis, 279-282

for snapping scapula syndrome, 279-282

for suprapectoral biceps tenodesis, 168, 174-175

for suprascapular nerve release, 228

radiography

for acromioclavicular joint dislocation, 73-74, 84

for Bankart lesions, 15

for bony Bankart repair, 149-150

for greater tuberosity fractures, 270

for Hill-Sachs lesions, 108, 113

for labral pathology, 287

for Latarjet stabilization, 200, 203

for posterior Bankart repair, 258

for rotator cuff injury, 97

for scapulothoracic bursitis, 279

for SLAP tears, 299-300

for snapping scapula syndrome, 279

for subscapularis injury, 236

for suprapectoral biceps tenodesis, 167

for suprascapular nerve compression, 221

Ramp test, for suprapectoral biceps tenodesis, 170

range of motion limitations, after Hill-Sachs remplissage, 118-119

rasps

for posterior Bankart repair, 262

for scapular access, 282

release (surprise) test, 14

relocation test, 14, 286

remplissage

for Bankart repair, 21-22

for Hill-Sachs lesions, 107-121

for Latarjet stabilization, 201

Rengachary classification, of suprascapular notch variants, 222

retrograde suturing, for subscapularis injury, 236

revision shoulder stabilization, 39-48

complications of, 47

imaging for, 41-42

indications for, 40-41

Latarjet stabilization for, 199-217

physical findings and, 41

positioning and portals for, 42

postoperative protocol for, 47

procedure for, 42-46

Revo-Southern California Orthopedic Institute knot, 5

Rockwood classification, of acromioclavicular joint dislocations, 71-73, 83-85

Roeder knot, 5

"roller wringer" effect, in subscapularis tears, 233

rotation

abnormalities of, in subscapularis injury, 235

limitation of, in adhesive capsulitis, 183

rotator cuff repair

vs. conservative treatment, 95

double-row, 133-145

extracellular matrix replacement for, 95-105

mobilization techniques for, 61-69

partial-thickness, 245-255

single-row, 49-60

transtendon, 245-255

rotator interval plication, 264

for Bankart repair, 24-25

for labral pathology, 292

Rowe classification, for Hill-Sachs lesions, 109

scapula, snapping, treatment of, 277-284

scapular artery, injury to, in scapulothoracic bursitis treatment, 283

scapular ligament, suprascapular nerve release at, 219-231

scapulothoracic bursitis, treatment of, 277-284

screw fixation
    for acromioclavicular joint repair, 89
    for bony Bankart repair, 148
    for glenoid bone block stabilization, 193-194
    for Latarjet stabilization, 212
    for suprapectoral biceps tenodesis, 168-169, 174-175

separated shoulder, 71. *See also* acromioclavicular joint, repair of

shavers
    for partial-thickness rotator cuff transtendon repair, 248-250
    for scapular access, 281-282

short-tailed interference knots, 97-103

shuttle sutures, for SLAP tear repair, 304-305

single-row construct, in bony Bankart repair, 158

single-row rotator cuff repair, 49-60

6-o'clock anchor placement, for revision arthroscopy, 44-45

SLAP (superior labral anteroposterior) tears
    classification of, 297
    with posterior extension, 309
    repair of, 297-311
        Latarjet stabilization, 200
        panlabral, 285-295

sliding knots, 5-7

snapping scapula syndrome, treatment of, 277-284

Southern California Orthopedic Institute row technique, 100

Spectrum crescent, 160

Speed's test
    for biceps disorders, 167
    for SLAP tears, 298

SpeedBridge technique, for rotator cuff repair, 137-139

SPIDER Limb Positioner, 287

spinal accessory nerve injury, in scapulothoracic bursitis treatment, 283

spinal needles
    for Latarjet stabilization, 208
    for partial-thickness rotator cuff transtendon repair, 247-250
    for posterior Bankart repair, 262
    for scapular access, 281-282
    for SLAP tear repair, 303
    for subscapularis repair, 238-239

for suprapectoral biceps tenodesis, 173

for suprascapular nerve release, 224-229

spinoglenoid ligament, release of, 228-229

spinoglenoid notch, suprascapular nerve release at, 219-231

"squeaky" shoulder, 27

"stabber-graspers," 8

stiffness
    after Bankart repair, 26
    after HAGL repair, 36
    after Latarjet stabilization, 214
    after pancapsular release, 186
    after panlabral repair, 292-293
    after partial-thickness rotator cuff transtendon repair, 253-254
    after posterior Bankart repair, 266

strength test, for SLAP tears, 298

Stryker notch view
    for Bankart lesions, 15
    for labral pathology, 287
    for suprascapular nerve compression, 221

subacromial bursectomy
    for greater tuberosity fracture repair, 272-273
    for rotator cuff repair, 52

subscapularis repair, extra-articular technique for, 233-244
    complications of, 24
    equipment for, 236-237
    imaging for, 236
    indications for, 234
    physical findings and, 234-235
    postoperative protocol for, 242
    procedure for, 237-242

subscapularis split, for Latarjet stabilization, 210-211

suicide portal creation, for anterior glenoid bone block stabilization, 193

sulcus sign
    for Bankart lesions, 16
    for Hill-Sachs lesions, 108
    in multidirectional instability, 123-124
    for posterior glenohumeral instability, 258

superior glenohumeral ligament, plication of, 264

superior labral anteroposterior repair, 297-311. *See also* SLAP (superior labral anteroposterior) tears
    complications of, 309
    equipment for, 300
    indications for, 298
    physical findings and, 298-299
    positioning and portals for, 300-304
    postoperative protocol for, 309
    procedure for, 304-309

superomedial angle resection, for scapulothoracic bursitis and snapping scapula syndrome, 277-284

super-sutures, 3, 5

suprapectoral biceps tenodesis, 165-179
 complications of, 175
 equipment for, 168-169
 history of, 165-166
 imaging for, 167
 indications for, 166
 physical findings and, 166
 positioning and portals for, 169
 postoperative protocol for, 175-176
 procedure for, 169-175

suprascapular artery, protection of, in suprascapular nerve release, 226-227

suprascapular nerve
 injury of, in Latarjet stabilization, 214
 release of, 219-231
  complications of, 230
  equipment for, 223
  imaging for, 221-222
  indications of, 219-220
  physical findings and, 220-221
  positioning and portals for, 223, 228
  postoperative protocol for, 229
  procedure for, 223-229

supraspinatus muscle, atrophy of, in suprascapular nerve compression, 219-231

Surgeon's Sixth Finger Knot Pusher, 140

suture(s)
 for acromioclavicular joint repair, 88-89
 through bone block, 161
 breakage of, 7-8
 tying. See knot-tying

suture anchors
 for Bankart repair, 20-24, 27, 46
 for bony Bankart repair, 151, 156-161
 for greater tuberosity fracture repair, 271
 for panlabral repair, 287, 290-292
 for partial-thickness rotator cuff transtendon repair, 250-251
 for posterior Bankart repair, 262-263
 for rotator cuff repair, 54-55, 102-103, 138, 141-142
 for SLAP tear repair, 303-309
 for subscapularis repair, 240-241
 types of, 54-55

Suture Lassos, 151

suture passing instruments, for bony Bankart repair, 151

suture retrievers
 for posterior Bankart repair, 263
 for SLAP tear repair, 307

suture shuttle, for subscapularis repair, 241

"suture stacks," 98

suture-bridge technique, for rotator cuff repair, 133-145

switching sticks or rods, 193
 for Latarjet stabilization, 207-212
 for subscapularis repair, 240

synovitis, in adhesive capsulitis, 181-188

tag stitch, for suprapectoral biceps tenodesis, 174

tears, rotator cuff, repair of. See rotator cuff repair

tendon grafts, for acromioclavicular joint repair, 86-90

Tennessee slider, 5, 6

tenodesis, suprapectoral biceps, 165-179

tenotomy, for suprapectoral biceps tenodesis, 174-175

testers, knot, 7

thawing stage, of adhesive capsulitis, 181

thrombosis, after subscapularis repair, 242

tissue elevators, for panlabral repair, 287

tissue preparation, in bony Bankart repair, 155

T-MAX Attachment, for Latarjet stabilization, 204

top hats, for Latarjet stabilization, 208

Tossy classification, of acromioclavicular joint dislocations, 71

traction stitches, 58, 239-240

training aids, for knot-tying, 7

transosseous tunnel, for greater tuberosity fracture repair, 269-276

trans-subscapularis portal, for revision arthroscopy, 45-46

transtendon rotator cuff repair, 245-255

transverse scapular ligament, suprascapular nerve release at, 219-231

triple-loaded anchor, for subscapularis repair, 240

TUBS classification, of multidirectional instability, 123

tunnel, for suprapectoral biceps tenodesis, 173

TunnelPro implant, 274

ultrasound
 for scapulothoracic bursitis, 279
 for snapping scapula syndrome, 279
 for subscapularis injury, 236
 for suprapectoral biceps tenodesis, 167

VAPR VUE Radiofrequency System, 168
vertical mattress sutures, for subscapularis repair,
    241-242

Weaver-Dunn procedure, 82
West Point view
    for Bankart lesions, 15
    for labral pathology, 287
Western Ontario Shoulder Instability index score,
    214-215

Weston knot, 5
winging, scapular, 278

Yergason's test, for SLAP tears, 298

Zanca view
    for acromioclavicular joint, 84
    for suprascapular nerve compression, 221